While the article below doesn't mention me by name, it does identify me with respect to the TV station KESQ and a local doctor kills breast cancer with unique procedure. Note the date 2015 but now in 2021 the results are in.

Topic: This is incredible!

Forum: Clinical Trials, Research News, Podcasts, and Study Results
—

Share your research articles, interpretations and experiences here. Let us know how these studies affect you and your decisions.

Posted on: Nov 1, 2015 09:59AM - edited Nov 1, 2015 09:59AM by ████████

████████ wrote:

http://www.kesq.com/news/local-doctor-kills-breast-cancer-with-unique-procedure/35985362

Sueris found this and I just had to create a thread on it hoping that many see this. This is a story on a breast cancer procedure that does not include chemotherapy, radiation nor surgery of course there can not be any spreading of the cancer for this to work. Time will tell if this procedure will truly be successful. If it is this guy will go down in history. The tumor stays with the person, it will be dead but it stays there, I wonder if over time a person's body will make it dissolve? The medical system will loose thousands of dollars on treatment but I think women will want to get tested more often so this procedure would be available to them, not to say that getting screened more often insures that the cancer will be found before it spreads. I also wonder if this procedure is applicable to other solid tumor cancers?

Make sure that you view what is on the second page which includes a small statement that the cancer must be found early. There are also additional videos, two which include statements about deaths from breast cancer.

LAVENDER IS THE NEW PINK

The following are a few of the patient letters I have received that will give you the flavor of how they feel toward me as my patients, knowing my true spirit.

Dr. Bretz,
We got your fax, and it was great. My plan is to make several copies so that I can give one to every doctor if needed. I have to say that when we left your office to make the 31/2 hour drive home, we felt like we had just been with an Eagle, and we were going back to the turkeys. Not a good feeling when you know your life is in these peoples' hands. (Actually my life is in God's hands, but you know what I mean). So, your report is going to be so helpful in guiding us and our doctor team to do the best course of treatment. I have a lot of peace about having the port put in and diving in with chemo. After reading your report, I don't know how the oncologist could disagree. We also loved how you began the report with ," We had the typical 3 hour discussion of anatomy, physiology, mammographic study and review........." We realize that probably no one else does that! As a matter of fact, you're the first person who has taken the time to even show me my mammogram and really explain things to me. Otherwise, I've done my own research, and had to ask many questions. You were wonderful yesterday by explaining everything to us as if we could handle the info and were "smart enough" to understand it.
I'm so glad I have you in my back pocket to guide me thru this valley. I will give you a blow by blow description of every appt I have.
As far as your idea, I'm not sure what you meant, except for possibly the cancer consultants of America, which looks like a great idea for sure. I will look into them and find out about costs associated. Otherwise everything else in your report seemed like we discussed yesterday. Am I missing something? You'll have to forgive me as my mind is so full of info and emotion.
Thank you again for being a part of my family's healing. My children and future grandchildren thank you too.
Blessings,
Danielle

Subject: Thank you!
From: Jeffrey Levine

Hi Phil:

A belated thank you for sending me a copy of your book which, like your life, is pedal to the medal—110 percent! This is a medical smackdown and I believe that's the way you want it. I need to carve out some time to work my way through the narrative, and then I'll get back to you with more detail.

However, based on what I've seen as a reporter, here's what sets you apart: If you believe in something, you're not waiting for permission. Cancer doesn't wait, nor do you. Really, it's hard to comprehend how awful it was for women suffering from the disease. It was a curse, a stigma, and a terrible secret. You gave women permission to life with and through their ordeal. No need to hide. Let's take it on and fight, if needs be, to the death!

OK, you broke a whole lot of china in the cabinet. Not everybody is on the same page with what you did and what you're doing. However, when all of this is codified, the doers are going to be remembered, not the folks who sat on the bench. When you're fighting a killer, you have to be all in. You're not playing it safe; you're playing to win.

You and I had some ups and downs, and, honestly, there were times when I doubted your approach. What I see now is that you do what the best doctors do—the laying on of hands in hope of healing. Tamoxifen, yes, is a breakthrough but compassion and empathy are powerful. Wanting recovery helps make it so. I remember talking to your patients and hearing the echoes of your inspiration.

Finally, your kind inscription to me is more than appreciated, and I'm delighted you put my thoughts about your achievements on the cover of your book. We did do good work together, and if it helped you make a difference, than an important purpose was served. Politics? Who cares? Saving Lives: We all care.

Very, very glad to know that "The Lone Ranger" is still fighting against the odds—not a task for the faint at heart, but you're up to it. Interesting that, apparently we are of the same faith. Not surprising! I'm waiting for the next chapter; it's sure to be suspenseful.

You know how every episode ends, someone asks, "Who was the masked man, anyway?" Then comes the answer: "That was the Lone Ranger!"

"Hi-Yo, Silver, away!"

With respect and friendship.

Jeff

You & Joan are such a wonderful gift to us & all you touch, you know how to dry our tears & bring great comfort back to us!

♔ Hallmark

www.hallmark.com

Please enjoy this gift to experience a wonderful evening with your bride & just sit back & relax a bit with a little sip...

Love,

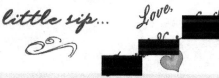

Card Studio

4/1/2016

Dear Dr. Bretz,
Your Lavender
Procedure not only
saved my life but it also
prevented the disfiguring
scars that result from a
lumpectomy (which is what was
recommended **THANKS** by an
oncologist). **FOR BEING** Your procedure
also spared **SO KIND.** me from
the horrendus effects of
chemo and radiation.

The experience of working with you and
Joan was so amazing because of the
personal and caring attention I was
given.

I will forever be grateful to you for
your expertise and your many years
of experience. Thanks again for
all you've done for me.

Sincerely ... D█

Dr. Bratz, Joan ~

Your kindness ~
   really made a difference...
Your thoughtfulness ~
   really touched my heart....
The gratitude I feel
   really can't be
     put into words.

I thank you from the bottom of
my heart for all the care,
compassion and wonderful advice
you have shown me throughout all
these years. I have trusted you
with the utmost confidence in
taking care of my medical needs.
I couldn't have felt more secure
in making the decisions I have
made without you. You have always

brought a sense of calm
when it came to facing some
medical challenges that
have met with another doctor.
You are a brilliant doctor
who always put women's health
at the forefront of your practice
and for that we all thank
you!
   I truly wish you &
Joan and wish you both
many blessings in the years
ahead!
   You have made a big
difference in many lives and
for that you should be very
proud!. Thank you for all you
have done for Brittany and
everyone's lives you have touched!
   With much love & gratitude~
     Desi

10/21

Dear Dr. Bretz,   Oct 13, '21
        First of all, I want to thank
you for taking care of me for "how
many years... are Countless" —

        From taking my breast implants
out when I knew they were making
me sick... Then in '05 when I had
breast cancer & you were there to
save me from disfiguement.

        From then on, you faithfully
checked me to make sure it did
not return!

        God has sent me YOU to care
for me & I personally believe He is
not done with you!

        You've always loved "The Lone-
ranger & you're NOT Alone in the

endorsement

Inbox

patricia

to philbretz

5:30 AM (2 hours ago)

I was referred to Dr Bretz, seeking information about cryoablation for my stage 1 breast cancer. I have been looking for alternatives to traditional treatment for several months now, feeling alone in this journey even though I have had several consults with other oncologists. I also underwent an expensive and ultimately completely ineffective month-long alternative treatment at a clinic in Arizona. Although I simply wanted a brief consultation regarding his experience using cryoablation, I received far more information regarding *all* of the possible treatments for my cancer than provided by the other doctors combined. I found Dr Bretz to be generous with his time and, by far, the doctor most concerned with my condition. Not only did he walk me though cryoablation, but also highlighted the risks and benefits of the other treatments that had been recommended with important details that none of the three other doctors had taken the time to provide, despite my requests. His compassionate guidance has been a breath of fresh air and equipped me with important information needed to make a difficult decision.
Best,

Patricia

September
2021

Dr. Bretz,

Here's wishing you every much deserved blessing as you move on into new endeavors.

Thank you, again, for saving my life (and sanity) (daily) over these past 32+ years. I have always known that no matter what you could fix me.. You never really needed to though because you did everything right in the first place.

Dr. and Joan - Always in my prayers - Bonnie Campbell

CLASS OF 1989

To reach me:

www.thelavenderproject.net
phil@thelavenderproject.net

Notice I didn't use Dr. Bretz, as by the time this book is published, I will no longer be a licensed physician in the State of California. I am unable to call myself doctor anymore after 40 years. I will not be able to comment on any particular case (like yours) because I would theoretically be practicing without a license. Regrettably, you should not send me any reports. This situation has cut deep and grieves me a great deal because I know how alone many of you feel having been diagnosed with breast cancer. However, assuming my website isn't taken down, there are multiple videos of the procedure incorporating years of follow-up so you know it's for real. All the videos are unscripted and spontaneous.

Aside from that, I'm very interested in your thoughts about the book. With publication of my paper and book, I can expect an outpouring of negative comments from my peers. However, one thing to keep in mind is whatever grievances one has with my methods, you can't overlook the patient outcomes. Does it matter how I got those outcomes with all FDA-approved technology? I thought we were all working together in the business of trying to cure breast cancer?

SACRIFICING AMERICA'S WOMEN

SACRIFICING AMERICA'S WOMEN

Defeating Breast Cancer
the Lavender Way/
Procedure

PHILLIP BRETZ, M.D.

I'm not an M.D. anymore just Mr. Why's that?

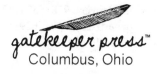
gatekeeper press™
Columbus, Ohio

DISCLAIMER

This book is about recent history as it unfolded. It is not meant to recommend, prescribe or otherwise direct anyone's medical care. It is for informational purposes only. I am no longer a doctor licensed to practice medicine and, therefore, can't give medical advice. The information contained in this book was written when I was a licensed M.D. You will read of cancer-free patients, eight years out from what I call the Lavender Way/Procedure. So far, there has been successful treatment of breast cancer without surgery, chemotherapy or radiation. It's about a 20-minute procedure with normal activity resumed immediately with the breasts appearing basically untouched. This book would be similar to reading an historical memoir from Dr. Jonas Salk (although I'm not in his league), the inventor of the polo vaccine. Having said that, I hope you find the book engaging and worth of your time. I can guarantee you it was worth my decades long fight to try to put breast cancer in the history books. I will forever miss the opportunity to care for my patients.

Sacrificing America's Women:
Defeating Breast Cancer the Lavender Way/Procedure

Published by Gatekeeper Press
2167 Stringtown Rd, Suite 109
Columbus, OH 43123-2989
www.GatekeeperPress.com

Library of Congress Control Number: 2021944686

ISBN (hardcover): 9781662914225
ISBN (paperback): 9781662914232
eISBN: 9781662914249

DEDICATION

I WOULD LIKE TO dedicate this work to my family and parents. This includes my wife of 52 years, Joan, and the children we were blessed with, Jason, Ashley, Christian, and Alexandra. They have been a joy to me. Nothing surpasses being present at each of their births, then helping your children through childhood, adolescence, coming of age and then seeing them take their place in society as responsible citizens. I would also like to dedicate this book to my family that have passed on including my father, mother, and my Aunt Florence, who helped raise me along with my mom when my father was taken from us when I was 12 years old.

One of the main reasons for writing this book was to propound my story for my grandsons, Oliver (Mr. O) and Harrison. I also dedicate this book to them.

Lastly, as you'll read, I made a promise to three women early on in my professional career that I couldn't save from breast cancer. I pledged to them I would continue the fight until I found an answer and along the way, be a voice for those who never had one and still don't. It will be up to you, the public, to bring in the verdict if I succeeded in my promise and if my voice means anything to anyone. Moreover, to see if collectively the women's voices of our great land will be heard and radical change takes place so we can preserve mind, body, and spirit of all women. You can't treat women with breast cancer like fixing a flat tire.

Phil, aka The Lone Ranger

Contents

The Road Not Taken -

The Road Not Taken
by:˙ Robert Frost

Two roads diverged in a yellow wood,
And sorry I could not travel both
And be one traveler, long I stood
And looked down one as far as I could
To where it bent in the undergrowth;

Then took the tother, as just as fair,
And having perhaps the better claim,
Because it was grassy ans wanted wear;
Though as for that the passing there
Had worn them really about the same,

And both that morning equally lay
In leaves no step had trodden black.
Oh, I kept the first for another day!
Yet knowing how way leads on to way,
I doubted if I should ever come back.

I shall be telling this with a sigh
Somewhere ages and ages˙hence:
Two roads diverged in a wood, and I -
I took the one less traveled by
And that has made all the difference.

This is an article by a publicist in Chicago who became one of my Lavender girls (and that's how they prefer to be known). If you are having trouble reading this, please Google "Fete Life Style Magazine October 2016" and scroll to page 40. She is now over five years out from Lavender and cancer free.

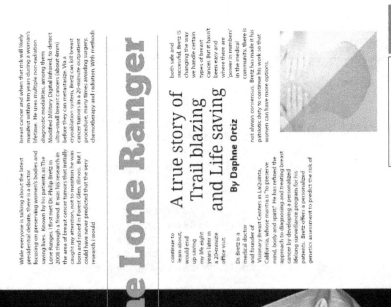

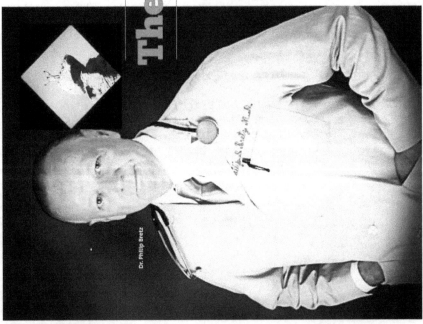

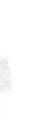

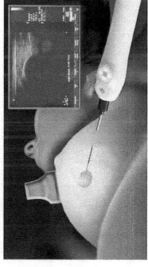

On December 21, 2015, a day after my 44th birthday, I was diagnosed with Grade 1 cancer classified as ER+/PR+ (Estrogen Receptor positive/ Progesterone Receptor positive) in two areas of my right breast. It was discovered during a routine checkup in November and further mammography and biopsy testing confirmed the results. Since I had already been seeing Dr. Bretz regularly for infrared scans (instead of mammograms), and researching his work for PR purposes, I was fully aware

of his successful treatment of specific types of breast cancer in women.

On Saturday, January 16, 2016, Dr. Bretz killed the tumor in my breast via cryoablation, which uses the application of extremely cold temperatures (cryo) to destroy diseased tissue (ablation) including cancer cells. The procedure was done in his office, took 20 minutes and consisted of a probe being inserted through the tumor and frozen with liquid nitrogen. This method of treatment effectively increases the kill zone to a much larger area surrounding the tumor,

requires no surgery or loss of breast tissue and recovery time is immediate. An hour later, we were toasting with a glass of wine at the restaurant across the street.

Dr. Bretz's surgical career spans over 30 years and includes being an integral part of the open heart surgical team at Eisenhower Memorial Hospital in Rancho Mirage, CA where they performed over 4000 open heart procedures (having lowest mortality rate in the country in

1983 and 1984), and pioneered techniques such as left ventricular reconstruction. He was privileged to be first assistant on First Lady Betty Ford's heart surgery before becoming the designated principal investigator for the National Surgical Adjuvant Breast Project (NSABP). His team successfully treated invasive breast cancer without surgery using just neo-adjuvant chemotherapy and radiation.

Among his many accomplishments, one of Bretz's significant achievements in research was authoring the country's first large-scale breast cancer prevention clinical trial using the drug Tamoxifen in 1990. He wrote a 400-page book on this experience called, Sacrificing America's Women. He was awarded the Carnegie Medal for heroism as well as two medals of excellence given by the commanding general of the 332nd Medical Brigade.

The National Cancer Institute predicts that breast cancer is set to double by 2030. That's over 400,000 cases and 80,000 deaths. I think it could be argued that America's women have never been in more perilous times; regarding breast cancer, not only because of the increase in numbers, but at the same time federal guidelines call for no mammograms below fifty and only every other year thereafter.

For me and the 28 other women Dr. Bretz has treated, cryoablation was the answer. Had I not known Dr. Bretz prior, chances are I would have listened to my doctor who offered no other option but immediate surgery.

Cryoablation for breast cancer treatment is currently offered at 25 centers nationwide and is FDA approved to treat benign and malignant tissue, including cancer cells. It costs around $2500 and is covered by most insurance plans. While it depends on the grade, stage and type of breast cancer, cryoablation needs to be talked about more! In a recent 5-year multicenter study sponsored by the National Cancer Institute, cryoablation showed a 100% success rate in early stage breast cancers less than 1cm and complete ablation of invasive ductal breast cancer tumors also known as D.C.I.S. or "Stage 0".

So while Trump and Clinton argue over the issues surrounding healthcare, Dr. Bretz is on to the solution. Seems to me this is the man who truly deserves OUR vote.

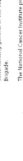

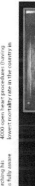

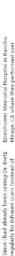

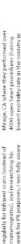

PREFACE

THROUGHOUT THIS BOOK, you'll learn why Lavender is the new pink.

Thank you for picking up my book. While the main concern is to relay my journey in trying to defeat breast cancer and addressing the consequences of my supposed misconduct (the public will be my judge), the other principal reason is to relay my life's story to my grandchildren. With the loss of my dad at age twelve, I never got to ask him anything about being a responsible adult. I have faced many obstacles in my life, and I want my grandchildren to know how I dealt with them and persevered. I've lived adventures enough for ten lifetimes. Remember, Lavender is the new pink but it's all up to you.

A word of WARNING. While most of the book tells a cool story, there are images that, to some, may be very disturbing that the public never sees. If you choose to see them, perhaps you'll know (with the aid of the book) why women are being sacrificed and are so afraid of the "system" that they would rather die than receive standard-of-care treatment. How dare the medical industrial complex create this type of environment. Herewithin is the story of how I change things for the better, the Lavender Way for ALL women.

PROLOGUE

THERE ARE A few reasons for putting my thoughts to pen. As a dedicated breast cancer surgeon and researcher, my entire life's work and pursuits have been taken away from me, and I want you to know why and how it may impact you. Breast cancer is a huge problem, but what if there was a relatively simple answer that is being systematically suppressed that would end this curse? What I mean by that is, what if there was a twenty-minute procedure performed outside the operating room (OR) and "system" that altogether omitted surgery, chemotherapy, and radiation, thus, in which case normal activity could be resumed immediately? Would that be of interest to you? Will it turn out that Occam's Razor theory is right concerning our fight to defeat breast cancer? If you'd like to know the truth, then read on.

Can you imagine everything you have worked for your entire life is now prohibited? It's not a good feeling. We shall deal with that issue later in the book, but I would like the public to make a determination; that is, to decide whether the action against me, which prevents me at the height of my career—when I would have been able to care for hundreds of women worldwide to avoid the horrendous breast cancer treatment that continues to be offered—was justified.

Another reason to write this book is that, I, like every surgeon worth his/her salt, have stories to tell that are compelling and, at times, heroic. Becoming a surgeon builds character. There is a company out my way called Granite. On each of their vehicles there is a bumper sticker and it says "CHARACTER MATTERS." You bet it does. Becoming a surgeon means reaching one of the loftiest plateaus, highly regarded, and most trusted positions humankind has to offer. A surgeon looks death in the face almost every day and prevents it. It's a story worth hearing.

There is a painting I like as it says it all. It depicts a patient lying on a gurney in supposed dire straits with the surgeon having his right hand on the patient's chest. The surgeon's left hand is on Death in the form of a skeleton who is kneeling trying to get to the patient but can't because the surgeon is there. That's how you often feel at times, and probably it's that feeling that keeps a surgeon going for decades. Early in my career I made a promise to three girls I couldn't save from breast cancer that I would continue the fight to find the answer to breast cancer until I found it. The following is the closest print I could find.

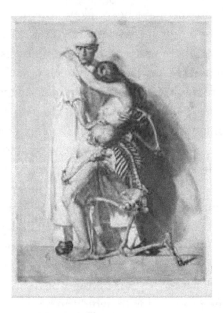

Another reason to write this book, considering the tumult we are all involved in currently with possible impending anarchy, is to relive with me how it felt to grow up in America in the fifties and sixties. It was an innocent time that will, I fear, never appear again. I want the reader to know me from my earliest childhood memories that shaped me and to know where my heart has been all along.

Before you make a final judgment on me, you must know what I have accomplished (if anything) was to try and protect women from unnecessary mutilation and death. I have done this by pioneering a new way to diagnose and treat breast cancer—the Lavender Way/Lavender Procedure. I would use all FDA-approved technology and didn't make anything up in my garage. I want women globally to know they are being sacrificed by a doctrine that refuses change. We are at a point now where a thing like "evidence-based medicine" has all but eviscerated the art of medicine, preventing any chance of a breakthrough. The question is just how important are ALL women?

I will also present my published paper that has the results of all my effort. As they say, the proof is in the pudding. You shall see that it is highly inflammatory toward the establishment. It has finally been published by two journals. You can go to *RAS Oncology and Therapy Journal* and click on "Oncology and Therapy," or to sciencerepository. org. Click on "Journal Surgical Case Reports." It sometimes takes a little doing but they are there. The paper will probably be in the archives section of each. Since my first amendment rights have not been taken away yet, I want you, the public, to know the truth.

I want women worldwide to know the Lavender Way/Lavender Procedure is real; you don't have to wait ten more years for further research (as is usually the case with any breakthrough announcement). After reading this book, you can judge for yourself if Lavender is being capriciously and actively suppressed. This action might well bear on you by denying women the possibility to avoid surgery, chemotherapy, and radiation. We just need someone in charge who has the guts to change the system.

In this age of supposed transparency, I want to acknowledge my sanction by a medical board and its consequences to my life's work. Again, the reader will decide like a jury of public opinion if I ever acted in a negligent manner or was in any way incompetent, reckless, unethical, or unprofessional. Did I not use my forty-plus years of experience as a surgeon to guide every decision I ever made for the total benefit of my patients? Should I be allowed to pursue my passion unrestricted, or do women want me to do something else?

Perhaps now is a good time to put the book down and view my TED TALK. Just search for "drbretztedtalk" on YouTube. This will give you the background if it hasn't been taken down like my website. At the end of the talk was supposed to be a video of the Lavender Procedure on an eighty-six-year-old who was told she needed a mastectomy, who is now ninety-two cancer-free in 2021. However, you will note I cry for the first minute-and-a-half or so, and I can assure you I'm a pretty tough guy. So, in the end, I ran out of time, no video, thus the reason for the link on the website. I cried because there is a big difference between wearing a pink ribbon and running a race for the cure (they have had over thirty years of running, and we still have the same 40,000-plus dying yearly from breast cancer), and being solely responsible for the thousands of lives of women who trust you. When those souls are on your shoulders, it's a different ballgame. And in that moment on stage when I knew I had an answer to breast cancer that could be implemented almost overnight and I was being snuffed out, yes, I cried.

When I look at anyone who has achieved any sort of accomplishments, I sometimes wonder what turn of events, at times seemingly at random, shaped a particular person into greatness. This book isn't about any importance or greatness I achieved, but as I look back (I'm seventy-five now), it became apparent that almost every step of the way, I was somehow molded into what I am today, not unlike most surgeons. I began my surgical training in the late 1970s, where the order of the day was extensive surgical resection (removing the diseased tissue, all of it). It was the *"Did you get it all?"* generation. Our motto was "For them, it's unresectable." Almost invariably back then, when we came out of the operating room to talk to the family, it was the second question besides, is she ok? "Did you get all the cancer, doc?" We always said yes, we did. That was correct for cancer we could see. Unfortunately, we were not fully aware of the concept of micro-metastasis or tumor biology, that is cancer that has spread, but it's so small we can't detect it and still can't in 2021. There was no genome. To be fair, back then, if you had cancer, the only real thing standing between you and the grave was the surgeon, as chemotherapy and radiation were in their infancy compared to what we have today. We would wheel a woman into the OR intact, and in an hour, would have the breast coming off with (depending on the surgeon) multiple hemostats clamping bleeders with some stats falling on the floor. I abhorred those surgeries and always thought there had to be a better way. I spent the better half of my surgical career chasing that elusive answer which would minimize treatment, and yet also not have women disfigured or globally dying of breast cancer. Part of the reason for writing this book is to let the reader decide if I came close to achieving my goal and if there was some force out there preventing what I learned from seeing the light of day.

What was it like becoming a surgeon in Chicago in the 1970s? Those were the days when, as residents, it was every other night in the hospital for five years, never knowing when you would get a chance to eat. There was a never-ending flow of very sick patients and it was unsaid but you just showed up day after day without regard to your personal responsibilities. It also served to weed out people who thought becoming a surgeon was a cake walk. One attending had us say, "You're too good to us, Master." That's how we were treated at times so I get today's distain for statements like that. We all suffer at some point.

The most prolonged surgery I was ever in was the first liver transplant in Illinois (26 hours). Dr. Peter Geis was the chief attending on the transplant service and taught us everything. Surgeons are like (or should be) the Seal Team 6 of medicine, caring yet relentless in the quest for the perfect surgery anytime, anywhere. With this new age of tolerance and blurring what is acceptable, and functionaries insinuating their way into our business, things have changed and not for the better. A paper stated that for every actual doctor now, there are fourteen functionaries at jobs that were completely manufactured and weren't needed up until we started to blur the lines. Why weren't they needed? Because doctors really were to be trusted, they showed up day after day, denying their families and their own well-being to care for people they didn't even know. Surgeons do this for decades. The guys I worked with at Eisenhower Memorial Hospital In Rancho Mirage, CA, really gave a damn about the patient, and the hospital, at the expense of themselves.

Now, actual doctors who attained a medical degree (an earned degree) are now lumped in with nurse practitioners (NPs) and physician assistants (PAs). In any dealings now with insurance companies, you will never find the word "doctor" used, just "provider." How dare they. How dare that doctors didn't stand up for themselves and put an end to that nonsense. Surgical residency for a general surgeon was usually five years. A recent paper said that about 50% of the current surgical residents at the end of their residency felt they were not competent to be turned out to the public and didn't actually have the skill to make life and death decisions day after day and decade after decade. They needed an extra year of "fellowship" training. Where did that come from? You can probably guess—functionaries demanding that surgical residents only work so many hours, etc. The problem with that is, at the end of the day and for the rest of their lives, surgeons are required to just be there without consideration to their own needs or the needs of their families. You must put in a full day's work, perhaps four or five surgeries, make rounds, then you're on emergency room (ER) call with cases demanding real expertise all night long, then start a new day at 7 a.m. having just finished a gunshot case at 4 a.m. Meanwhile, all the functionaries are nestled in their beds. We could change this back to the way surgeons used to be trained, of course, if someone in charge had the guts.

Among those in the list of positions I would immediately do away with are hospitalists. These people are basically hired guns to man the hospital whilst the attending is away. Different ones are there day and night and take over the management of patients. It becomes hard for the patient to know just who is in charge with so many different faces. One of the edicts I grew up with is a person should find a skilled doctor they can be proud of and relate to. So, if the time ever came when one had to be hospitalized, you wouldn't be dealing with some stranger. But that is exactly what has transpired with the implementation of hospitalists. Again, as in the case of PAs and NPs, jobs, including hospitalists, were not in existence when I was on staff. It was just you and the floor nurse. The more patients you had on her floor, the more experience you and the nurse had working together. You were confident in her ability to carry out what needed to be done (because you taught her how to care for your patients) and what she would do in a particular instance. An example is the taping of a nasogastric tube. I often saw it taped to the nose. If it's there for days, it tends to cause ulcerations on the nares. If you tape it to the upper lip, that doesn't happen. Our nurses were people who lived in the area, were proud of their jobs and the hospital, and gave a damn. "Per diem" hired hands, flying in from someplace back East for the winter, don't have the same commitment.

I can remember any number of times, but especially with the "Bird Lady," when I would spend the entire night in the intensive care unit (ICU) managing patient care.

16 - THE DESERT SUN, Palm Springs, Calif.—Thursday, January 8, 1981

Multiple-organ failure

EMC doctor, equipment saves life

(EDITOR'S NOTE: This story was written by John Milburn, a local public relations consultant and former newspaperman. This is a story about a sturdier, 41-year-old woman with a fondness for breeding cattle at her Santa Rosa Mountains ranch, who was obligated to go on a 3,000-calorie diet — the hard way. On a damp evening several months ago, she was deliberately run over by a car of "joyriders" as she jogged along Highway 74 near Anza. Clinically, she experienced three to four "deaths" during the next several weeks of hospitalization at Eisenhower Medical Center in Rancho Mirage. Only sophisticated medical equipment, a physician skilled in trauma, other doctors and support personnel could pull her through during her 38-day ordeal.

RANCHO MIRAGE: "Go home and feed your beefalo." To Velva Eddy, housewife and mother of two, those were the sweetest words she ever heard.

For nearly two months, she lay near death as a result of severe colon injuries, shock-lung complicated by pneumonia, critical cardiac arrythmia, renal failure, fractured spine and shattered pelvis.

"If I'm ever going to see a miracle, this is the one," commented Dr. Phillip Bretz, surgeon and EMC trauma expert who was Mrs. Eddy's primary physician following her May accident. "She should have died many times," he added.

For a relatively small population, the Coachella Valley experiences an unusual occurrence of trauma cases, the physician noted. A majority of trauma cases in large cities are gunshot or stab wounds, he explained. Locally, however, it's traffic accidents — truck drivers falling asleep on the Interstate, vehicles careening off cliffs on tortuous Palms to Pines Highway 74, drivers "boiled" and entering desert spa cities at excessive speed, and so on.

Fortunately for Mrs. Eddy, EMC is trauma-ready. Mrs. Eddy had the severest type of trauma: Multiple-organ failure.

Before her hospital discharge, the patient would undergo the intensive care of Drs. Bretz, surgeon; Ronald Snelder, pulmonary expert; Richard Stone, nephrologist; Jack Sternlieb, open-heart surgeon; and Phil Shaver, cardiologist. Support services including pharmacy and dietary were also deeply involved along with round-the-clock nursing care.

After arriving at the emergency room, Mrs. Eddy was rushed to surgery for the most critical trauma detected, a massive necrosis of the large bowel. Such a condition raises a 90 percent mortality factor.

The next crisis was shock-lung followed by superimposed pneumonia. Each chest cavity required a chest tube and the maximum pressure setting the respirator could generate over an extended period. Prognosis: 80 percent mortality rate (partially due to long-term, high-oxygen concentration) through mechanical means.

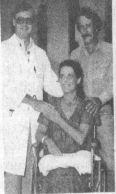

ESCAPES DEATH — Velva Eddy of Anza, who narrowly escaped death several times while hospitalized with major-trauma injuries, departs Eisenhower Medical Center with new husband Guy, as a speedy convalescence.

The next insult to her body was kidney failure as a result of overwhelming sepsis (spread of infection). The mortality rate here was 70-75 percent. She required extended hemodialysis (artificial kidney.)

In short, Mrs. Eddy incurred "multiple-organ failure" of the most severe kind.

"In such instances, one thing leads to another; it snowballs and it almost leads to the demise of the patient," he said.

But Mrs. Eddy clung precariously to life. For the first several weeks, she maintained, "I never slept once. The doctors said my mind was alert, though I couldn't speak. I just felt if I went to sleep, I'd never wake up."

Nutrition-wise, the patient was again in near fatal peril. Without hyper-alimentation (concentrated glucose and amino acids solution) her nutrient-starved body would have begun consuming its own muscles. The hyper-alimentation team was able to keep her alive, plus provide nutrients with which to build on, by means of a 3,000-calorie daily diet introduced through her subclavian vein.

She faced yet another crisis: Three cardiac arrests which each brought emergency physician visits from the Desert Cardiology Group. Mrs. Eddy continued to have severe

abdominal infection and her white count was approaching 40,000 (as opposed to about 10,000 normal), signaling inability to fight off the sepsis, exacerbated by inability to sustain her blood pressure.

By this time, she was on multiple, maximal-dose medication for the blood pressure problem. Bretz was "more concerned than ever about her survivability."

As Bretz lay awake one night trying to think of something that could bring her back, it suddenly came to him . . . "Intra-aortic balloon pump." Dr. Jack Sternlieb (Heart Institute of the Desert) who uses the pump in open heart surgery would have the key to her "second heart." To Bretz's knowledge, Sternlieb had not used the intra-aortic balloon pump in a multiple-organ failure patient.

After explaining Mrs. Eddy's case, Bretz and Sternlieb were in surgery at 3 a.m., giving her a temporary second heart. Sternlieb inserted the balloon, and one more battle in the war for patient survival was won.

"Even though we were still fighting the sepsis problem, over a period of time we were able to wean her from the blood pressure medication. Inch by inch she came back."

Still immobilized by chest, neck and abdominal tubes, Mrs. Eddy found the door to speech. Her first words: "Hi. I want to tell my husband how much I love him."

Her blood proteins improved, she no longer required kidney dialysis. And she could now talk.

"I truly believe that Dr. Bretz saved my life," Mrs. Eddy said. "I think every doctor in the hospital was here to see me. I've been treated royally, just royally."

Bretz continued: "This has been a case where many unusual things were done. It was the only way to save this life. Multiple-organ failure on the basis of sepsis has a near 100 percent mortality factor." Hence, a miracle appeared to unfold on behalf of a steel-willed individual.

"Not only did Mrs. Eddy come back, she came back as a whole person," he added.

Mrs. Eddy is able to walk and is now home with her family. Other than the psychological "nightmares" she recalls, Mrs. Eddy's only medical exigency is recovery from surgical alteration of her abdominal wall.

"I'll be looking for steady progress in her recovery" is Mrs. Eddy's benign prognosis by her doctor.

Meanwhile, whe will be able to continue mating black angus cows to buffaloes, poducing "beefaloes."

"That's what Dr. Bretz told me to do," Mrs. Eddy smiled. "He said, 'Go home and feed your beefalo . . . and put some meat on your bones.'"

She was my first foray into publication, *The National Inquirer.* I couldn't believe it. At the time, Eisenhower Memorial Hospital (my hospital) was trying to become "the" designated trauma center for the Coachella Valley. With the outcome of the "Bird Lady" requiring a team effort, I was asked to give an interview to a magazine. I didn't know it was *The National Inquirer.* While I'm sure there are still doctors who do spend all night in the ICU managing patients, I don't see that as routine anymore. Don't worry, the hospitalists will take care of it. In some respects, medicine is no different than any other walk of life. As soon as you take away that critical bond of just you and the nurse and insinuate functionaries, then by nature, people slack off because it is human nature.

On top of that, when functionaries manufacture unending regulations in the name of quality assurance, doctors now spend about 50% or more of their time making sure the Ts are crossed and Is dotted in their electronic medical record, and that's a problem. It's no longer whether you cared for the patient properly and perhaps saved a life; it's if your electronic medical record (EMR) is complete with the right wording and codes. I just downloaded a paper from Doximity that says the burnout rate for doctors, while always high, now approaches half of the doctors in our great country, "often due to increased administrative tasks, EHR issues and lack of workplace support."

As you will read later, it's not just me. Just correct it by doing away with all this regulatory nonsense. What the hell kind of doctors are we minting that need such supervision? Make it so doctors are happy and want to get up in the morning to help you and don't have their faces staring at a computer screen, but actually have time to examine you properly (that is touch you), care, and interact. You just need the right people with the guts and vision to make the decisions that affect you and your family. That's one of the reasons I ran for Congress, which I will talk about later as well.

My grievances continue with the status quo (taking away more individuality) in lieu of a "team." Everything now has to be a "comprehensive decision" where the attending doctor must essentially kowtow to the desires of the "team." The hell with that. Again, in my day, if I needed a consult, I just called the doctor and they, without fail, responded every time. A colleague recently told me that he stopped for a "curbside consult" with a doctor he had known for years, and the guy said he wasn't on call, that my friend should call their office. In my day, a good surgeon was like an astronaut, trained to handle the most severe life-threatening circumstances, much more involved training than any functionary could imagine. The guys I practiced with at Eisenhower for decades would drop everything they were doing (like Dr. Randy Blakely) to help you if you asked. As a breast surgeon, I can't and never did depend on a computer program to tell me what I should do.

This is a perfect spot for a pun; breast care is a hands-on enterprise, not staring into some computer screen increasingly detached from the patient. I lost count of the times my patients have come in complaining now that their doctor never touches them anymore (let alone listen to their carotid artery for a bruit); they just stare into the screen and ask questions as if that is real doctoring. As I finished my time as an active surgeon (thirty years' worth) at Eisenhower Memorial Hospital, I noted that as soon as computers were brought into the OR, the nursing staff changed their priorities. The priority went from the patient to making sure they had all the things properly checked off that the functionaries had required for surgery to proceed, as if before, we were operating aimlessly amid incompetence.

I always made sure I was there for every woman as she was wheeled into the OR and held their hand. I held their hand while on the gurney and helped transfer them to the OR bed, and held their hand until they were intubated and put to sleep. It's the one thing they always remembered. It helped a great deal to diminish their fears and let them know I was in charge.

You can ask yourself truthfully if you get enough time with your doctor; do they really know you, care for you, and are there for you? If not, who are we to blame? Who could change things for the better when doctors practiced the "art of medicine," were called doctors, respected, and took orders from no one? Why? Because they went to medical school, did a full residency, and, in the past, we counted on them to know what they had to learn and use that knowledge to provide care second to none. That's what the docs at Eisenhower did for years. What went horribly wrong? I hope you know the answer by now—one last burr under my saddle. When I first started in 1979, I never heard from insurance companies, period. The only time was when they would send a check. Now I (like every doctor) am just inundated with faxes. I receive multiple pages daily from some with new edicts being laid down that you must abide by or else. They even have insurance people calling the patient and, at times, I'm notified a "provider" will interview my patient at their home about care received.

Next, I suppose some agencies will be calling children at their homes to inquire about how their parents are treating them. You see how this creeps in. It gets back to what kind of doctors are we putting out there now that need that sort of surveillance? Good doctors are hard to find, and with the increasing shortage, functionaries will have destroyed medicine as it was practiced for eons. Hippocrates would turn over in his grave. We will end this discussion with a quote from him. "There are, in fact, two things, science and opinion; the former begets knowledge and the latter ignorance." I might add to that and say, "a misguided false sense of authoritarianism."

Real doctors know the science; functionaries think they know it. Enough. Let's see what made me who I am today.

My very last reason for writing this book is that I want my grandchildren to know about me, my efforts, shortcomings, and perseverance. I want them to know how to deal with life.

It's challenging to put any highlights of my life in some sort of chronological order. Some things I remember more easily. I remember my dad bringing me a machine gun that fired caps and I must have been about eight years old—just a thing a guy would recall. Remember, folks, it was a different time. I'm sure the taste of WWII remained in him as it probably did almost every man who served in WWII. My dad was a Seabee (the Navy's 53rd Construction Battalion), attached to the 1st Marines in Guadalcanal, New Caledonia, Bougainville, Kwajalein, Eniwetok, Saipan, and Guam. And I'm sure, like hundreds of thousands of sons of those battle-hardened warriors, safe gun practices were passed along to the next generation. As generations came along, this practice diminished but was rooted in guys like me. I also remember climbing the big sand piles at his building sites and him having me go up on the car lift in the gas stations he built after the war.

I also remember him giving me a dime if I could broad jump the cracks in the sidewalks. In 1956, he had a phone in his 1953 Buick convertible (white with red leather) pictured below. Next to it is the side of our house in the winter. Talk about idyllic place for a kid to play in.

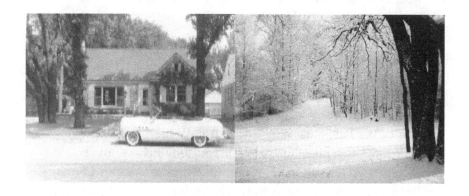

I called my mother as the first call. That phone took up nearly all the trunk space.

I also remember the one hunting trip we went on before his untimely accidental death at age fifty-one; I was twelve. I will write now about those things that impacted my life, again in no particular order. It somehow all worked together to make me who I am today. Ultimately, years later when I found my destiny in helping women with breast cancer, I would love engaging people in foreign countries (some of whom were former enemies and perhaps still are) to bring them the Lavender Way and make the world safer. You will judge if I made any difference for the women of the world. The book you are reading is only half the story.

Sacrificing America's Women II is the entire documented saga of how I came up with the idea of a large-scale breast cancer prevention clinical trial (the first of its kind) using the drug Tamoxifen, and subsequent adventures with the Federal Drug Administration (FDA), White House, erstwhile Soviet Union, Congressional hearings, and the obfuscation that took place there. It's also a story of how your tax dollars are spent by the powers that be, and how honest work gets crushed in favor of the cabal. SAW II made me feel like a cross between James Bond and Huck Finn. In your judgement of me, remember I didn't have to do any of that stuff. I could have just gone to the office every day and then at 5 p.m., gone home, no harm no foul. But I opened the book that on its cover said, "Don't open this book unless you want to change the world." It was a fire started in Chicago of a quest to do more and to push the envelope every day. That quest came with consequences as not everyone is pleased with my conduct. But I answer to a higher authority and below that the women of the world.

I've come from caring for my first patients that were six baby opossums whose mother had been hit by a car, to hopefully treating breast cancer in the least invasive way possible so that a cure is within reach with the Lavender Way/Procedure. While I never use the word "cure," I have patients who are seven-and-a-half years out and cancer-free. See how all this came to be and what kind of a doctor I became.

Come back with me now to those thrilling days of yesteryear, the Lone Ranger rides again!

Photo of my Mom and Dad

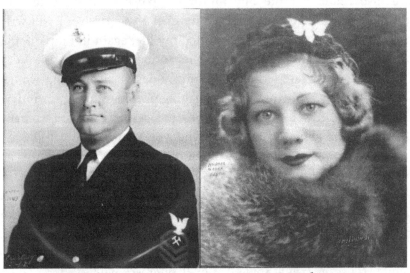

Born July 4, 1906   Born March 1, 1903
Died December 12, 1957   Died August 14, 1996

Before WWII and years before I came along, my dad was a supervisor for Sinclair Oil covering the State of Wisconsin. During the war, he served as a Chief Warrant Officer attached to the 53rd Naval Construction Battalion (otherwise known as the Seabees) in the South Pacific. His unit was attached to the First Marines starting with Guadalcanal. The Seabees were responsible for building living quarters, air fields, and the rest of the buildings and roads that would constitute an operational military base. In all these islands, they started with just jungle. In the Solomon Islands, they encountered native headhunters. The Japanese killed them and the Americans let them wear uniforms complete with sergeant stripes. The headhunters would go out and frequently bring back Japanese heads. After the war, Mom and Dad settled in Forest Glen on the outskirts of Chicago where my Dad developed a successful business building gas stations, Superior Pump Service. As you will read, he was killed in a work-related accident when I was twelve.

My Mom then had the task of raising me along with my Aunt Florence (her sister), who lived with us. She was a wonderful mother and Aunt Florence was a wonderful aunt; they got me started in a modeling career, made sure I had a higher education, and made sure there was always a chocolate cake or lemon meringue pie for me to eat. They made sure I went to North Park Academy (a college prep school in Chicago). Later they moved out to the Palm Springs area of Southern California.

At the age ninety-one my mom fell and broke a hip. I can still remember the sound. For the last six months of her life, while her brain was fine, she was in a wheelchair and I transferred her to bed each night. I had a joke that I would see her in the morning and if not, I'd see her in Chicago where my dad was buried. She told me she never wanted to make another trip to the hospital. She died in her sleep.

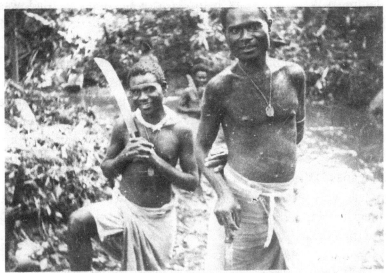

Bouganville natives ready for action

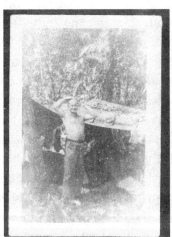

John, The Chief, after 81 days
in this Fox-hole on Guadalcanal
On the back he wrote: Show this
to Dick DuBois, I want to make
him jealous. Can you see my curly
locks? If you can it is news to me
because I couldn't.

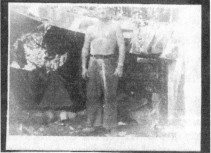

On the back John Wrote: Note the Asiatic
jewelry, also the 34 waist and the new cut
on the pant legs. Made the bracelets from
metal of Jap Zero Planes and Submarines.
April 22, 1944 - Guadalcanal

CHAPTER 1

HOW GROWING UP IN CHICAGO LAID THE FOUNDATION

I GREW UP IN Forest Glen and went to the two-room schoolhouse set in the woods along the North Branch of the Chicago River. A prairie surrounded it. I used to put snakes in Ms. Plegge's, my first-grade teacher's, desk. She would say, "Phillip, there's another snake in my desk." Below is one of those snakes.

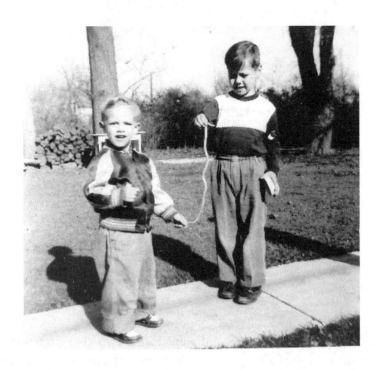

I thought, gee, there are other guys, like Richard, Stevie, Joey, but somehow, she always knew I was the perpetrator. Nowadays, I would be referred for psychological counseling and probably medicated. We would build forts either in the trees or dig them in the prairie. We didn't wash our hands every ten minutes. In our dug-out forts, we would put candles in holes in the wall. It was very dangerous as the roofs of the fort and bedding were made of prairie grass. No matter, no one ever got hurt because we weren't stupid. We also used to shoot arrows straight up in the air and dodged them as they came down. Now that was stupid, but very fun. Like in *A Christmas Story,* "You'll shoot your eye out, kid."

This schoolhouse went to the third grade. I could walk home for lunch and watch Uncle Johnnie Coons and Two Ton Baker on TV. At age eight, Ms. Plegge inexplicably endowed me with the responsibility of becoming a patrol boy. I've been protecting people ever since. I guarded kids as they crossed the street (especially the girls). I also had a monkey named Ginger (a ringtail capuchin). My two-room school house is seen below.

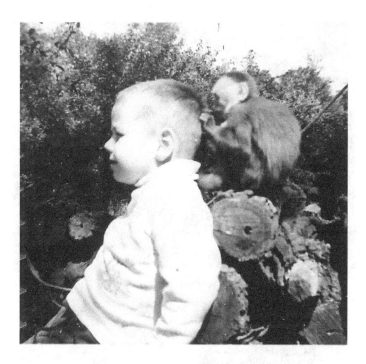

FARNSWORTH-BRANCH-SCHOOL

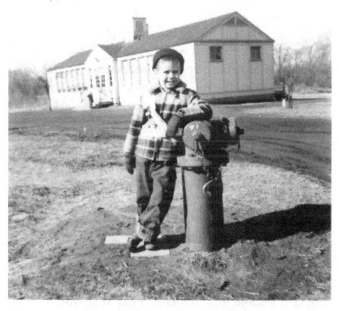

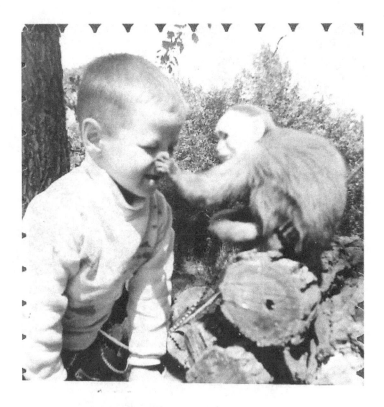

My dad and I built Ginger a big cage in the basement. I would sometimes take him to school on my shoulder for the kids to see. When he got older, he wouldn't come to anyone except my mother. Marlin Perkins (the director of Lincoln Park Zoo and original Wild Kingdom man) had a local TV program in Chicago called *Zoo Parade*. My dad talked to him about taking Ginger, and they did. *Zoo Parade* aired on Saturday mornings in Chicago and Marlin would have Ginger on his shoulder. My dad and I would go down and see Ginger living with other ringtails.

Next to Ginger's cage was Bushman's. Bushman was one of the first silverbacks to be raised in captivity. When he was young, they would walk him around the zoo in diapers. In his prime, he was six-foot-two and he weighed close to 600 pounds. They would let me go around back to give Ginger a PB and J sandwich. Today that would be prohibited because of all sorts of legal entanglements instead of people letting the right thing happen. After a couple of times of Bushman watching the goings-on, he would stick out his hand when he saw me. My mom would make extra, and I used to throw the sandwich to him. He is now stuffed and on display in the Field Museum in Chicago. He still looks very imposing and to think he was kind of my friend.

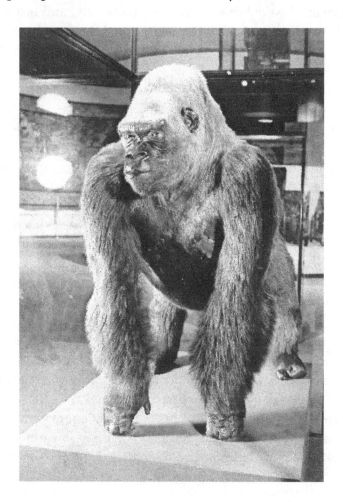

When I got older, my friends and I (Steve Power and Richard Hilke—RIP) would walk to Farnsworth, a typical Chicago public school (just like in *A Christmas Story*). It was a four-mile walk, and again, I became a patrol boy. This carried a lot more responsibility than the two-room schoolhouse location as it was on a busy Chicago street, Elston Avenue. In the winter it was bitter cold, but we were there. I was so cold I used to go into the gas station that was on the same corner to warm up. It was my first introduction to nude women in garter belts, etc., in the calendar they always had. I rose to the rank of lieutenant. I would line up my men (about six) and inspect their patrol belts as we had rallies on Fridays and the patrol boys would carry in the flags. Chicago had heavy snowstorms and when the side streets were of a certain thickness of snow, my friends and I would skitch—that's what we called grabbing onto the rear bumper of a car and letting it pull you down the street.

Those were the days during the Cold War with the Soviet Union when we all learned to "duck and cover" under our desks if we saw the flash of the atomic bomb. Or if you were riding your bike and saw the flash, you would crouch by a nearby wall. In Chicago, out on Edens Expressway, the military had six Nike missiles set to go, pointing straight up. Years later (the story told in Sacrificing America's Women Part II, coming soon), I would travel to the Soviet Union in part to try and make the world safer. Instead of butting heads with the USSR, I figured we could talk and get together to promote trust and friendship, working on a common problem like breast cancer. I was right!

As a kid growing up in Chicago, I can't leave out Riverview Park. It was probably the largest amusement park in the world until Disneyland opened. I still remember the first TV show on the opening of Disneyland and, of course, we were all jealous. When I was dating my future wife, I took her to Riverview and made sure we rode in the Tunnel of Love. None of your business what happened in there. We even had our picture taken in an old Model T that had a sign that said, "Off to California."

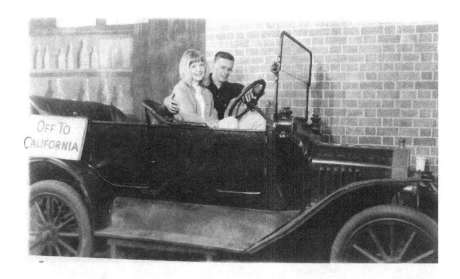

How prophetic. My two favorite attractions were the Aladdin's Castle and the Rotor. Upon entering Aladdin's Castle, there was a maze of screen doors. It took a long time to figure out. The Rotor was cool as it spun you around so fast you could (while spinning) stretch out on just your feet if you didn't weigh a lot. Also, the girl's dresses tended to go way up. The floor dropped out from under you.

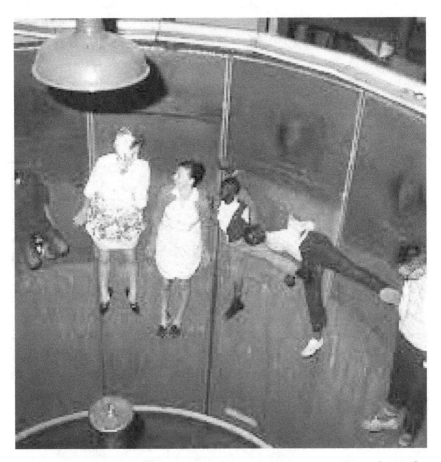

We rode all the roller coasters from the Silver Streak to the Bobs. Every kid in Chicago looked forward to Riverview when school let out for summer vacation. You can Google it to view historical pictures.

Almost every day after school we would play baseball at the nearby park or bike along the Chicago River. Sometimes we would put pennies on the railroad track to have them flattened. One time one of the guys had some Parliament cigarettes, and we smoked them. That was the last time I put a cigarette in my mouth.

However, I did occasionally smoke my dad's pipe once a week while I watched *Jim Thomas Outdoors*, pretending I was some sort of outdoorsman. There were fairly big hills leading from the park's picnic grounds down to the paths along the river. One day we (I) decided I would go down the hill on the bike with "no hands." It wasn't only that; I decided to hold two lit candles, one in each hand. I made it down the hill okay; however, two paths forked around a large oak tree at the bottom, and I went right into it. I think I saw stars.

If you see me and look closely, you will see I carry the result of that impact to this day as a small bump on my forehead's right side. Maybe it knocked some sense into me, or some would argue out of me. This is an example of how early on, I wasn't going to conduct my life in the standard way, toeing the party line, as it were. Below you can see the oak tree in the middle. The path around it that was on the right is now overgrown. If you look closely, you can see the scar on the tree the bike and my forehead made (ha).

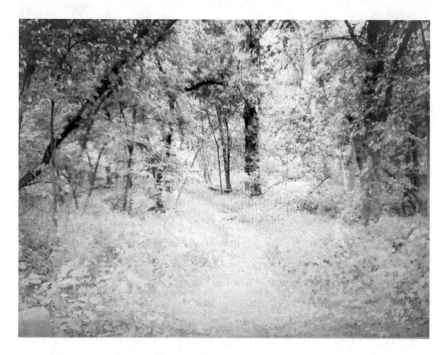

Below is a mother's worse nightmare, a prelude to the bike incident. Speaking of the bike incident, below is a photo of me and my cousin Gary in Minnesota, taken near the farm that we visited for many years, taking the Hiawatha train from Chicago. Some people probably think

I should carry that sign around with me now. And my mother is taking the photo. What the hell?

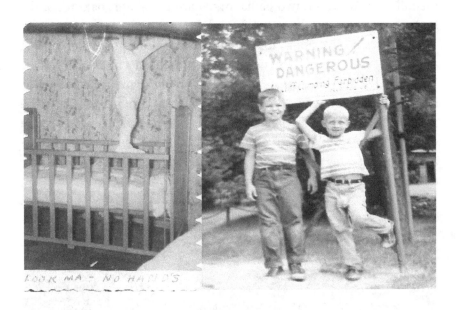

We had forest on two sides of our house, and there were several large oak trees in the front yard. In the fall, Steve (our next-door neighbor) and I used to rake the front yards and make a huge pile of leaves in the alley. The piles were so big you could jump into them and not get hurt. When we finished raking, we would throw potatoes in and have a big bonfire. Of course, now that would be against the law for air pollution. It was a different time, folks. In the winter, we would all go down to the river and shovel the snow off so we could ice skate. It was like a scene out of a Norman Rockwell painting with the snow clinging to the branches. The ice would crackle if you were at a thin spot.

In the winter, I'd have a fun time taping walnuts to the living room window about a foot or so up from the ledge. The squirrels would come and have to jump a little, and then they would hang on the nuts until they dropped. During the rest of the year, if I went out front with nuts, they would crawl up my leg and end up on my shoulder and eat nuts out of my hand. Although wild, they never tried to bite me.

Sometimes I would take my dad's fishing tackle down to the river (North Branch of the Chicago), but never caught anything. However, that was my first introduction to contraception. Almost always there were broken-off branches from all the trees lying in the water. Inevitably, there would be a condom stuck on a limb. Because it was against the current, it would be stretched out to a foot or more. I didn't know what they were then. On a more innocent note, when they were flowering, I would climb one of the many lilac trees and bring home a bouquet to my mom.

Almost every day upon coming home from school, my mom would have either a cake (usually chocolate) or my favorite lemon meringue pie. All the kids would have a piece. Being from Chicago, we ate meat, potatoes, gravy, and a hell of a lot of it. She was a great cook, and my family and I still have her recipe book. Joan (my wife of 52 years of putting up with me), who is a great chef as well, will once in a while go to it, especially for my mom's German potato salad.

There was a corner store in Forest Glen. Usually, after we played baseball, we would scout the area for discarded Coke bottles. If we found five worth two cents each, we could run to that store and get a cold replacement.

On Wednesday nights my friends and I (after dinner) would run down to the park and sit on the wooden fence. Why? We were waiting for the Chicago Outlaws, who held meetings there. My cousin Dick was a card-carrying member, as it were. He was their artist. He was the one who painted their motorcycles and painted the skull and pistons on the back of their leather jackets. I was treated like a big shot by my friends as I had a family member in the Outlaws. The cops would usually stop by but never stayed. As we sat on the fence, it took probably a good five minutes for them all to pass by, and the sound was deafening. Sometimes Dick would go on long trips. One time, he went to Florida and on the way back, caught a cottonmouth.

Dick had the thing living in a moss-covered area with branches mimicking its habitat near the ceiling of his bedroom. Don't know what eventually happened there. He also had some guinea pigs living in the basement, but he had built a little conduit of pipe so they could go outside at will. His motorcycle was a Harley and painted purple with a spider and web on the front fender. Along with the white saddlebags, it was quite a show, especially when he wore one of several wigs.

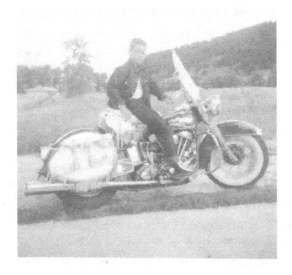

He ended up a stellar citizen, though, owning Bretz VW, Porsche/ Audi and Bretz Toyota. Before moving to California, Dick lived in Sycamore, Illinois, the birthplace of barbed wire and the Kishwaukee River named by the Potowatomi Native Americans. I believe it's the only river that flows north. In Sycamore, he started Bretz Volkswagen. He had a banana tree growing in the showroom and a guy from Haiti came in the middle of winter and stopped dead in his tracks, saying, "Ah, banana tree." He had a macaw and an original Ford F40. It was deafening when those six Weber carburetors kicked in. Later, when I was in my surgical residency at Loyola, Joan and I were invited to his birthday dinner. I was working thirty-six hours straight with one night off in those days, so I was plenty tired. How tired? Well, I ended up falling asleep on top of my lobster.

All throughout these adventures, I also worked as a model and actor throughout grammar school and partly into high school. My mom entered me in a baby beauty contest when I was six months old. I won first place. My first job based on that win was walking live up and down in the front window of John Allen studios in Chicago. From there I got my Screen Actors Guild card and began a successful modeling career.

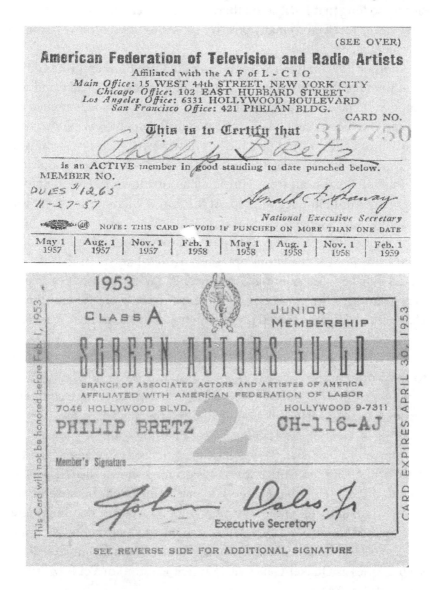

I would work for various studios that shot the Sears or Spiegel catalog. I appeared in the Chicago Tribune many times and on live TV in prime time modeling for National Clothing. I remember one time on live TV they didn't get the sleeve length on the suit right, but it was live, and there were no other suits around. They sent me out with sleeves so long that I just stood there flapping them, unsure what to do. They never received so many positive calls into the station regarding a commercial.

Another time on live TV was during the Rose Bowl and I was doing a commercial for Sunbeam. I was seen with the piece of cake and was supposed to take a big bite out of it. Well, the guy who cued me cued me too early so I took that bite off camera and all you saw was me chewing.

My mom and I would take the bus downtown when I was younger. As I grew, I would take the bus by myself. Sometimes I took the Milwaukee Road train from Forest Glen downtown to Union Station where my Aunt Florence worked. At the Forest Glen station, there was a building so passengers could stand inside. At one end was a pot belly stove with a pile of wood next to it. On snowy or cold days, you could start a fire to heat the room up. They trusted back then that people would behave in an honorable manner. We were fresh out of World War II and it didn't make any difference if you were Republican or Democrat; everyone wanted peace with no disruptions, or so it seemed to me.

Having lost many lives, we all knew what it took to bring freedom to the world and preserve ours. Like I said, it was a different time. I remember one cold snowy night when I had finished modeling and made my way to Michigan Avenue to catch the bus home, I saw a man standing in front of the Tribune Tower building with the snow falling in front of TV cameras. It was Jack Brickhouse (for many years, the voice of the Chicago Cubs). It was his evening show called "The Man on the Street." He would interview passersby. Well, because of the snow, wind, and cold, there wasn't anyone except me standing there, so he talked to me. As I grew, I became, as some agencies called me, "Chicago's Golden Boy." I would be on TV a lot doing commercials for such entities as Quaker Oats (with Sargent Preston) or Pet Ritz Frozen Pies with Red Skeleton.

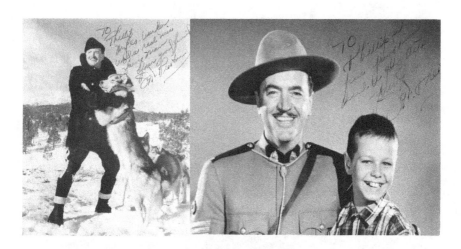

My biggest (almost) claim to fame was when I was a finalist for the TV show in the late fifties called *Father Knows Best*.

They had auditions and there were hundreds of kids trying out for the part of Bud. It turned out that of all of them, I was one of the three selected from Chicago. Because it would be shot in California and my dad's business was going so well in Chicago, it was decided I wouldn't fly out. Billy Gray got the part. Billy also had the kid part in "The Day the Earth Stood Still," one of my favorite films. That was 1951 and years later, when I successfully bid on a Lone Ranger item, we went to Profiles in History to pick it up. They had Gort's helmet and I got to put it on. Fast forward to when I started my surgical residency, Joan and I would park and stare at the house on Woodbine and Le Moyne, hoping we could buy it.

I was able to use the money I made from modeling to buy that house at 1202 Woodbine, Oak Park, Illinois. It was featured in a magazine as the Santa Claus house.

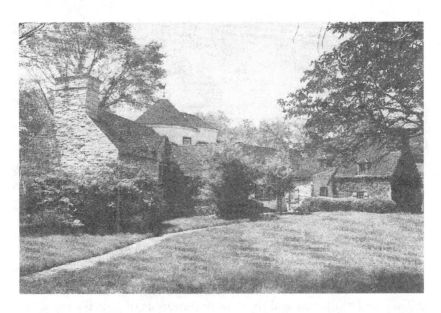

Library   Dining room   Kitchen

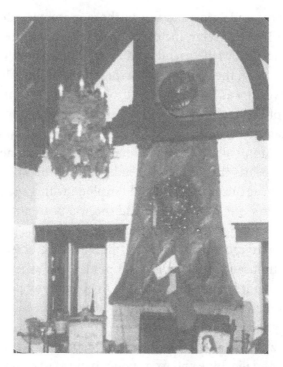

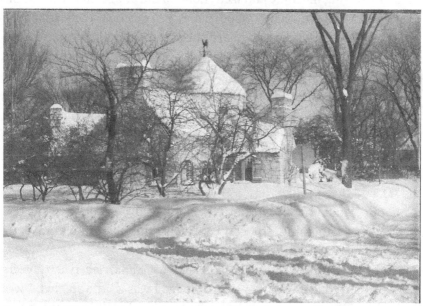

There was so much joy and fun in those grammar school days, so many stories I wish to relay, including a weekend escapade going to the theater. Each Saturday my friends and I would see a show, usually a war or horror movie, at the Gateway or Portage. One of the things I used to do at Farnsworth was in the library; I would read Popular Mechanics. In the back of the book were ads for all sorts of things boys would like, like Cushman motorbikes, WHAM-O Slingshots and among the ads was one for 'Atomic Pearls.' These came in a little container filled with sawdust. The pearls (like BBs) were embedded in the sawdust. Well, if you threw one against a wall, it would explode with a big flash. At the Gateway Theater one day, I got up and threw a pearl at the side of the screen, and the flash was blinding and huge.

It was a pretty good throw since I didn't hit the screen, causing a big fire and thousands in damages. No matter, the usher grabbed me, and I was brought to the office and had to give up my pearls, but they didn't, for some reason, call the cops. They just said I couldn't go there anymore. I waited a couple of weeks and went back without a problem. Another crazy thing we did was to take a spool of thread from our mother's sewing machine and fix a rubber band at one end. Then at the other end, we would insert a wooden match. You could then launch the match, and if it landed on any hard surface, it would light up. We had to make this stuff up as there were no video games and cartoons were only shown on Saturday mornings. We were plenty happy though.

I remember when air conditioning came out. When Sputnik was launched by the Soviet Union, my dad got me up at 4 a.m. to stand on the overpass on Edens Expressway to see it. Speaking of Edens, I also remember when that opened up. Years later during my surgical residence, I remember the first time liquid soap came out. One of the nurses said it looks like, "jiz." I also remember when credit cards first came out. Since there was minimal automation, if you were in line to purchase something, the cashier had to thumb through an ever-enlarging book with denied numbers.

As an only child (my mom and dad were married twenty years before I showed up), I should acknowledge I was a little spoiled. I was part of the "Boomer Generation" after World War II. Everything was great, normal in many ways, and peaceful throughout my childhood. Little did I know that Christmas of 1956 would be my last with my dad and my family intact.

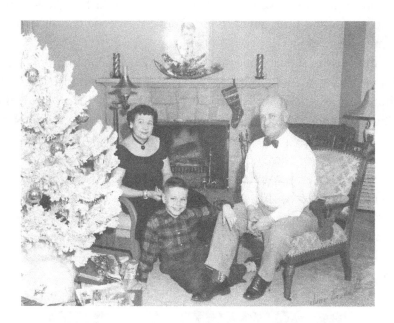

Until one day I came home from school December 12, 1957 (eighth grade), and the doorbell rang. It was Gene Travelstead (my dad's foreman). He was telling my mom that my dad had been killed in an accident. I was twelve.

While I wasn't there, in building gas stations, the gas you put in your car comes from huge tanks about 30 feet long by 10 feet wide. When you put the tank in the ground, you have to make sure the spout points straight up. While the hole is dug by a big scoop crane, to get the tank just right, you had to get down there with a shovel and finesse the final resting place. I guess he shouted to the crane driver to go forward, and instead, he went backward, crushing him. He probably died of pneumothorax from the crush injury. Not good. That was the first big blow in my life; there would be others.

My life was forever altered from what it would have been had he lived. He had just signed the contract to build Sunoco gas stations. He went all through World War II in the South Pacific without a scratch (except partial hearing loss from the big guns aboard ship). While I didn't appreciate it as such at age twelve, I loved him. He was bigger than life. I'm almost sure if he had lived, I would have followed in his footsteps and built gas stations. Apparently, G-D had other plans for me.

I still miss him every day, and every day, I touch a picture of him with me sitting on his lap. Upon graduation from Farnsworth Grammar School, my mother enrolled me in North Park Academy instead of going to Schurz High School, where all my friends ended up. North Park was a college prep school, and for the most part, the kids who attended were very smart, much smarter than me.

Growing up, I always had three birthday parties. One with the kids at school, another with my friends (in costume as my birthday was close to Halloween), and lastly, with my mom and dad's friends. On those occasions at the adult party, I sensed an opportunity and got out my shoe shine kit and made a little money shining shoes. With those parties it meant three cakes total.

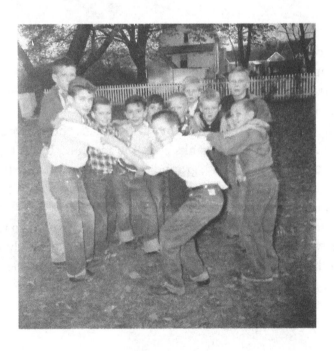

After my dad was killed, we got a dog, a chihuahua, and named him Poncho after Poncho on the Cisco Kid TV show. When we went to see the puppies, he was the only one to come to me. He was a joy, as all my pets have been, including Ginger, Racky (Racoon), Mimi, Chou Chou (poodles), Fleury (cat), Red, Mim, Mary (all cats), Arnold (red-tailed boa), Howie (Great Pyrenees, see below), named after Howie Long the defensive end for the Raiders, Wylie, and Chico (Wylie and Chico are rescue dogs we still have). Here is Howie learning to shake hands and Poncho below.

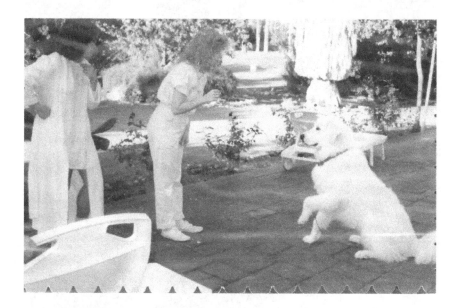

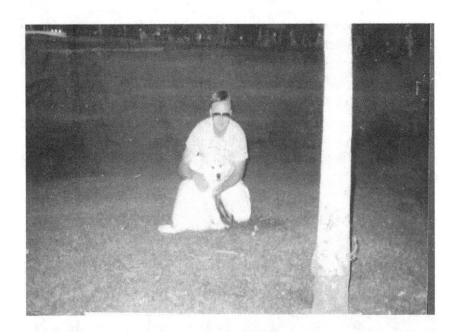

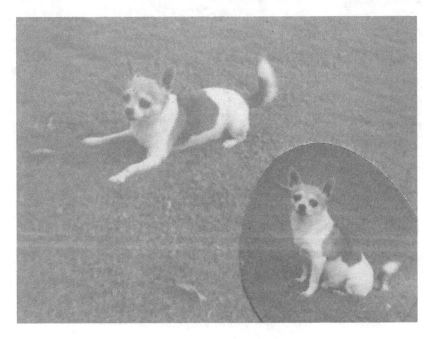

Here are a couple of photos of Howie

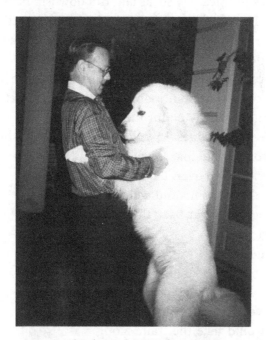

No doubt ordering dog treats

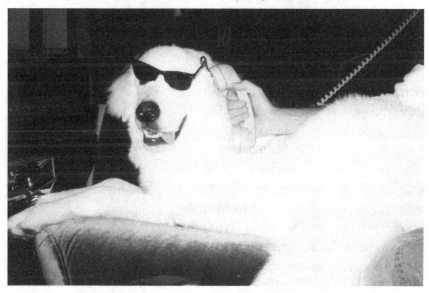

Every night Poncho slept by my feet under the covers. In the morning, he would steal my socks and run downstairs. A friend of the family had built my bedroom of knotty pine up in the attic. It occupied the entire floor including a full bath. I had a half nude mermaid etched on my shower door; it was almost like a log cabin.

Denny Joyce, the son of one of my dad's friends, gave me a poster of a stripper he knew, and I put it on the back of my closet door. Denny was a squadron leader flying for the Marines and later flew for many years for American Airlines. I recall when Denny got a brand new red 1955 Chevy convertible that his parents, Eddy and Marie, drove over to our house one night to take my mom and dad for a ride. Acquiring a new car back then was an event to celebrate.

During the summer, we would catch fireflies and nightcrawlers if we were going fishing. My Aunt Florence had a friend who lived in Long Lake, Illinois. Stevie and I would take the train, along with our freshly caught nightcrawlers, and we'd get to fish from a rowboat along the canal. We always caught a lot of bullhead.

I was a Cub and Boy Scout (still remember the pledges) and almost earned a 'life' badge just below Eagle. I hiked the Blackhawk Trail and still have the medal. I had a great time in Scouts, and I still have the Christmas ornaments I made in Cub Scouts. I remember we would send new recruits out to get a left-handed sky hook from surrounding camps. While my dad was alive, he bought new trucks for his business, Superior Pump Service. He named the big truck "Little Phil."

Wednesday, August 2, 1961

Here's a news item that certainly BEARS reporting. PHIL BRETZ, 5533 Forest Glen, has added something new to his list of sports. Besides water-skiing, skin-diving and fishing, he has taken up wrestling.

He has been spending his weekends with his cousin up at Burlington, Wis.; on Saturday night they all went to town because the circus had arrived. Among the many sideshows there was a special feature: a 6 foot, 380 pound bear waiting for someone to wrestle with him.

PHIL, who plans another canoe trip into northern Canada the first of August, thought he could use the experience, and having attended a number of wrestling matches the past season, wanted to try one of the many wrestling holds.

PHIL entered the ring and very cautiously approached the bear. When he saw his chance, he made a leap and put a headhold on the bear. PHIL held his ground until MR. BEAR decided he was being taken. The bear shook himself and threw PHIL to the ropes.

PHIL was soon back on his feet and again attempted to tackle the bear but this time the animule' put the famous bearhug on PHIL and after a struggle PHIL finally freed himself.

It was exciting while it lasted and PHIL stayed with the bear for six minutes.

As I said, this story BEARS reporting.

—0—

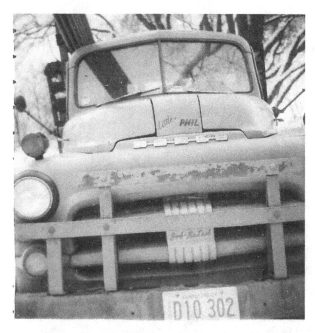

When we went to pick it up, I rode in the back and climbed the wood railings. Nowadays, that would be child endangerment. My generation was the last not to have to wear helmets, knee, or elbow pads to prevent injury. Now, of course, I wear a helmet while riding my Madone. We were just free back then without ever-increasing regulations creeping in slowly. I'm not saying protective gear is bad. But there are limits to where they begin to interfere with just enjoying life.

After my dad was killed, Mr. Istok, who lived two doors down from us, frequently took me fishing. We would go at night to Foster Avenue Jetty on Lake Michigan and fish for perch. We would get hot dogs at the stands, and we usually caught several perch to eat. He taught me how to tie a fisherman's knot, which I still use today. Jason and I used that knot (I taught him) to catch two large 48-inch muskies during our trip to Century Lodge in Ontario, Canada, in 2017. What was neat was that the very spot I caught my muskie (with a homemade lure) was the very spot my brother-in-law fished not fifteen minutes before. You never know. Who's is bigger? I contend mine is. But it should be every father's wish your son gets the big one.

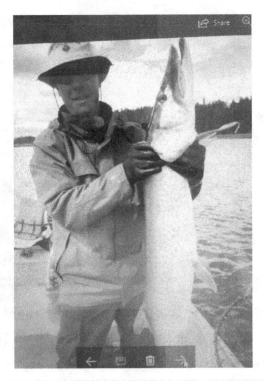

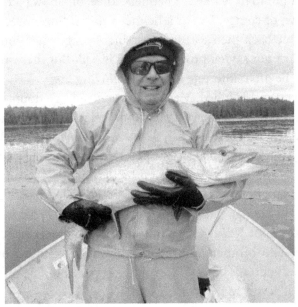

From fourth to sixth grade, I went to a Catholic School at the Queen of All Saints Basilica. The nuns were our teachers, and they wore traditional black nun uniforms. They also had long leather straps hanging from their waist and would threaten to rap you on the hands if you did something out of turn. That's how we learned to listen. On Fridays they would have mass in the afternoon, and all the kids would go except Robert Coleman (who I would reunite with at North Park Academy) and me. He and I had to sit out in the hall as we were Protestants. On Christmas Eve we always went to midnight mass at Queen of All Saints.

While at Queen of All Saints, I met Dennis Anheier. His father was in the Secret Service and ran President Truman's detachment. His dad, Harry, was tall and can be seen in photos standing behind Truman at the Potsdam Conference with Winston Churchill and Stalin. He was secret service to three presidents. Near Dennis's house there was a factory where they made toy soldiers. We would climb into the trash containers to scrounge for plastic war toys.

Sometimes I would ride the bus to cousin Ronnie's house (Aunt Hazel's son, my mom's sister), and at one point, we made a soapbox car out of a large can. I would push him; he would drive. Much later, when I was in high school, he and I raced his Ford Fairlane at Union Grove dragstrip in Wisconsin. We won the nationals in F stock automatic. I thought I was a big shot. Below is the soapbox.

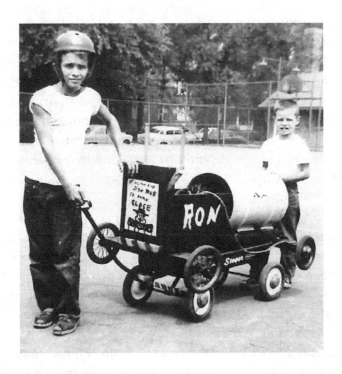

On the cover of Newsweek Magazine, February 12, 1945, is my Uncle Clarence (Ronnie's father) with his Thompson machine gun (in the foreground) leaning against the tank. It is one of the iconic photos of World War II and appeared in Ken Burns' book "The War." He was in the Thunderbird Division, 45th Infantry. He landed in Sicily, Anzio, France and fought his way into Germany at times under General Patton.

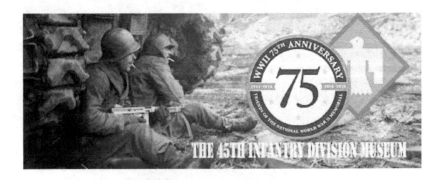

The Thunderbird division liberated the concentration camp Dachau. Uncle Clarence was awarded the Bronze Star. I'm proud to say he was my uncle.

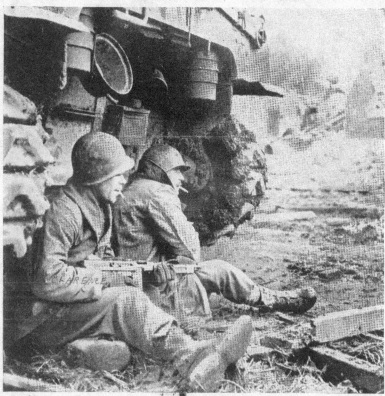

Newsweek

FEBRUARY 12, 1945   15c

THE MAGAZINE OF NEWS SIGNIFICANCE

CLARENCE TROY   In the West: Ready for the Kill

I started at North Park Academy (NPA) in the fall of 1959. I went out for sports as I was pretty good. It seemed to level the playing field with all those smart kids around me. It was a different environment geared toward accomplishment for sure. As time went on, I lettered in football (my nickname was "Crusher"), swimming (captain), and track (captain) and could run the 440 in 50 seconds flat, well off world record pace but could hang with most.

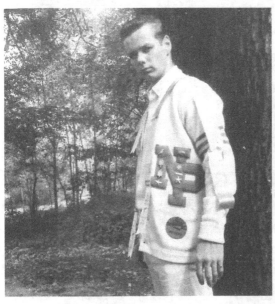 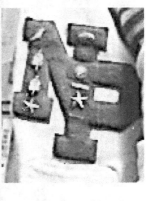

In my training for football, I would do sit-ups with a 50-pound weight behind my head and do fifty. On my seventeenth birthday after football practice, I did 1,000 sit-ups. The team watched me do it.

Getting in touch with the great outdoors started with visits to Ely, Minnesota. Coach Ted Headstrand (RIP) at North Park had a cabin up there. He used to take about ten guys up there for a canoe trip. We would canoe along the Boundary Waters between the US and Canada. It was Basswood Lake, and we would pitch tents and fry fish we had caught during the day. It was a great time. I must have gone about three times, and one time I bought a wolf skin to hang in my room.

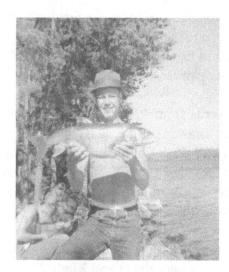

Another time, Coach took just me and Doug Johnson up, and Doug and I made a wayside (clearing bushes and trees) where cars could stop. We put up a sign, WAYSIDE BY PHIL AND DOUG. On one trip, I climbed a big waterfall. Speaking of signs, my dad, a supervisor for Sinclair Oil Company, helped a farmer hang the brass ball in Antioch, Illinois. It's still called Brass Ball Corner. We used to drive by it going to the cabin at Honey Lake in Burlington, Wisconsin.

Without fail, I must reiterate the bear wrestling saga of legend. One time we were at the Burlington County Fair, when we walked by this wrestling ring. As we did, a guy started to bark out, "Who will wrestle the bear and win a free dinner?" You had to stay for three rounds. We looked over, and there was a cart moving back and forth, it looked like the bear was inside. Before a few seconds passed, Stan (my cousin) yelled out, "This guy will fight the bear!" as he pointed to me. When he got the bear out of the cart, it stood up on his hind legs (just like in *The Great Outdoors* with John Candy). The bear had a muzzle on but had claws. I remember going to him and trying to give him a bear hug, but he was too big. I only lasted less than a round but I did it, see documentation in the newspaper article.

At the time, Stan (he married Darlyn, Aunt Hazel's daughter) bought a gas station (Cities Service later Citgo) with Ron Jaworski out in Northfield Woods. He purchased his first house, a three bedroom, two bath ranch for $15,000. Decades later, I would buy a lot for our home at Thunderbird Country Club, 1.5 acres for $275,000.

That was a lot to pay back in 1980 just for the land. It was an acre-and-a-half on the sixth green, seventh tee at Thunderbird Country Club about 300 yards from President Ford. Lucille Ball lived right across the fairway. I never got the hang of studying hard until I met Bernie Lerner at North Park College in my junior year. Then it was too late. Mr. Safstrum, my algebra teacher at North Park Academy, said he never saw me carrying any homework when I left school. Which, in all honesty, was probably true.

I just did enough to get Cs or a hook; as Bernie said, that would make me eligible for sports. During that time, I would take the bus on Fridays to Aunt Hazel's on Elston and Kimball, miles away from my house. Stan would pick me up there, and I would work at the gas station all weekend. On Saturday nights, he and I would stay up and watch wrestling (Buddy Rogers or Hay Stack Calhoun), or we'd walk on a path in the back of his house to a pond where we would fish.

One night I drank too much and laid on the bathroom floor all night. I remember we had gas price wars, and we would try and undercut the competition. We had a sign that said "Gas 25 Cents." I would change oil and tires and do tune-ups. On New Year's Eve, we had Jack Daniels bottles and would pour shots for our customers (which was probably highly illegal).

During that time, I got a new shotgun specifically for skeet shooting, a Browning over and under. Ron Jaworski and I would often go out to Hilldale Gun Club and shoot skeet. Hilldale was a cool place. You would park on a hill just on grass because there was no parking lot. Inside it was like a lodge. They had a huge fireplace and wood paneling. I remember the world champion skeet shooter was there. He had two German shorthaired pointers. They would walk on either side of him and he would shoot skeet from the hip. I did manage to shoot twenty-five straight and got my patch. I still have my Hilldale vest. I never managed to shoot fifty straight, though.

Also at that time, I got a reloading set and would reload my shotgun shells. One time I drove up to Wisconsin where a friend of the family had a hunting farm and I shot ring-neck pheasants. Aunt Florence prepared them.

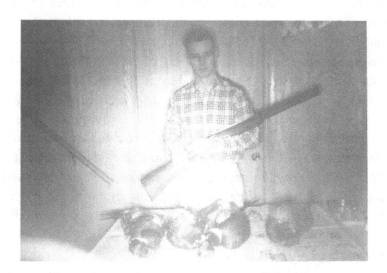

During the gas station days, Stan bought a lot at Honey Lake (near Burlington, Wisconsin), where some friends of Aunt Hazel's had had a cabin for years just inside the border of Wisconsin near Lake Geneva. Stan, Ron Jaworski, and I built a cabin from scratch. We would go fishing along the nearby river. We had three spots and we would always catch many bullhead.

We would nail them to the tree, skin them, and fry them. The fishing spots were like a jungle. We would water ski on Honey Lake and swim in Del Monte Lake right outside the cabin. One time Stan and I were out there in my canoe and I asked him if he had his wallet on him, and before he could think, he said, "no." I rocked the canoe until we tipped over. We'd do stuff like that all the time.

Stan had bought a little "bug," as Aunt Hazel would say, actually a Renault. On the way back, he pulled over and let me drive. It was the first time I drove, no license. It must have been in my first or second year in high school. One time I had to drive home by myself, having ridden with my cousin Ronnie to Great Lakes Naval Yard after his leave expired, no license then either. I was probably about thirteen. It was in Ronnie's Ford Fairlane blue convertible, and thankfully I didn't get caught. Ronnie and I used to drive out to Skips. I forgot exactly where it was but on North Avenue, Melrose Park? It was called the Fiesta Restaurant, but everyone knew it as Skips. It was a real hangout. Guys would drive from all over to show off their cars and drag race.

Before Stan married my cousin Darlyn, he was in the Navy and was the air traffic controller at the now decommissioned Glenview Naval Air station. Because it was in a residential area (Glenview), he would request all jets to be at least 2,000 feet in the air by the runway's end. The Blue Angles would, at times, fly in. They wouldn't land one at a time but in threes. When they departed, he would remind them to be at least at flight level 2000 by the end of the runway for noise abatement. They would take off three at a time, throw in the afterburners, climb straight up to 20,000 feet and then call into the tower requesting permission to cross the runway threshold.

Sometimes I would play basketball on the path by the side of our house. My dad had put up a backboard there. Here is a photo of my bedroom at 5533.

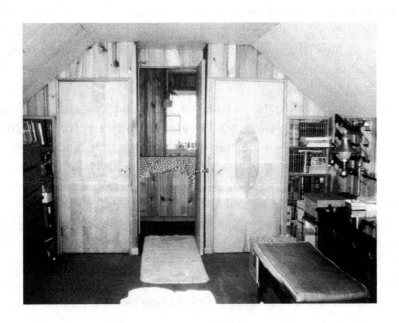

And while I think about it, in my estimation, it doesn't take a village to raise a child. It takes two loving parents who have a foundation, work ethic, and a moral compass. Or, in my case, after my dad was killed, a strong woman who had to do the work of two. A great example, watching the Olympics from Tokyo, are the families of Simone Biles, Suni Lee (her dad in a wheelchair), Caeleb Dressel, or Katie Ledecky. Every one of those kids thanked their parents for getting them to that lofty position in life of being an Olympic athlete. Their family TV spots should be an inspiration to all families (a real supportive nucleus) on what can be achieved with proper upbringing (assuming the kid doesn't put snakes in their teacher's desk!).

CHAPTER 2
NORTH PARK ACADEMY– NORTH PARK COLLEGE

B ACK AT NORTH Park Academy, I would walk to the bus at Foster and Elston. It was about a mile-and-a-half walk. In my first year, I was still modeling. I had to leave football practice for that a few times. I guess I pretty much hung by myself until my prowess in sports attracted some attention. As time went on, there were the big three: me, Gino, and Gerry. Here is Gino and I on the track team. I'm handing off the baton.

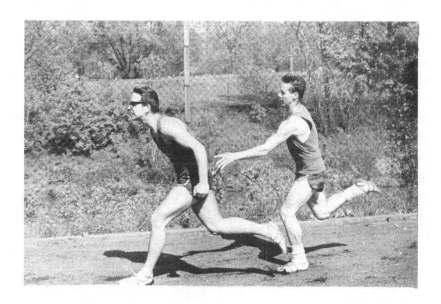

On one occasion, we were downtown and walking around. In the distance, we saw a sign going around; I think the same sign is seen in the movie *Running Scared*. It said "Jesus Saves." Being from North Park, a Swedish Covenant School where there was no dancing and no proms, just banquets, we decided to walk to see what was going on at Jesus Saves. Halfway there, we stumbled into the Rialto Theater, a strip joint. We went in and enjoyed the show. In the last act, Fay Starr came out and stripped. Taking her panties off, she yelled out, "Who wants um?" Of course, we stood up and raised our hands along with others. She rolled them in a ball and threw them out, and Gerry (about six-foot-two) stuck his arm out and grabbed them. They were red, and in ballpoint pen written in the crotch was, "Come back again, baby, I love you, Fay Starr."

We went home after that, and I get a call at about 11 p.m. from Gerry to come to get the panties. His dad was a pastor and he was afraid his mother would smell them as they were loaded with perfume. I get over there, and Gerry's room was on the second floor. He opened the window and threw them out. They floated all the way down past the window where I could see his father sitting. I prayed all the way down for him not to look out the window. It was like a scene out of *Animal House*.

Another time at North Park Academy, we were in typing class. During lunch I had gone there to type the paragraph we would type to see how many words we could type per minute with the least number of errors. The teacher would use the same paragraph, so I typed, I think, a little over 60 words letter by letter with one finger and hid the paper. At the start of the class, we put the typewriter covers on our heads like nuns. It drew a big laugh. During class, I was typing like mad and just switched the pages. But the best part was Gerry got so frustrated, he picked up the typewriter and said, "I'm throwing it out the window." We were on the third floor. The teacher panicked and said, "Please don't." He hung the thing out the window but didn't throw it out. That also got a big laugh.

When I got my driver's license, things changed. My car (my Dad's 1957 Olds convertible) came to be known as the "Pink Lady." It never hurt to have pretty girls want to wash her. Note the personalized license plates, PB 5533, my home address.

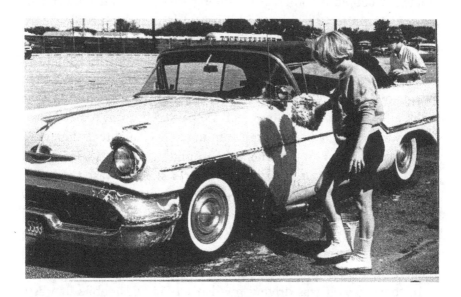

On the weekends the guys would drive late at night to Jakes. It was a greasy spoon on Touhy Avenue that served delicious silver dollar pancakes. But my life changed the day I saw Joan. It was the middle of August, and I was going into my senior year at NPA. I had just come back from football practice and showered in the locker room in the school's basement. As I bounded up the stairs, I was about to burst through the door when I saw her coming toward me. I stopped dead. I forget what I said to myself, but it was something like, "You have to open the door for this one." I waited until she almost reached the door, and I opened it and held it for her. As I recall, she blew right by me almost without recognition. I checked out her legs (wearing shorts) and everything else. She was going to the bookstore. I was hooked. I knew in ten seconds I wanted to be with her my entire life.

How do I do that? It is what the French call, *Je ne sais quoi* or "that certain something," which is indefinable. Joan was the most beautiful girl I had ever seen or would ever see. Even at seventy-five now she still looks outstanding. My playboy days were over.

To be quite honest, I was kind of a whiz as my experience with the girls grew, and I knew what I wanted. Before Joan came on the scene, I dated a couple of other girls, among them AB and CD. Initials changed to protect the innocent! These girls were both really smart, like Latin Honor Society smart. CD was a math genius. If she only knew I couldn't add two plus two. I think they were after my body and just wanted to see what dating a jock was like. I don't really know, except they enjoyed their time with me, and I never got any complaints. One night, after I took AB out to dinner, we parked in front of her house. Lucky for me her dad didn't come out to see his daughter being taken advantage of, or was it the other way around? That night was the first time I successfully put my hand up a girl's skirt. It wasn't just that accomplishment for a novice, but using the same hand, I somehow worked my way up her back to unhook her bra, also, a first. Luckily, I didn't know how to do anything else; otherwise, we would have been in trouble. In the meantime, my tongue felt like it was being reshaped. What a night, a real learning experience.

In those days, I was driving my dad's 1957 Oldsmobile. It was a convertible, all pink with a white and black interior. She became known as the notorious "Pink Lady." I put spotlights on her, side skirts, and what they called "lake pipes." Dating AB and CD went a long way to refining my expertise in managing women's needs, shall we say. When Joan came on the scene, AB came up to her in the locker room and told her to watch out because Phillip really knew how to make a girl hot. Oh well, Joan didn't listen, I guess. And how could I not recall ZZ, (initials changed again) bringing me coffee and donuts in the morning? The only trouble was (not that that was any trouble), I was still in bed undressed. It was like every guy's dream, a cute girl wearing boots and a miniskirt wakes you up with coffee and donuts. I should add, she drove a Corvette, white with a red interior. I still don't know if she was trying to get me to dump Joan or just what was on her agenda?

Those were the days. At the risk of making my kids fall asleep (since they have heard this many times) after school started, I set out trying to find out who my future wife was. It didn't take me long. It turned out she lived all the time about a mile-and-a-half away, but on the other side of Cicero Avenue, the highbrow side. By that I mean, she got to go to public school in Sauganash, which was all lannon stone. On the other side of Cicero, where I lived at 5533 N. Forest Glen, Chicago, Illinois, we went to a regular Chicago public school just like in *A Christmas Story*. I somehow found out that her birthday was coming up. It was a cold September night. I walked over to 5941 N. Knox and peeked into the window like a peeping tom.

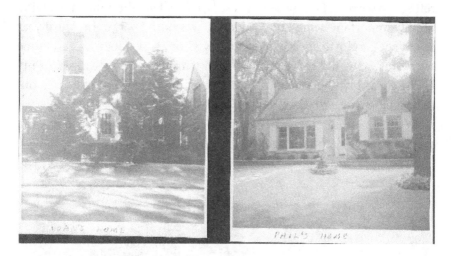

I was uninvited, and she didn't know I was coming. I waited until she had opened her presents and they had cake. Then I rang the doorbell. She came to the door, and I introduced myself. I didn't know if she knew who I was or not. Gee, I thought everyone at North Park Academy knew I was part of the big three, me, Gino, and Gerry. Wait, I just asked Joan if she knew who I was? She said days before I had, without saying a word, put my hand on hers on the railing going up to class, nice move (you have to know the nuances). She remembers thinking I was cute.

Back at the party, she let me in. On Saturday nights after our dates, the guys would dump off the girls and come to my house and play cards. Remember the red panties? I had put them on a board I had painted red, and everyone would touch them. I told the girls at the party that all the guys were over at my house, so they all left, and Joan and I were alone. I didn't try anything; we just sat and watched *House on Haunted Hill* with Vincent Price. And that was the end for me. As I said, I knew in the first ten seconds, and fifty-two-plus years and four kids later, I still know.

At North Park Academy I lettered in football, swimming (captain), and track (captain). I think Joan just wanted to wear my letter sweater. I still have the sweater, which Ashley and Alexandra (my daughters) refused to wear on Halloween. As I said, I didn't get the hang of studying or how important being knowledgeable was until I was in the third year of college at North Park College (now University). Joan would come over, and we would carve pumpkins or trim the Christmas tree, or my favorite was I would tell her we were going to a party, and it turned out to be a party for two. Looking back, it was the best of times.

When I turned eighteen, my mom had sent in for a Playboy Club card for me. You couldn't get one until you were twenty-one.

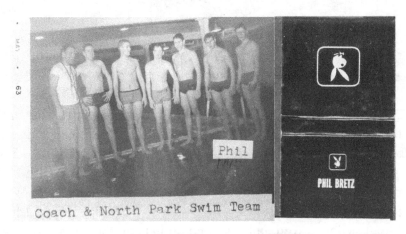

Coach & North Park Swim Team

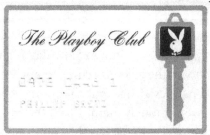

But having one was prima facie evidence you were 21. Joan and I would drive downtown to a nightclub called Mr. Kelly's on Rush Street, have dinner, and see comedians like Shelly Berman and Bob Newhart. Then we would walk over to Walton where the Playboy Club was, and bingo, we were let in without question because I had the magic card. I also had matches with the Playboy insignia and my name. Bigshot. The club was a multistory vintage mansion, and you climbed on stairs that were narrow, just able to pass people on the way. When you came in, they put your name up. Late in the evening, they would have a midnight buffet of scrambled eggs, sausage, etc., with a live jazz band playing in the background. We would drive home late at night on Lake Shore Drive along Lake Michigan.

Those were the days in Chicago when Playboy had bought the old Palmolive Building at the entrance to Michigan Avenue and had PLAYBOY atop the building in big letters. The spotlight rotated right as you entered Michigan Avenue Also, I used to watch *Playboy After Dark.* It was also the time of the "Big Bunny." That was Hugh Hefner's jet, a DC-9, painted black with the bunny logo on the tail. Its call numbers were 950PB. I thought the letters stood for Phil Bretz. Other times we would eat at Chez Paul or Club on 39, which was on the thirty-ninth floor of some building I can't remember the name of. They had arranged along the windows, single file, big red leather swivel chairs. It was an idyllic time. It was Chicago. By the way, the Big Bunny ended up in a children's playground in Queretaro, Mexico, sans wings and engines, of course. Probably a most fitting end to let children play on her. Below is the Big Bunny in all her glory and her resting place.

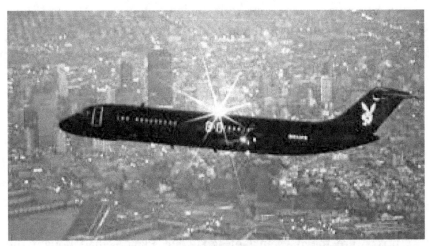

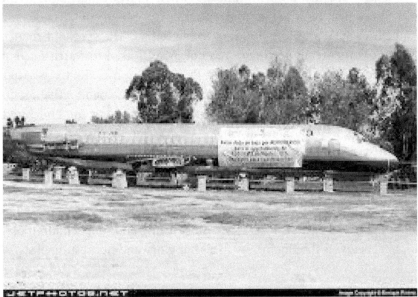

I was a pretty jealous guy when it came to Joan, obviously owing to my own insecurity. I remember one time when she was sitting in class, and this guy sat next to her. It wasn't by accident, I figured he was trying to make headway. I was so pissed I turned around and put my fist through the hall door window. It had chicken wire in it, so it didn't shatter. But that stunt landed me in the principal's office, where I explained I was showing a friend a football move. (My nickname was "Crusher"). Joan was elected homecoming queen at North Park Academy, when I was in my freshman year at North Park College. Below is that moment in time.

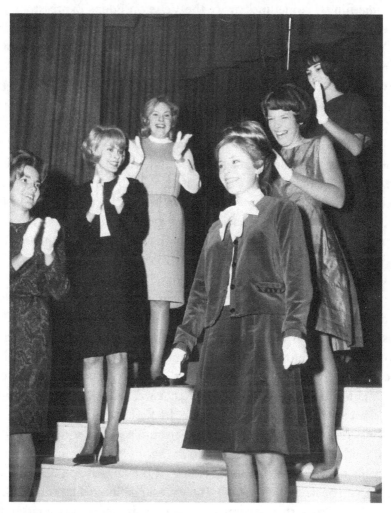

It was a tradition that the King and Queen kissed at halftime. The King came over to me and asked for permission. I said, "Enjoy yourself." Joan dumped me a couple of times when I was in college, thus the nursing school episode at Swedish Covenant Hospital and the anatomy labs.

Another episode, which we still laugh about to this day, is the guy in the lime green Dodge Dart. I don't know how I knew she was going on a date with this guy, probably from Pam. But when I was pissed off at something, I sometimes drove the Vette on Edens Expressway. Just serendipitously, as I pulled off the cloverleaf, I was right behind him. So, I opened up the "lake pipes" from the dash and gunned the motor. I knew he could hear it. When I did that at the college, you could hear it two blocks away. I think he is still shaking from that encounter. But sometimes now, when things don't go right, I tell Joan she wouldn't be in this fix if she had married the guy in the Dart.

But all in all, persistence on my part won out. When a couple is making their vows before a congregation and G-D, they have no idea the curveballs that life can throw at them. About a year before our 50th wedding anniversary, we were invited to attend Joan's cousin's wedding of his daughter back in Chicago. As we were talking with Joan's relatives, Bill Feind said, "I was battle-tested." I suppose Joan and I both were, as was he and his wife Kathleen.

Once I came onto the radar with Joan, I suppose you could say we were going steady. While we didn't know it, the time at North Park Academy was part of what would be called "the good old days." It was a time I often would like to go back to, and it was a time when most people got along because it was mostly carefree. I remember Mr. Safstrum stopping our algebra class to hear the blastoff of America's first man into space, Alan Shepard. That was May 5, 1961, just about five days after Yuri Gargarin became the first human into space from the erstwhile USSR. Yuri would die in an auto accident some years later. I just read astronaut Scott Kelly's book *Endurance* (very intriguing).

In his book Scott talks about riding to the launch pad at Star City, Russia, to be launched to the International Space Station (ISS). A tradition follows that several hundred yards before arriving at the launch site, the bus pulls over and all the astronauts get out and pee on the right back tire. They do it for good luck as Yuri had his bus stop to pee. Poor Alan Shepard, did he just have to go in his suit? The rocket ride I'm sure made up for it.

I remember once having won my two individual events at a swim meet (100-yard breaststroke and 100-yard butterfly) and I was anxious to tell Joan. I didn't stop enough at a stop sign and was pulled over by the Chicago Police. I explained the situation and asked if I could take care of it right there. The cost was $2.00, all I had on me. Another story I recall at North Park Academy was one time during track (I ran the 440 in 50 seconds flat), as I came around the final turn, it was like I was just starting to run, a second wind came upon me. It was the only time throughout high school or college that I felt I was in the ZONE. The image below is that race that I won.

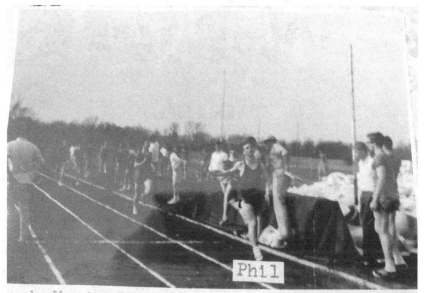

ack Meet, Lake Forest Academy, May 196

Here are the Band of Brothers, we were ready to take on the world, or so we thought.

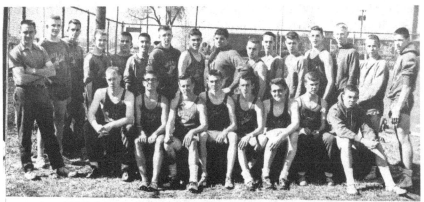

1st row, L-R-G. Ewald, D. Ginosi, P. Bretz, B. Albrecht, P. Stenmark, H. Doden, J. Deer, J. Douglass. 2nd row--Coach McCarrell, B. Lindquist, J. Comunale, W. Eifler, R. Mack, P. Warton, J. Mc-Clurkin, D. Keren, J. Kussy, R. Handschuh, L. Fleckles, R. Larson, J. Lindberg, B. Swanson, W. Suska, J. Furnoff.

TRACK & FIELD

For homecoming, we always had floats stationed throughout the campus. Our senior float was called "Beat'em or Bust." It was a covered wagon made of colored crepe paper, and the wheels turned (motorized). But at the time of the judging, the wheels wouldn't turn. Four of us hid behind the wheels and turned them. I don't remember if we won or not.

Before moving on to North Park College, I must acknowledge three individuals who helped shape my future in terms of persistence and believing in G-D almighty. They are Mr. Swanson (RIP), my English teacher at North Park Academy, who taught me how to articulate a complete sentence, although he didn't know it at the time. AT (RIP), our biology teacher who lit the candle of interest in science that propelled me into pre-med, and Rev. Magnuson (RIP), who instilled spiritual values in me that last until this day. He was like a second father to me, and I remember him in my prayers every night.

Rev. Magnuson married Joan and me on June 27, 1969, at 6 p.m. That's Rev. Magnuson on the right.

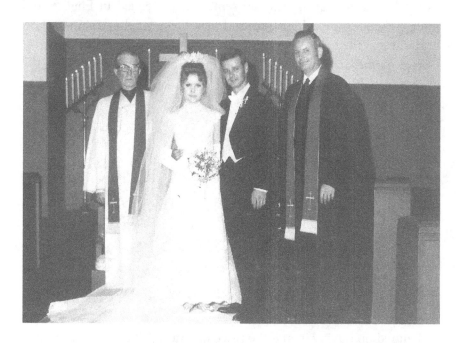

There was one point there where I felt I could be a darn good minister and briefly set my sights on North Park's Seminary School. That lasted until I met Bernie and his family, and then I was convinced I should become a surgeon.

I was a jock and cared more about Joan than my GPA. I did manage to maintain a 2.0 plus GPA, which allowed my participation in sports. Besides, my future had been planned, or so I thought. I was to go into the construction business with a guy who was with my dad as a Seabee in Guadalcanal. This was out in Palm Springs, California. However, I realized that a college education was something I needed. I, of course, applied to North Park College (now University). I remember my interview with Dean Olson. He said that I wouldn't hire a contractor to build my house that didn't have the right tools. Translating it meant that an underachiever like me grade-wise shouldn't be allowed into college.

I guess because I went to North Park Academy, he allowed me to take summer courses at North Park College. If I got a B or better, he would let me in starting the fall semester. I enrolled in English and Biology. I got Bs (I think) in both and was allowed in the freshman class, beginning in the fall of 1963. As freshmen, we had to wear beanies.

Here comes my black 1963 split-window Vette (Stingray). Note the license plate PB 5533.

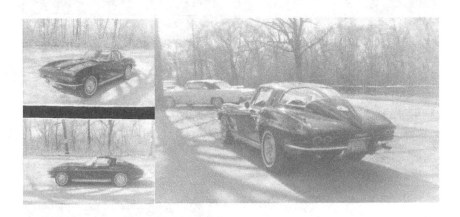

I ended up buying it, and the price tag was $3,400.00. Now, if I still owned it, the price would be around $100,000. It had a 456 rear-end (gear ratio), and if I popped the clutch, it was so fast off the line that the cigarette lighter would fly out.

While at North Park College, Bill Sarring and I put in dash-operated cutouts. That meant that from the dashboard of the Vette, I could pull the handles out and the exhaust would be coming directly out of the manifold. It was very very loud but also very very cool. One day when we were at Road America in Wisconsin where Ernie and Joan's dad were racing, I came over a hill on this country road and the stop sign was out. I went directly across the road into a ditch. The horn's button popped off and cut my nose pretty bad. Blood was all over, but I didn't lose consciousness. It healed up well. At the end of my college days, when I thought I would be going into the Air Force as a pilot, I sold the Vette. Mistake, I should have kept it.

At North Park College I went out for football, which was short-lived.

However, I did go out for swimming and track, which I lettered in both two years in a row. In fact, just like Clark Griswald, I took third in the state my senior year in the 200-yard butterfly in the College Conference of Illinois. I remember one incident where MOC (men off campus) carried a VW into the library. There were also so-called "panty raids," which I only heard about.

I hit it off with my biology professor Mr. Tofte. He taught the first ecology class, as there had been no such thing before at North Park College. With Mr. Tofte's two sons, we constructed an RC track in their basement. We had a great time racing RC cars. A memorable field trip he took the class on was to Coal City just outside Chicago, a place where you can find fossils and dinosaur bones.

As time went on, he appointed me his lab assistant. One perk was I was able to teach the nursing class at Swedish Covenant Hospital. The hospital was about four miles away, and the nurses were pretty much off the radar and sequestered. There were a couple of nurses that I hit it off with, and we used to ride around in the Vette. Nothing serious, though. It was at a time when Joan had dumped me for some reason, which remains unclear? I majored in biology and psychology. As I advanced in years, I enrolled in cell physiology.

There were only four people in the class. One of the perks in this class was that I got to go to Fermilab in Batavia, Illinois. It is a big cyclotron. It's where they smash protons together to find ever smaller components of the atom like quarks and gluons. They also have the only herd of albino deer. They were snow-white, and very cool to see. It was named after Enrico Fermi, and years later, I would read about the Fermi Paradox. He just asked, with so many stars and planets capable of developing life, where are they? One had to have clearance to get in and you were issued a badge.

During this time around 1966 we had a home in Palm Springs. My mother (at my request) brought back (on the plane) a big female black widow complete with egg. It was a different time. Just like when I was growing up, we didn't have helmets or knee and elbow pads to protect us from a fall. We learned (sometimes the hard way) not to fall. Being a big shot lab assistant, I had my own office. I had the black widow in there and put flies, etc., for her to eat. One morning I came in to find hundreds of black widow babies running all over my desk. While the top of her glass aquarium had a screen, the babies just went right through. We had to close the place down and had it fumigated.

While I was in college, I took care of my Uncle Nels' (through marriage) yacht. It was a 50+ footer based at Belmont Harbor in Chicago on Lake Shore Drive, just outside the downtown Chicago proper. It had relatively few slips, and there was a long waiting list to moor your boat there. It also happened to be in the neighborhood where a lot of flight attendants lived. They would ride their bikes along the shore and look at the yachts. One thing led to another, and pretty soon, I had them lying on the boat in their bikinis. I never did more than that. Joan would also grace the boat in her bikini. I could hardly get any work done. Uncle Nels would always say the same thing when he intermittently came, "How ya doing boy? G-d damn weather."

About this time, Steve, my next-door neighbor, had earned his pilot's license. He took me for a ride, and I was hooked on flying. I began to fly from Sky Harbor and Jerry Zucha (sp?) was my instructor. After a few sessions, I remember taxiing out to the runway, and he jumped out of the plane and told me to take off and land. I remember the call letters of the Cessna 150, 4670X.

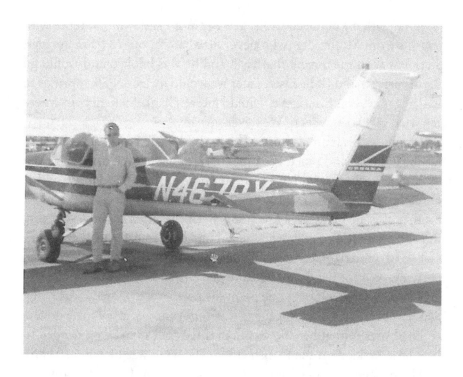

I also remember how fast it took off without the extra weight of Jerry in the co-pilot seat. I landed successfully. From there, I was able to practice on my own and do several cross-country flights to obtain my necessary forty hours of instruction. During this time, Sky Harbor had a Cessna Skymaster. It was a twin-engine front and back or a push puller.

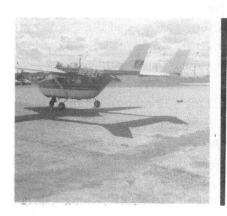
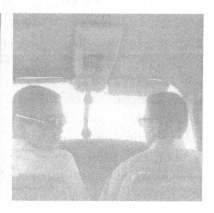

Jerry, with me at the controls, flew my mom and Aunt Florence with cousins from Minnesota (who never flew before) out to Palm Springs. Stan flew with me during that visit, and he was hooked and would go for his private and IR licenses. Later we would fly from Palm Springs to Las Vegas several times. We would land at Giant Rock airstrip where reported UFOs were seen. We never saw any.

I suppose this is an ideal time to bring in Bernie Lerner. I can't recall just how Bernie and I met. We probably sat next to each other in a class sometime at the beginning of my junior year at North Park College. He came from a Jewish family and his dad was a surgeon and his older brother was in medical school, and Bernie wanted to be a surgeon, thus he majored in pre-med. His dad had him transfer to North Park College from Arizona State as he felt Bernie was exposed to too much partying. We hit it off and became good friends. Both of us liked to golf, so we golfed a lot. At one point, he used to tell people I was Doug Sander's brother. Doug was the first flamboyantly dressed male golfer.

I'll always remember the less than three-foot putt Doug needed to beat Jack Nicklaus at the British Open. The wind was blowing so hard, and he pushed the put—his one chance at a major. I can't imagine the agony. The Lerners lived in upscale Highland Park, Illinois. I would be invited up there often, and during Passover, they would have me there for the seder. They gave me my own yarmulka and tallit. I still have both. I would have to ask, "Why is this night different from all others?" I think they were hoping I would defect.

Dr. Lerner was a great guy. If we had two tests the same day, he would write us lying letters to delay the one test as all these tests were necessary for our final grades and getting into medical school. The problem with me, though, was that I wasn't an A student. Yes, I did pull As in my final year, but it's too late for any medical school to see it. Dr. Lerner used to take Bernie and me on rounds on Saturdays. He would outfit us with white jackets (like we were doctors or at least in medical school), and we would see patients he had operated on. Those were the days when doctors were called doctors (an earned title), not providers. Now all doctors have been demoted by functionaries who haven't so much as used a Band-Aid but see fit to tell doctors what they can and cannot do. Those were also the days when a surgeon walked down the hall and everyone got out of the way. And at the end of the hall, the nurses had coffee and donuts waiting. This exposure made me study more and respect the medical profession. Dr. Lerner gave me a five-dollar bill and told me to keep it so I'd never go broke. I still have it. Bernie got married to Judy, and I was probably the only *goy* there.

One time after Bernie was in medical school, he called me to come down to Cook County Hospital. There, the unofficial motto was "see one, do one, teach one." I was a senior at North Park College. When I got down there, he put a white jacket and scrubs on me to watch him deliver a baby. They had women lined up in a hallway, ready to deliver. They all had small aluminum bowls with masks filled with Trilene. They could inhale it during painful contractions. I watched Bernie deliver a couple of babies, and while watching a third, a nurse tapped me on the shoulder and said there was a patient "crowning" in the next room. I had to come and deliver her baby. By the time I scrubbed and gowned, I could see the baby's head. It was her seventh baby. I just stood there and caught it as she pushed it out. A nurse clamped the cord, and I handed the baby off.

Bernie finished at North Park College sooner than I did. He got into Chicago Medical School, which is now part of the Rosalind Franklin University, but it was stand-alone back then.

During this time, the Vietnam War (undeclared) was raging. While I had a 2S deferment from Selective Service, I also had a high draft number from the lottery, around 265. This meant I could finish college. As my time at North Park College was coming to a close, and I had applied unsuccessfully to several medical schools, it became clear I would go into the military. I think my GPA was around 3.2 but that was my last year. I was gung-ho as I wanted to go into the Air Force as a pilot. I took the officer's training exam, and they sent me to Chanute Air Force base in Rantoul, Illinois, for my flight physical. I was eighteen. I had my own officer's quarters and got to sit in the jets. The food was all you could eat and good. I was ready to sign up. I came home and in the mailbox was my acceptance letter to medical school in Guadalajara, Mexico, at the Universidad Autonoma de Guadalajara. Ironically, one of the reasons I didn't get into a US medical school was my D in Spanish. Now I would have to learn medicine in Spanish. Years later I would use my fluency in Spanish to care for the indigent at Dr. Koka's in San Jacinto, California.

People talk about the good old days. Only baby boomers know the good old days. Kids have no idea, they just know what they see on TV and from their history lessons. We didn't know it then but growing up and living in Chicago in the 50s and 60s, in fact, were the good old days. While I'm not a fanatical reader of the Bible, I know that there are multiple times in the Bible, for instance, the supposed Israelites were enslaved for about 400 years. That meant that several generations of them saw nothing but toil and drudgery every day of their lives. There is a Bible verse in Romans Chapter 1 verse 18-35 that says, in essence, "G-D permits unrighteous behavior" and I wonder if we are in a time when that behavior will persist for generations? I'm deeply sorry it has come to that in the United States of America. We all should be helping each other to keep America strong and free.

CHAPTER 3

MEDICAL SCHOOL AT UAG AND GETTING MARRIED

THE QUESTION WAS what to do with my life, be a jet jockey, or go to medical school. My cousin Cam, who had been a Lieutenant in the Army and was now a high-powered corporate lawyer doing international labor relations, sat me down and told me I should go to medical school. He said my dad would have wanted that. So off I went to Guadalajara. I remember that first flight. I left from Palm Springs to LAX, then Mexicana to GDL. I met a guy on the plane and having no hotel reservations myself, I followed him downtown to The Felix Hotel. There, in a run-down room, I had cockroaches running across the desk. The next morning I somehow made my way to the university offices and met a couple of other gringos. Stuart Chisholm, who would end up renting a house with me, was one. All the gringos had to take and pass a Spanish class before they let you in. It was two months long. Joan came down for part of it just to test the waters. She was the only blond in GDL.

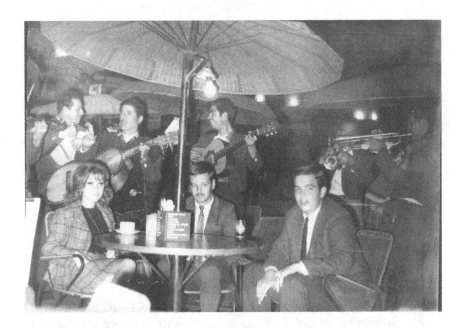

One day we drove to Puerto Vallarta. We must have been crazy as we were lucky not to meet up with bandidos. We stayed at the Posada Vallarta and had papaya for the first time. We rented a small fishing boat from two kids. They took us out beyond the sight of shore, and we were hooking fish so big they always broke the line. We also saw a huge manta ray, bigger than the boat, as it swam under us.

Joan didn't stay the whole time so I could study. I passed the test and started medical school in January 1969. The school was located in Lomas Del Valle. They were still building it, and as we sat in class, guys would be going up a ladder with bricks on their heads. Also, there were armed guards at the entrance. I found out later that there was this huge rivalry between the state-run school and the Autonoma. One time I was driving past the state school, and there was a large white sheet with a saying written in blood that said (as best I can remember), "Lo que escrito en sangre se permanece." or, "What is written in blood lasts."

I became friends with one of the administrators of the school named Gil Martinez. He taught me dirty words in Spanish like "Via a la mierda," or "go to the shit." I think he wanted to practice his English.

We also had a friend, Pedro, at a place called Tourist Servicios located on Minerva Circle just on the main drag going into town. Tourists Servicios was where we got our mail. Stuart and I stumbled on a really cool house at 1350 Mar Amarillo (Yellow Sea).

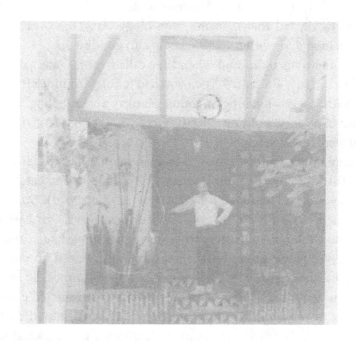

It was located in Lomas Del Country, one of the sectors in GDL. We searched out restaurants that wouldn't make us sick. Among them was one in Chaplita that served fried chicken in a basket with fries, called, *pollo a la canasta.*

There was a steak house run by a gringo called The Cattleman. The restaurant was on the first floor, and the family lived on the second. It was good food and sometimes you were entertained with someone shouting from upstairs and throwing a chair down the stairs. Toward the end of my years there, they built a sort of mall, and a Denny's opened. It was like a little bit of home. After my first night at the Felix, I stayed at the Gran Hotel with the Tyrol restaurant right across the street. It was clean and cheap. I stayed there about two weeks before finding 1350 Mar Amarillo.

Luckily the textbooks they used were the same as in English—like Guyton's Physiology. We could read the English text and just know that's what the Spanish meant. But we spent the first six months whispering, "What did he say?"

The UAG (Universidad Autonoma de Guadalajara) didn't like Hippies (a US fad then). In my physiology class, the professors sat behind a long desk with a velvet curtain surrounding it.

They had binoculars, and when they called your name, you had to stand up and say "Presente." Then you had to turn around, letting them see if your hair was too long or your sideburns were too long. If so, you had two choices. Go out on the patio and get your hair cut right then, or you were out of school.

Our anatomy professor used to bring human bones to class, and he would throw a bone out into the class. Someone had to catch it. If it came to you, you had to tell the class, *Que es?* (what is it), *Donde esta?* (where is it), and *Para que serve?* (what does it do). Our cardiology prof would call for volunteers to discuss something like aortic valve stenosis. We would study for the next day, and we put up our hands and talked about aortic stenosis. After a couple of times, he wouldn't call on us anymore, saying he knew we knew the topic. We were off the hook. In surgery, the Shub brothers had an edge as their father was a surgeon. The professor let them demonstrate on an anesthetized dog how to open the abdomen. We all had a turn. During my time, someone came up to me and said, the dog's owner is here watching. The dog survived, and so did I.

The 1968 Olympics from Mexico were on and the bicycle race came right past our house. I had a desk made, and most days were spent just reading textbooks month after month. While there were plenty of cute girls at school that gave the term miniskirt a new definition, I never ventured there. Below is my graduating class. Ostensibly, these young ladies are now "doctors." Please, a little decorum with the hemlines. On the other hand (ha).

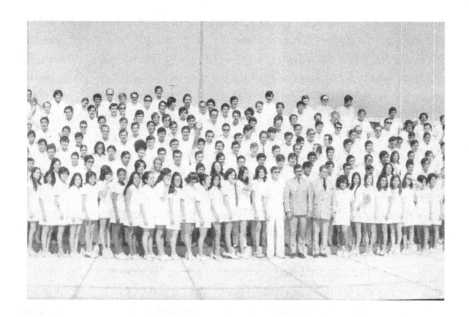

I didn't want to get married until I knew I could hack medical school. Otherwise, it was a government-paid trip to Vietnam. As a student, you had to have what they called an FM 9. It was like a passport. As a student, you couldn't leave Mexico for more than ninety days. Every time you left, it was recorded. Our vacation of summer, Christmas, and Easter were more than the allotted time. So, here's what we did. To get out, we would drive to Texas, getting to the frontier, as they called it, about 30 miles before the US Border. We made sure we got there around 3 a.m. It was usually a small shack with one light bulb hanging. We would stop the car, and one or two guys would get in the trunk. The remaining guy would go in and present the deputy on duty with a bottle of liquor. This worked every time. Now we were out, how do you get back in as a student without your FM 9 to present? We would have one of our stateside friends with the same features get a Tourist Card. Chuck Tonge usually got mine. The Tourist Card had no photos and that worked every time. Once in, another guy would use the card to get out.

As an international student, you were required to not only study medicine in Spanish but also take and pass exams in Mexican law, history, and geography. This is something the US should do, so those entering get to know our land and what it stands for. We made several Mexican friends who would come over for, say, Thanksgiving. I would make a pavo (turkey). One night we went to the movies (all English subtitles) to see *The Good, the Bad, and the Ugly*, which had just come out. In the movie, there were a couple of scenes where a guy would have bullets across his chest. In the end, when the lights went on, we got up, and in back of us was a guy with bullets across his chest looking like he rode out of the movie only he wasn't acting. He got on his horse and rode away. GDL back then was different.

A pizza joint opened up and it was a big hit. Another big hit was Helados (ice cream) Bing. There was always a kid shining shoes there. My cousin Dick came down one time and we went to a newly opened high-end restaurant that had on their matches, "For people who knows and loves good food." We couldn't help smiling at that. One night Joan and I came out of the theater to find my car had been stolen. It took a month to find it. After the first semester, when I knew I could make it, Joan and I decided to get married. Actually, Joan decided for me that we should get married. We set a date of June 27, 1969. On Valentine's Day that year, Joan's best friend, Pam, got married to Chuck, and I flew up for the wedding.

I remember flying back to the states via Mexico City, and we hopped on a new DC-10. It was the first time we saw luggage bins. Before, your luggage was just sat there in plain sight on overhead racks. I got home in plenty of time for my wedding. Bernie was my best man. He came over early the morning of, and we took pictures in the backyard. The night before, I had my bachelor party at the Playboy Club, and they had my name right up top. From there, we went to someplace called the Chesterfield Club. Then we all went to Uncle Nels' boat for more drinks. Here is a photo of me lying down after my bachelor party, and it's double-exposed. That's what I felt like.

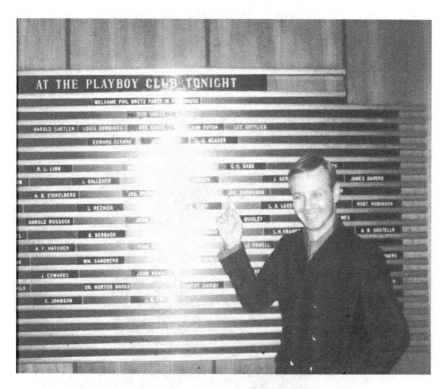

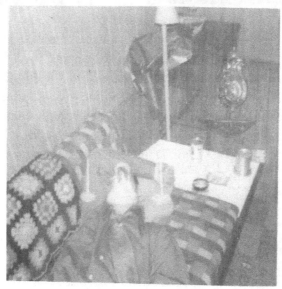

I don't know who got to the church first, Joan or me. Rev. Magnuson and Joan's pastor Rev. Richard both showed up. After the night before, I couldn't believe I was standing. I got a look at my bride walking down the aisle, and she was stunning.

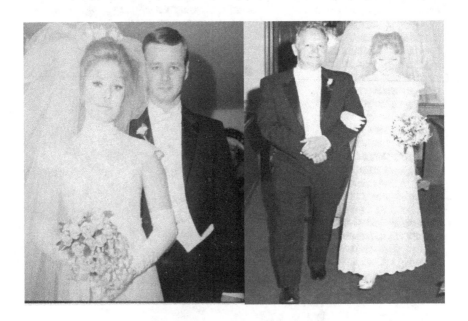

As I recollect, somewhere during that ceremony, I "plighted my troth." Now fifty-two years later, I'm just realizing what that meant. I would do it all over again though in a heartbeat. The question is, would Joan do it all over again or go with the lime green Dodge Dart? Our reception was at Evanston Country Club, where Joan's dad was a long-standing member. It was great. Bernie had a surprise for us. Both Frank Sinatra and Chicago's Mayor Daly sent us telegrams and their best wishes.

CLASS OF SERVICE

This is a fast message unless its deferred character is indicated by the proper symbol.

WESTERN UNION
TELEGRAM

SYMBOLS

DL=Day Letter
NL=Night Letter
LT=International Letter Telegr

The filing time shown in the date line on domestic telegrams is LOCAL TIME at point of origin. Time of receipt is LOCAL TIME at point of destination

1217P EST JUN 27 69 DEA290 BC159 NK227

NN NCB124 CGN NL PDF MO NQB NEW YORK NY 26

MR AND MRS PHILLIP BRETZ, DLY .75

DLR 530PM JUN 27 EVANSTON GOLF CLUB 4401 DEMPSTER ST SKOKIE ILL
ILL

DEAR JOAN AND PHILLIP. MY VERY BEST WISHES TO BOTH OF YOU
FOR GOOD HEALTH AND HAPPINESS. MAY YOUR WEDDING DAY BE A JOYOUS
OCCASION AND ONE TO BE LONG REMEMBERED. WITH WARMEST REGARDS
    FRANK SINATRA

(1125).

CLASS OF SERVICE

This is a fast message unless its deferred character is indicated by the proper symbol.

WESTERN UNION
TELEGRAM

SYMBOLS

DL=Day Letter
NL=Night Letter
LT=International Letter Telegr

The filing time shown in the date line on domestic telegrams is LOCAL TIME at point of origin. Time of receipt is LOCAL TIME at point of destination

1124A EST JUN 27 69 DEB635 CTF125

VCC BCA015 GX PDB BC CHICAGO ILL 27 1043A CDT

MR AND MRS PHILLIP DE EVANS BRETZ, DELIVER 7:30 PM, DLY 75

    EVANSTON GOLF CLUB 4401 DEMPSTER ST SKOKIE ILL

MRS DALEY JOINS ME IN SENDING CONGRATULATIONS TO YOU BOTH ON
THIS YOUR WEDDING DAY. MAY THE COMING YEARS BRING YOU
YOU HEALTH AND HAPPINESS AS YOU BEGIN MARRIED
LIFE TOGETHER
    RICHARD J DALEY MAYOR

(1047).

It was quite a night, and at least I didn't step on my bride's feet during our first dance (clumsy as I am). I went as far up her leg lifting her dress as I could to retrieve her garter for me to throw.

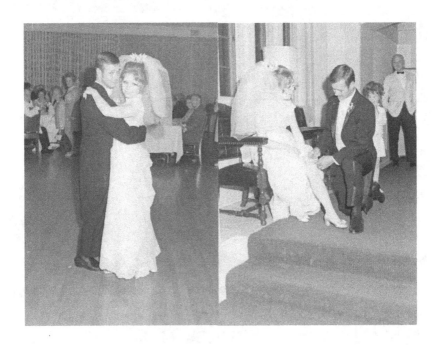

I believe we were the last ones to leave, and we headed downtown where Joan had made all the arrangements for our first night together as husband and wife at the Knickerbocker Hotel. We checked in, and when we got up to our room, there were twin beds. Oh well, we had fun anyway. The following morning, I dragged our luggage down Michigan Avenue and checked into the Continental Hotel. I think I had the audacity to check in as Dr. and Mrs. Bretz. That afternoon we tried to eat at Jacques, and I got thrown out because I had no tie.

Two days later, we were on the plane to New York and then on to Europe. We had the pleasure of visiting England, Italy, Switzerland, and France. We saw the changing of the guard at Buckingham Palace and went to the London Playboy Club. Going to Italy was like going back in time. Joan got thrown out of St. Peter's because her dress was too short, but I liked it.

Then in Venice, she got yelled at because she was wearing a crochet-knit dress, but I loved that one even more. Switzerland was very peaceful; we took a chair lift along the Jungfrau Mountain; it was astounding, just like my new bride.

One night we were having dinner at the Hotel Montana dining room overlooking Lake Geneva, when the waiters brought out a cheese dessert cart. The only cheese I recognized was the Swiss cheese with its holes. I said, "I'll have the Swiss cheese." The waiter replied with, "Sir, they're all Swiss cheeses." When we were in Naples at dinner, they came out with sliver domed trays with our entree underneath. We had ordered squab, as I thought it would be like a Rock Cornish game hen.

When they removed the silver cover, the squab was lying on its back with feet up in the air and the head intact. It might have been a little larger than a sparrow. In England, it was really quiet during dinner at the hotel, and I think I have more ice in my fridge back home than in all of England. You could almost hear a pin drop, very proper in England. During that eventful evening for all humankind, July 20, 1969, when Neil Armstrong and Buzz Aldrin landed on the lunar surface, Joan and I looked at the moon while having dinner on a Bateaux-Mouches boat floating down the Seine in Paris. It was a great honeymoon.

In years hence, we would be fortunate enough to travel to Europe to present papers of my work. In September, it was back to GDL, and most days were spent studying all day after school and into the night. There was no question American medical students were, for the most part, self-taught. I put in my time and initially Joan stayed home. When Christmas rolled around, the movie theaters would play ads with a Christmas theme, and then we knew it was a sign of our going back soon. Eventually, Joan came down and stayed for prolonged periods.

Long about the third year, there was a buzz about being able to take the National Boards. The purpose being if you passed, you had a real chance of transferring into a stateside medical school. In addition, there was a facility in New York in Manhattan called the French and Poly Clinic that had a prep course.

Nelson Shub (RIP), his brother Steve (RIP), and a couple more guys and I decided we should try it, so we registered for classes in GDL then left (on someone else's tourist card). I stayed at my cousin Cam's house in Ramsey, New Jersey, on weekends. I remember the first plane trip to Manhattan. New York City was covered with clouds. The only thing I could see on our approach was the two twin towers of the World Trade Center coming through the cloud cover.

We stayed at a hotel just off Broadway and 42nd Street across from a theater. Walking along Broadway was the first time I ever heard anybody talking to themselves. We ate at Nathan's and the Flame a lot. There was a Howard Johnsons on the corner and I ordered a chocolate sundae. It came with chocolate ice cream. Back in Chicago, a chocolate sundae was vanilla ice cream with chocolate syrup. I was seeing a lot of girls in nice fur coats. There were ads on TV that you could buy one for not much money. I went up to one of the girls, and before I could ask where she purchased her coat, she asked me if I wanted to go out.

Back at French Poly Clinic, I noted any person with MD on his/her license plate could park where they wanted, period, a nice perk. We had an excellent anatomy class and teacher, where I learned a lot, unlike GDL, where the first thing they did in our anatomy class was to hand us a saw so we could saw the cadaver in half from the head down. There were no organs inside. Again, I spent most of the time reading. I think the classes lasted for about six weeks. When we finished, I came home and waited for the National Board Exam. I took it and then we went to Palm Springs.

After a while, I got a call from the dean at Rush Medical, and he said while I passed multiple parts, I didn't pass every part, so he couldn't let me transfer. It was a tremendous blow. That meant I had to go back to GDL. I wondered if I could even re-enroll as I had enrolled in classes but never showed up. To this day, I don't know how, but we were given the opportunity of taking what they called "examenes extraordanario." I somehow passed all of those and entered my senior year.

Just before graduation, some men came down from various medical schools in the US. They had started what they called the Fifth Pathway.

It was a route to becoming a doctor in the US for American citizens. Without it, one had to spend a year after graduation in Mexico doing what they called a Guardia. Basically, you were out on your own in some remote village, providing care for a year to get your Titulo and practice in Mexico. In the end, though, we received an MD degree allowing us to sign up for the Fifth Pathway. See my diploma below.

I can't tell the good people of Mexico, and more specifically the people at the UAG, how grateful I am for their accepting me into medical school when my own country said no. I hope they are happy with my outcome, as they were the ones who really started my quest to help women. I can never thank you enough.

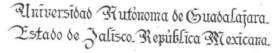

Universidad Autónoma de Guadalajara. Estado de Jalisco. República Mexicana.

A todos aquéllos que estas letras vieren comunicamos:

El Rector de la Universidad, el Director y Cuerpo de Profesores de la Escu de Medicina, de conformidad con los Tribunales de Exámenes, hacen constar que:

Phillip De Ivans Bretz

por el tiempo acostumbrado y sujeto a las pruebas semestrales cursó y aprobó los tudios previstos en el plan oficial vigente para la carrera de:

Médico Cirujano

En consecuencia se le ha dado todo derecho, honor y dignidad que a tal carr corresponde.

En testimonio de lo cual se expide este Diploma sellado por la Universidad dia 24 de mayo de 1973.

El Rector de la U. A. de G.

El Director de la Escuela de Medicina

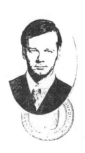

CHAPTER 4

FIFTH PATHWAY AT RUTGERS AND SURGICAL RESIDENCY AT LOYOLA

I HAD A PRODUCTIVE talk with the men from Coney Island Hospital in New York, where I was to serve a year internship. Graduation time came around, and having passed all my final classes, my mother flew down for the ceremony. That final year I had moved to 44 Moscu, a brand new building. Gil Martinez (the official from the school) showed my mother and me around the sights in GDL. We had a great time. I had bought some antique Thonet bentwood furniture. They were cane chairs and settees, and they carried the original stamp from Austria. We still have them. Joan, by then, was pregnant from my trip home around Easter, so she remained stateside just in case. We spent the final days packing and the night of graduation, we all were dressed in tuxedos. We all took the Hippocratic Oath, and finally, they called my name. It was a moment of great satisfaction that I had accomplished something extraordinary in completing medical school in a foreign language. I'm sure my mother was inwardly elated. I graduated twenty-seventh in a class of about 120.

The day came when I would say goodbye to GDL, and we boarded the plane. When we landed in Texas, I knelt and kissed the ground. I was so happy to be back in the USA. Back home they had a big party for Joan and me. And then, soon it was time to go to New York.

Joan and I set out for Coney Island. Upon arriving, it was like culture shock the way the houses looked and the state of the hospital. There was some kind of protest outside, and we managed to find a parking space and went in. Joan used the bathroom and came out crying as there were no faucets. She was beside herself. So, without seeking out anyone, we just got in the car and headed west. I knew there was a Fifth Pathway-sponsored program by Rutgers at Muhlenberg Hospital in Plainfield, New Jersey (see the next photo). We arrived there, and I just walked in and got to Dr. Johnson, the Director of the Fifth Pathway program there. I told him the story, and by the grace of G-D, he welcomed us.

COLLEGE OF MEDICINE AND DENTISTRY OF NEW JERSEY

RUTGERS MEDICAL SCHOOL
University Heights
Piscataway, New Jersey 08851

OFFICE OF THE DEAN

April 27, 1973

Mr. Phillip D. Bretz
APDO 1-631
Guadalajara, Jalisco
MEXICO

Dear Mr. Bretz:

We are happy to inform you that you have been accepted to the Fifth Channel Program in New Jersey beginning September 10. You have been assigned to Muhlenberg Hospital and should be hearing from them shortly. This is a firm acceptance, contingent upon your taking the American Medical Screening Examination (M.S.E.) in order that you get credit for having been in the Fifth Channel Program.

We will still need your advance registration and the other credentials we have requested (transcripts and letters of recommendation). Please let us hear from you as soon as possible.

Very truly yours,

W. Edward McGough, M.D.
Associate Dean and Director,
Fifth Channel Program in N. J.

WEMcG/jrs

It was a much different feeling than Coney Island (no offense). We found an apartment at 1106 Park Avenue. We went back home and packed a U-Haul. Pam and Chuck drove out with us and were a great help.

I started my internship, and from day one (as I knew I was playing catch-up), I absorbed everything like a sponge. My first rotation was with a really cool guy named Earl O'Neil, a thoracic surgeon. He was very busy. He had just hired a young surgeon out of his residency. Those days, if we were called to put in a central line, we would do it in the patient's room. This would be prohibited today. Dr. O'Neil knew I wanted to be a surgeon, so after a couple of cases, he guided my hands to learn how to sew and handle tissue. Then one night while doing an appendix, he let me do the whole thing. Word spread that I had accomplished this feat. My nickname became "the Silver Knife." It became known if anyone wanted a cutdown (where you cut the skin to place an IV line), they called me. I became pretty proficient at this. I was liking my profession. All the time we were in GDL, we had no TV. Now we had purchased a small one, and I could see *Monday Night Football* with Dandy Don Meredith singing *Old Blue Dog* with Howard Cosell and Frank Gifford giving their colorful commentary.

I looked forward to every day to learn something new in order to save lives. Dr. O'Neil's partner (a young surgeon) and I would go around when called to put in a central line (when an arm IV was not available) at the patient's bedside. Now that would lead to corrective action by a host of functionaries. I remember one case when Dr. O'Neil was performing a mastectomy, and he pointed to a structure and asked me if I knew what it was. I knew it was a nerve but didn't know which one. The anesthesiologist started ringing a bell, which didn't help stupid me. It was the long thoracic nerve of Bell. It controls motor movements to the serratus anterior muscle. Injury during a mastectomy causes a winged scapula.

Joan was pregnant with Jason, and soon it was time for his appearance. Dr. Kreitzer was in charge. During his birth, Dr. Kreitzer stuck electrodes in his scalp to monitor. I can't recall for what; it was experimental. I don't remember Joan having a lot of trouble. We had enrolled in Lamaze classes. I think I recall telling her to find her focal point; (big help I was).

Seeing your firstborn instills a feeling that can only be summed up as something miraculous. I gave out cigars to everyone, which was the custom back then. I still have them and the other kids' cigars—what a joy to have my little Jason. I used to change his diaper on the table that had a light. I would turn it on by saying the word, "light," which, consequently, at six months was his first word. We had brought up a custom-made brass bed from GDL, which served as his first bed. My experience at Muhlenberg was very extensive at seeing what a surgeon could do and seeing the side of complications.

One time I was called for a cutdown during a code. While I can't remember the exact sequence, the resident gave the patient IV digitalis (short-acting). Within a couple of minutes, the patient's heart rate went from almost 200 blocked down to zero, and we couldn't revive him. Being a doctor, I learned early on you have to learn and cope with bad outcomes even though you meant the best and tried your best. Eventually, I came to the realization that anyone who criticizes a doctor for a bad result should step up to the plate and do better. Can you imagine the guilt a doctor must carry all his or her days for an unintended bad result? And each doctor knows that every patient carries the potential for a disaster for whatever reason. It's a much easier life to sell balloons at Disneyland. And surgeons carry that realization with them all the days of their lives, for people they don't even know. Some fun.

All too soon, it was time to take the National Boards and enter the "match program" for a surgical residency. Our taking the National Boards as Fifth Pathway enrollees wouldn't officially count. Why wouldn't it count, I wondered? Was it just that we were being put in our place as second-class citizens? I passed all parts. By this time, Bernie was at Loyola University in Maywood, Illinois, where his brother Eli had gone, and they set up an interview for me. I went and actually interviewed with a couple more surgical programs. At Loyola, I met with Dr. Jack Pickleman himself, a foreign medical graduate (FMG) from McGill in Canada. Although programs are not supposed to tell a candidate if or how they will place their name on the matching agenda, he said if I put Loyola first, he would put me first. I didn't ask why, and to this day, I don't know why he did that (divine intervention)? Before finishing at Muhlenberg, I gave a grand rounds.

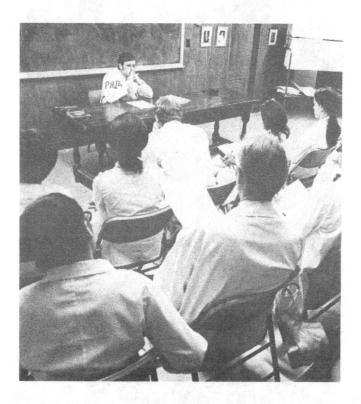

No question, I needed that time in the Fifth Pathway, and I remain grateful for Rutgers, Muhlenberg, and Dr. Johnson (RIP), for giving me the opportunity. I remember getting the acceptance letter in the mail from Loyola. I was overjoyed that all the work thus far had paid off. I was with the big boys. There is a current TV show called *Chicago Med*. During the next five years, I would be in Chicago Med along with the other residents of all the programs in Chicago. Patients like the one below while I was on the burn unit honed my skills. They don't let you undertake this kind of responsibility unless they know you're up to it in more ways than one.

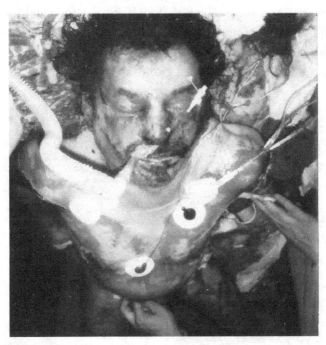

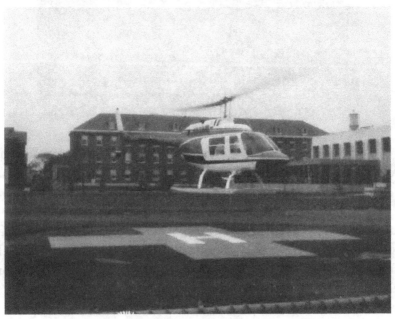

Below is my acceptance letter from Loyola. You'll note it is for only one calendar year and any further years (five in total) would be at the concurrence of the Department Chairman. In this case it was Robert Freeark. No question I would be with the big boys now and had to earn my keep, as it were. And while the focus of the lens was not as acute as it would be in my chief resident year, you would be watched like a hawk to judge almost daily if you belonged or not. You will also note the salary of $11,000 at a time now when the guys I went to college with were securing positions as vice presidents of banks. Like every other doctor, I would be behind that eight ball initially. It would take years to catch up. But the important thing was it was all coming together. But one item still needed to be checked off. That was me passing the two-day FLEX exam, which newly minted foreign medical graduates had to pass to obtain a license anywhere in the states. If I didn't pass it, all would be lost. All those years of studying and my surgical residency all gone. Doctors have a lot riding on many things and many hurdles they have to clear just to keep their head above water. And now the real fun would start of being able to be taught enough to save lives right and left.

FOSTER G. McGAW HOSPITAL
LOYOLA UNIVERSITY OF CHICAGO
2160 South First Avenue, Maywood, Illinois 60153   312 531-3000

March 8, 1974

Phillip D. Bretz, M. D.

Building 1
Plainfield, New Jersey 07060

Dear Doctor Bretz:

Upon the recommendation of Doctor Freeark, Chairman of the Department
of Surgery, I am pleased to inform you that you have been accepted for post
doctoral training in Loyola University Affiliated Hospitals.

The appointment is for one calendar year and is to begin on July 1, 1974.
Subsequent appointments for the completion of your specialty training will be at
your election with the concurrence of the Chairman of the Department of
Surgery. Release from this contract at a date earlier than the expiration can be
obtained only with the approval of the Chairman of the Department of Surgery.
The Chairman of the Department of Surgery may terminate this contract for failure
to fulfill the duties required of housestaff or failure to make satisfactory
progress in the required training program.   Action to terminate this contract
by the Departmental Chairman may be subject to review by the Housestaff
Committee of the Medical-Dental Staff.

This appointment is at the first year post graduate level and has an annual
stipend of $11,000. The institution will provide malpractice insurance for insti-
tutional practice. The institution will pay for one half of the hospitalization
premium for either individual or family coverage for all housestaff enrolling in
our group plan. Two weeks of vacation for first year post graduates and three
weeks of vacation for each year of training thereafter will be granted during this
contract period. Leave for educational purposes is up to the discretion of the
Departmental Chairman.

The hours of duty, the rotation to affiliating institutions and services and the on
call hours or days vary from department to department and are determined by the
Departmental Chairman. The Departmental Chairman with his faculty establishes
the educationl program for each program of specialty training. These programs
may be modified from time to time as requirements dictate.

I remember well my first day at Loyola. Actually, I started at Hines
VA, the largest VA in the country. It is located on the same campus as
Loyola in Maywood, Illinois. I was the SOD, or Surgical Officer of the
Day. It was a baptism of fire in the ER. My first patient nearly died. He
was brought in by ambulance near death from a bee sting (of all things).

I shot him with epinephrine and gave him O2, and he came back. It was a miracle. My residency in general surgery would last five years with every other night in the hospital and constant surveillance by the attending surgeons questioning your every move and order. It was a pyramid program. We started with seventeen and ended with seven. Not everyone could hack it.

You'll note every other night in the hospital. This encompasses a full day's work, including surgeries, admission history and physicals, and rounds with every attending who admitted patients on your service. Then your night started being on call for every surgical patient and every patient in the hospital that needed surgical attention. You had a little room, just enough for a twin bed and a small desk. Sleep was intermittent at best; as Loyola being a Level 1 trauma center, there was always someone in the ER. All too soon, morning came around, and you had to make rounds on your patients and review any labs or imaging studies *before* the attendings came in. And, since I don't want to forget this part, our Chairman of the Department of Surgery was Dr. Robert J. Freeark. He distinguished himself for developing the concept of nationwide trauma centers and founded the first trauma center at Cook County Hospital in Chicago on March 16, 1966. He did that in conjunction with Dr. Robert Baker, who stayed at Cook County to develop one of the first blood banks and Dr. Freeark was recruited to Loyola.

Joan and I were still living at Forest Glen when I started at Loyola. One of the first nights, I got a call from Phil Rice, the chief resident, to come in as we had a case. It was about 3 a.m. It was a fairly long way to Loyola, which meant we had to find a place to live soon. We looked around and found the house of houses. If I became a millionaire, I wouldn't want another home. It was in Oak Park on the corner of Le Moyne and Woodbine. To be specific 1202 Woodbine. It was a copy of a house in Scotland by the architect Jerome Cerny. Cerny did about four homes in Oak Park. An obstetrician built the house.

The cathedral style living room had a massive fireplace and a custom chandelier. It depicted an obstetrician in his horse-drawn cart chasing a stork carrying a baby. Off the living room was a winding stairway leading to the turret bedroom. In it was a small window where you could look out through the massive hand-hewn beams into the living room. There was an exercise room above the garage that you had to climb a rope to get to. It had a small library with its own fireplace. On the corner were large flowering trees. It gave me joy just to cut the grass. In the small garden out back were roses transplanted from a home at Pickets Charge (during the Civil War). After Joan and I saw Woodbine and made an offer, we parked outside and just looked at it, hoping it would be ours. We were so happy when our offer was accepted at $80,000. I used the money I made modeling to pay for half of it. What a joy that house was. It was the first house Ashley (my oldest daughter) was brought home to.

Back at Loyola I was holding my own and enjoying becoming a surgeon. As a first-year resident, you rarely saw any actual surgery being performed. The reason was the primary surgeon had the best view, but across from him was the first assistant (junior resident) with the same view, but those two blocked everything. The first surgery I did was at Hines. It was a bilateral inguinal hernia. Rice and Charlie Voss (Rice teaching Voss) were on one side and myself and the attending on the other.

I had prepared; I looked at a hundred pictures. I can tell you when it came time to make the incision, it was very difficult. Unlike a line drawn with a pencil, once you drop the knife, you can't erase that incision. The attending said, "We're slow but poor."

That bastard. Having arrived at the time when I can perform almost any surgery from gunshot wounds, to assist in heart surgery, the last thing I would do is degrade a budding surgeon. Why? Because any surgeon who has been in the operating theater has been up to his/her ass in alligators plenty of times, no matter how good you are. Because you are violating a human body that is very dynamic, not changing spark plugs in an inanimate object like an engine. Any surgeon that says he/she hasn't been up to their ass in alligators is a liar. When I became chief resident, the first thing I said to my junior resident, intern, and medical students was, "We are going to make some mistakes; the trick is to learn and not repeat them." At the end of the day, we are all on the same team and support each other as your time for bad news will come. We are not treating some rash; people will die right under us on the operating table if we don't execute properly 100% every time. We play the Superbowl every day with every patient, especially those with cancer.

This might be a good time to bring up the issue of surgical training. Like I said, from day one, we all were in the hospital every other night for five years, those that made it through. Indeed, you never knew if you were going to get dinner or any lunch. You put in a full day's work, starting with reviewing labs and rounding (before the attendings came in), then it was off to the OR for a full day of a surgical tour de force. Then it was admission time for new patients and history and physicals and getting them into the chart. Then, if you were lucky and not on call for the ER, which for our Level 1 trauma center was always bringing in an accident, you could choke down dinner before your beeper went off.

Or in one case I remember a patient coming to the ER with an open abdominal incision with lap sponges stuffed in the wound as the surgeon from another hospital didn't know what to do or how to fix the problem. Then you were basically up most of the night since you were the only surgical person in the hospital. There was no shower. You were up at dawn to review labs and do rounds. It was the same routine. Then after another full day's work, you could go home, but you were always on call if your service had emergency surgery. This went on year after year and weeded people out.

Fast forward after my residency, some resident sued for "break time" and to limit the number of hours a program could make you work. If and when you ever need emergency surgery because of an accident or the like, you sure as hell want a surgeon who has been through hell and back and not someone who had limited hours and cupcakes on breaks.

The fact is the life of a surgeon is constant exhaustion. That's why the topic of burnout is so timely. The other fact is you want your surgeon to be like a member of Seal Team 6 and not a sluggard who made it through because of cupcake time. A surgeon's life is brutal, period, and if I were in charge, things would change. There was an article in *General Surgery News* in which the author said, "Ignorance is no substitute for experience." Meaning no cupcakes. The other fact is when a surgeon is finally out in the community, when that surgeon is on ER call for a week, he/she is on call 24/7, including any major cases that the surgeon has. There are no "rest" periods. So, getting used to limited hours during your residency when you should be learning difficult surgeries is no help when people are betting their lives on your ability. When you're in private practice and on ER call, you can't call in and tell them you are too tired. As soon as we (as a country) started to blur black and white, that's when the trouble started.

I can't omit an article appearing in *General Surgery News* in January 2017 authored by David V. Cossman, MD. In this article, he is initially dreaming about making surgery great again. I think it sums up the situation nicely, and I quote, "When I'm elected, the 80-hour workweek for residents is history. Ignorance is more dangerous than fatigue. I like the 'timeout'—it stays. If interns and residents are looking for a safe space with a level playing field, they should stay at Harvard and Yale. Pimping residents will be legal again. Teaching isn't bullying. Doctors will repossess what was rightfully theirs but taken away by Big Government and special interests that have picked their pockets in the name of cost, quality, and access—none of which has happened. The doctor-patient relationship will be restored. Teams won't take care of patients. Neither will physician assistants, nurse practitioners, practice extenders, or any form of med level yet to be invented. Hospitalists will be looking for work." That about sums it up. See, I'm not the only one. The trouble is, few read things like this article (certainly the public never sees this). No one does anything about this to make medicine better for all.

As I got older and had years of experience under my belt, I realized that whatever they taught us fundamentally, it was to understand what a huge responsibility we as surgeons had to perform 100% every time, no excuses. People depended on us to save them. And we were taught indirectly to keep our thoughts to ourselves and not lash out at any patient or colleague. They taught us to be humble. A surgeon is only as good as his/her last surgery.

Getting back to the attending who said, "We're slow but poor," after the surgery, he sat me down and told me I should think about going into dermatology. I'll let history decide if I should have become a dermatologist or not. Needless to say, his conduct toward me was not how I treated fledgling surgeons once I knew how to operate. As the years passed, we were whittled down from our starting number of seventeen, wherein my chief resident year we were seven.

I forget the exact timeline, but during the first year at Loyola, I had to take the Federal Licensure Exam (FLEX). Traditionally, FMGs would take the ECFMG before entering into a US residency, I don't know why the FLEX. Perhaps it was the Fifth Pathway program? The whole ball of wax was riding on that exam. Suppose I didn't pass it, no license to practice, no residency, no nothing, and many years of studying for naught. It was a two-day exam. I remember Joan calling me to tell me I passed as the letter came while I was at work.

What a load off my mind. It meant I was good to go. In the "Short Stories" section, I have discussed a few stories that will give you an inkling of my later years at Loyola. As the years passed, each year rolled around, we seemed to lose people (my fellow surgical residents) for reasons I was not privy to. We were heading into our supposed chief resident year. No one said anything to me, and I remember Jim Wielgolewski calling me to tell me I was on the boss's service (Dr. Freeark) right out of the chute. What an honor, I had made it.

I think Dr. John G. Raffensperger, the Chairman of the Department of Surgery at Children's Memorial, may have had a talk with Dr. Freeark on my behalf. My rotation at Children's was my last as a junior resident before the chief resident year. I had enjoyed my time at Children's and felt I was ready for anything. I was starting to piss vinegar, as we say in the trade. By this time, I had finished my rotation at Henrotin Hospital (now defunct). We named Henrotin the "little" Cook County as you were the only surgical resident, and we had our share of trauma from downtown Chicago. There was a case that haunts me to this day. A fellow was brought into the ER coding with multiple gunshot wounds in the chest and abdomen.

I was by myself, and with all things to do like start a central line for fluids and blood, draw blood, and intubate him, I may have inserted the

ET tube into the esophagus. He was in CPR mode on arrival. He didn't make it, and I still mention him in my prayers every night.

Like I said, being a surgeon on the initial side of the learning curve endows you with guilt beyond what an average person should ever have to live with. But you have to get up the next day and possibly do it all over again, hoping that next time you save a life. As I said, it's much easier just selling balloons at Disneyland, where the worst thing that can happen is all the balloons float away, and everyone claps.

I had been given the chief resident's beeper, and I showed up early my first day to do rounds, etc., when I got a call. My junior resident was in the ER with abdominal pain. Great. I went down and examined him. I thought he had a kidney stone, and we ordered an IVP (intravenous pyelogram), something that outlines the kidneys and ureter but something they probably don't do anymore. That was it, so he was out of commission for a little while. That made it a little more challenging to do big cases with the intern who had no idea how to assist correctly. Dr. Pickleman had a saying, "He who controls the sucker, controls the case," meaning the assistant could suck blood and schmutz out of the line of sight of the surgeon without being told. That's assuming one knew how to use the sucker. A good assistant can make a mediocre surgeon look tremendous and vice versa. A good assistant can make a mediocre surgeon look great (for anyone watching) like surgery is so easy. It isn't. There shouldn't be any mediocre surgeons, right?

Before I interviewed at Loyola, I interviewed at a hospital where the Chairman of the Department showed three other prospective surgeons around. I remember him saying, "I can teach a monkey to do surgery." I beg to differ. Being a surgeon and knowing you have the skill to cut into someone, remove a diseased part, and put them back together again so they can hardly tell you where, is, I think, an innate gift. It's almost like a sprinter, born to run. Sometimes when I see the results of a lot of breast surgery, I think that yeah, there must have been a monkey performing that obliterative surgery.

Years hence, when I opened the first Comprehensive Breast Center in the Coachella Valley and one of the first in the country in 1988, the mantra was and is "to preserve mind, body, and spirit." I wanted those girls I was privileged to operate on to be able to look in the mirror ten days or ten years down the line and say, "I can't even tell that guy was there." It's that good if the surgeon wants it. If that isn't a priority, then disfigurement is the result. That's why when we discuss the Lavender Way, one of the prerequisites for our breast doctors would be to preserve, mind, and spirit all the time.

During my fourth year, I was elected the Vice President of the Charles B. Puestow Surgical Society. Dr. Puestow was an Army surgeon and invented the Puestow Procedure or lateral pancreaticojejunostomy. It's a surgical procedure for chronic pancreatitis. The main pancreatic duct is opened from the head to the tail.

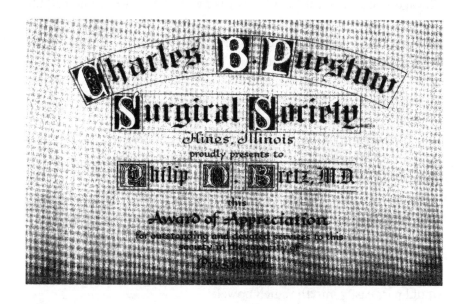

The jejunum (proximal small bowel) is anastomosed to it, so the pancreatic fluid (aiding in digestion) flows directly into the small bowel instead of being blocked by the multiple constrictions of the pancreatic duct by the chronic inflammation. It was an honor. It was a more significant honor to be elected President in my chief resident year. During my chief resident year, I felt like I could be a good surgeon. At Hines, I developed what came to be called the "Palm

Springs hernia." It was repairing an inguinal hernia through a one-inch incision.

By this time, my mother and Aunt Florence had had a home in Palm Springs, California, for some years. Originally, one of my dad's friends from World War II ended up in Palm Springs building houses. I was going to join his construction business before I met Bernie and got interested in becoming a surgeon. During this time, Eisenhower Medical Center (EMC) in Rancho Mirage was being built with money from Bob Hope, his friends, including Hazel Wright (a fellow Chicagoan), Walter Probst, Peter Kiewit, and proceeds from the Bob Hope Desert Classic. The desert was growing, pushing eastward from Palm Springs. I remember most of it as just desert. Joan and I had had enough of Chicago winters, and if I could get on staff at EMC, we would call the desert home.

One time, I was teaching the junior resident how to do a Palm Springs hernia (my invention), and the boss came in, and said, "G-d damn it Bretz, you can't teach somebody how to do a hernia like that, make an incision from the anterior superior iliac crest to the pubic bone and show him the anatomy."

Later, when my rotation with Dr. Freeark ended, I rotated to Hines VA, but continued to perfect the Palm Springs hernia. Another time on the boss's service, I was doing a sub-total gastrectomy on a stomach cancer patient. Dr. Freeark came in and looked over my shoulder, and asked me if I wanted him to critique my performance. "Oh yes, sir, and I also wish to have a hole in my head." You can't imagine the tension with your reputation being on the line because everyone was listening. As it turned out, he liked the angle I had on the gastric pouch so food would pass easily into the small bowel.

Yes, I was being trained very well to take on anything if I had to. One of the last cases I did with Dr. Freeark was a trauma case. During the case (with him assisting me), while repairing the small bowel, the patient's liver had been injured, but I thought it would heal on its own. He said, "I want you to resect the liver." So, he taught me how to resect the liver even though that liver could probably have been left alone. This moment of teaching by the master would come in handy when at EMC a young boy was brought into the ER having been injured by a homemade bomb that blew part of his liver and diaphragm away, and he survived. That case at EMC propelled my reputation as a go-to surgeon. As time progressed at EMC, seven physicians on staff had me operate on themselves or a family member.

That's probably the highest respect one can get when they entrust themselves or their family members to your surgical expertise. As doctors, they could have gone anywhere, like the Mayo Clinic or the like. That made me feel good. It felt so good that I got dedicated license plates for my car: EMC SURG.

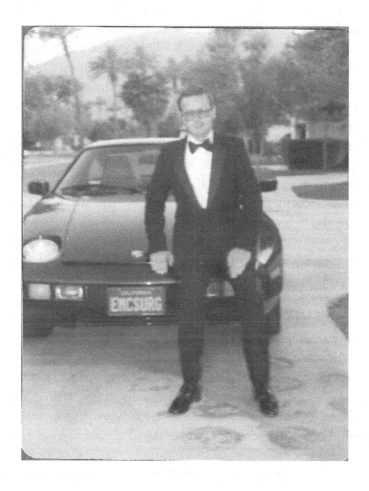

That took balls if I do say so myself. There are a few more stories from Loyola that are in the "Short Stories" section of this book I won't repeat here.

But one time I was assisting one of the cardiac surgeons, Dr. Moran, and it was a long case. Sometimes on those long cardiac cases, they start to bleed, and it's hard to stop because they have been heparinized so long while on the heart-lung machine. I thought nothing like fresh blood being able to clot. Things weren't going too well, and I asked the patient's blood type. It was type A, my blood type. I asked Dr. Moran if I could give blood and bring it back, and he thought it was a great idea. So, I ran over to the blood bank. They called ahead, explaining the situation, and were ready for me. They took the pint of whole blood, I ran back with it and continued to assist while my blood was being pumped into the patient. It was kind of miraculous; the bleeding stopped. I got a nice letter from Dr. Moran about that initiative, (see "Short Stories"). I was pissing vinegar and felt like I had really been trained very well. At Hines, banding of hemorrhoids had just come out, and I remember "beating the bushes" as we used to say, going around all the floors and talking to patients about the procedure. We got many takers. Some people might think the care at a veterans hospital is somehow second rate. But as far as I was concerned, the reason I was able to be trained as a surgeon and help people was their sacrifice allowed our country to be free, and I saw to it their care under my watch was on par or better than anywhere. That's why I put a hole in the wall when I didn't get what I wanted right away to help a vet who needed help right then, not two hours from then.

I had two rotations on the open-heart service, and Dr. Roque Pifarre, the chairman of the department, wanted me to do a cardiac fellowship. In 1984 he would perform the first heart transplant in Loyola's history. After Mexico and five years of every other night in the hospital, Joan would have killed me, although I thought about it. Cardiac surgery is just a different kettle of fish than general surgery. In general surgery, often you have to move things like the colon or small bowel around in sweeping movements.

In cardiac surgery, you're operating on sometimes 1-millimeter vessels wearing "loops" to magnify your field of vision. If you pull a suture through a 1mm vessel, it's not good. Everything is very exact. If I'd stayed on to become a cardiac surgeon, it almost certainly would have meant staying at a university, probably Loyola. I really wanted to be on my own and enjoyed trauma cases and the like. Plus, Joan and I were looking forward to Palm Springs. The fact that the "Rock" asked me to be part of his team meant a lot about how far I had come in those five years.

My first daughter, Ashley, was born in 1976, and we brought her home to Woodbine in Oak Park, Illinois. Almost as soon as she could walk, she was an entertainer. She ended up in school plays and wanted to be a "thespian." Immediately after high school, she went off to Harvard to study theater. It was the first time she would be away from us and on her own. She did very well, of course. Even the Russians who were there with the Stanislaviski's system taught in Russia wanted to take her back to study with them. I'm convinced, had she not met and married Justin, she would probably have a great career on Broadway or the silver screen. Jason and I played golf with Justin and his dad, Roger. I told his dad that whatever happens between Ashley and Justin was fine with me as I thought Justin and Ashley were a good match. I knew they were in love with each other. In any case, she and Justin are now married for over eleven years and have two great children, Oliver and Harrison. They flip houses in Seattle. Google *The House of Stiles*. You can look for Mr. O. (what Joan and I call our grandson) to be some professional athlete in the future. At age eleven, he can throw a fastball around 60 mph. Five-year-old Harry, their younger son, could become a doctor as he looks forward to me sending him slides/images of cases we then discuss. We'll see if my predictions come true.

When the kids got engaged, I told our guests to be at the house before 7 p.m. I told them I had a friend at NASA that would have the ISS tweak its orbit to fly right over the house in honor of Ashley and Justin. Their jaws dropped when the ISS flew right over. They were amazed. I didn't tell them I had the app to tell me that the space station just happened to be on that orbit at that time.

But at Loyola, I remember attending The Chicago Surgical Society and presenting cases. It was a massive building of stone and paneled wood, just like in the movies. Residents from all the programs in Chicago would present interesting cases. While I was looking forward to completing my residency, I had become very comfortable, and I felt as though I fit in and had gained a reputation as a damn good surgeon. All too soon, we were nearing the end. Traditionally, there was a party where they would give out our certificates. Mine said that I had faithfully and successfully completed my residency in General Surgery from July 1, 1974, to June 30, 1979.

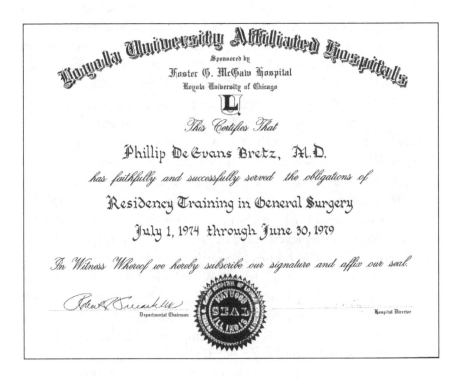

Let's look at that statement a little closer, as it has a bearing on my future. By examining the few paragraphs I've written, you get an inkling of just how tough it is to become a surgeon. The process starts as early as high school, where a lot of graduates are trying to get not just into a college but a good college where entrance into medical school might be easier. Let's look at the path.

So now you finish high school and get into a respectable real college/ university. That process just weeded out all those who didn't achieve academically and were prevented from attending college, like me almost. Now you're in college, and you enroll in pre-med. Nowadays, this includes not only organic and inorganic chemistry but calculus.

These daunting classes will weed out a bunch more. Perfect time for this old joke. Do you know what a lawyer is? It's someone who couldn't get into medical school. Was Shakespeare right? If you went to college, you'd know why I said that, and you don't have to look up Henry VI, Part 2, Act IV, Scene 2. Now you are getting good grades in tough courses, and the Medical College Admission Test (MCAT) is coming. Without a good score on MCAT, you will probably not get into medical school. Now by some unexplained miracle, you are admitted to medical school. Having achieved this, you have left behind untold numbers of medical school wannabees. Do you see a pattern here?

The further you go up the ladder, the more rarefied the air is. Meaning, with each rung of the ladder you advance, you have left a lot of people behind.

During medical school, you are on different rotations like family practice, dermatology, and thoracic surgery. That's assuming you make it past your first year, and a few don't. That leaves more people behind. Well, without a word being spoken, you get a sense of the pecking order in medicine. You don't get the same feeling of awe doing a rotation on family practice taking care of blood pressure and caring for diabetes as you do on a trauma rotation where everything is split-second life and death decisions made by you. Only a chosen few get to be placed in that position of life and death. They are people who have the stamina, guts, and skill to pull off the impossible. Looking back at EMC covering the ER, when I was called to care for multiple stab wounds to the victim's chest and abdomen, it was no accident I pulled that guy through. That was when about 200 people were waiting for me after I, unbeknownst, saved the King of the Gypsies. My training at Loyola enabled me to pull that off and many others. Note there is no "evidence-based medicine" when you're trying to stop otherwise fatal bleeding. I never saw any functionaries in the trauma OR; wonder why? You should know by now.

So, you have had rotations (because you made it through into advanced years in medical school), and you like the challenge of becoming a surgeon, and you decide that's what you want to be. Okay, so now you're finished with medical school and apply for a surgical residency. Luck is with you, and your interview goes well, and you match with a high-powered university program like Loyola. You now find yourself in a pyramid program, which means that we started with seventeen, and we finished with seven. One guy did all four years and was told he couldn't do his chief resident year. What? Can you imagine the devastation?

You made it into a surgical residency and in your rotations, you visit thoracic surgery, neurosurgery, and transplant. Now there lies the pinnacle. That's at least two more years after you successfully complete your general surgery residency.

Now we are at the meat of the entire process, which, including high school, is nineteen years, including an internship if you did it like me. Now what? Well, we come to Board Certification and what that entails and means. After you get your General Surgery certificate that has on it "faithfully and successfully," your chairman has to recommend you to the Board. Yes, your chairman has to recommend you to sit for the Boards. One very brilliant resident had to do another year as he couldn't operate his way out of a paper bag. The American Board of Surgery (ABS) is a private organization and sets its own standards. The certification exam consists of two parts, a written exam (qualifying exam) and an oral exam (certifying) exam given by multiple examiners.

The way it works is staff members from, say Loyola, would provide the exam for guys from the Mayo Clinic or the like and vice versa. A doctor's Board Certificate is good for ten years, at which time he/she must re-certify. I never had a problem with that concept. What I had a problem with was the hierarchy that determined a time limit to your certification, who grandfathered themselves to lifelong status of certification. They never had to take another exam. You just don't take the qualifying exam (written exam) the day after you complete your residency; it's usually a year after or thereabouts. You had to submit all your cases, and they decided after your chairman's recommendation, whether you tallied enough major cases, about 200. In my day, you had three attempts, and if you weren't successful, you had to do another year, somehow, of residency. It is not the Board's concern that there aren't open places for you. In addition, by the time you reach the Board Certification level, you need to start earning a living.

That means, for instance, in my case, I made about $17,000 a year as Chief Resident. The guys I left college with were already vice presidents of banks. And once you are out on your own, you begin to have colossal overhead, including malpractice, office rent, help, and probably a mortgage so you have a home and can raise a family. You didn't have to pay for malpractice during your residency. Also, I might add again, which makes no difference to the Board, is that the people who give the exam are usually employed by their hospital and never have to worry about any of the things like malpractice that the surgeons who are out on their own must. Malpractice can reach astronomical levels like about $150,000 yearly for an obstetrics doctor. While we're on the subject, because car insurance rates drop if you have no accidents (according to commercials), why isn't it fair to drop the rates of doctors who don't get sued? That's many thousands of dollars before you can even open your door to see patients. Those academic surgeons, who generally look down on surgeons out in the community, never have to meet a payroll; they just pick up their check every two weeks. Or better yet, it is probably delivered to them, or directly deposited. Generally, if you are recommended to the Board, any hospital you apply to accepts you, and you have three years to become Board-certified. The vernacular is that you're "Board-eligible" until then.

Another interesting fact is the American Board of Surgery never actually sends some senior surgeons to watch you perform surgery. Forgive me, but that's a little like the FAA asking you questions about flying but not sending you up in the wild blue yonder with an FAA-certified examiner seeing to it you can actually handle the aircraft safely? Remember, I said that at one of the places I interviewed the boss said, "I can teach a monkey to operate." Years later, having earned my bones, I say no, you can't teach a monkey to perform flawless surgery. Furthermore, for five years you have been scrutinized ten ways from Sunday each and every day (*by the very people who give the boards*). And after those five years, the people whose job it is to weed out incompetent surgeon wannabees have pronounced you faithful and successful.

Back to my own journey; I passed the written (qualifying) exam and scheduled myself for the oral (certification) exam. It is a day-long exercise of questions by people you have never met. I remember in each of my three attempts to certify, I answered every question without much hesitation. Never once did I say, "I don't know." While I don't remember any of those surgeons or where they were from, I do remember one, Dr. Bernard Fisher (RIP). He was the Director of the National Surgical Adjuvant Breast Project (NSABP), the largest research group in the world. I assume he torpedoed me, but I'll never know. Years later, he would send me several letters when I authored our country's first large-scale breast cancer prevention clinical trial, and his letter to me, in part, says, "I (meaning Dr. Bretz) should be commended for what I have done."

NSABP

NATIONAL SURGICAL ADJUVANT
BREAST AND BOWEL PROJECT

3550 Terrace Street • Room 914
Pittsburgh, PA 15261
412/648-9720
FAX 412/648-1912

Bernard Fisher, M.D.
Chairman

OPERATIONS OFFICE
Bernard Fisher, M.D.
Director
Norman Wolmark, M.D.
Deputy Director, Medical
D. Lawrence Wickerham, M.D.
Deputy Director, Administration
Joan C. Oash, M.A.
Assistant Dir., Fiscal Affairs
Mary Ketner, R.N.
Assistant Dir., Clinical Affairs

August 7, 1991

Phillip D. Bretz, M.D.
Founder-Director
Desert Breast Institute
39-800 Bob Hope Drive, Suite 3
Rancho Mirage, CA 92270

Dear Phil:

Please accept my apology for not replying sooner to your inquiry about your possible participation in the NSABP Breast Cancer Prevention Trial. At the time I received your letter, I did not yet have all the information necessary to formulate a response.

Much, if not most, of the interest that has been generated regarding the implementation of a prevention trial came from your groundbreaking efforts, and I think you are to be commended for what you have attempted to do.

During the last year we have been actively engaged in the development of what I hope will be considered an appropriate study. We have not yet received final approval, but we are hoping to do so in the near future.

We will soon be sending out an RFA, and I hope your proposal will be acceptable to the selection committee. They will be interested primarily in those institutions that are willing to make a commitment to NSABP activities in general, as well as to the prevention trial. For further procedural information, please call Gladys Hurst at (412) 648-2066 or, for medical information, Mary Ketner at (412) 648-9597.

I hope you will keep in touch with me and that, from time to time, we may discuss further our mutual interest in this endeavor.

Sincerely,

Bernard Fisher, M.D.

BF:gdh

Part of my problem was I really had no time to study or attend courses as they're offered now. They are mock certifying exams by people who have just gone through and relay the questions, so the prospective examinees actually have real questions and are more prepared. Loyola, for its part, never discussed a word to any of us on how to answer questions or how to comport ourselves. Knowing what

I know now, I think it would be difficult not to certify me. But I was up to my ass in alligators with ten or more patients in the hospital with no time to study. Patients like the "Bird Lady" occupied all my time; it was relentless. No excuses, though.

What I can't reconcile to this day is, here I was on my own, no help by an attending to fall back on and taking on major gastrointestinal (GI) bleeds, cancers, gunshots, and other trauma very successfully. Many people would think I shouldn't have been able to do that or at least that's the impression. I was building a reputation at the hospital that I was a go-to surgeon. That's why seven physician staff members chose me to operate on them or their family member. Now these guys who don't know me or anything about me (except maybe that I graduated from medical school in Mexico) are saying I'm incompetent, and not worthy; how can this be? Oh, the American Board of Surgery will never say you're incompetent although they know damn well that's what others will think and act on. I earned my bones on cases like Betty Ford, the bomb boy, and the two-year-old with appendicitis that would have died if I had made the wrong decision. I don't want to say that they didn't (back then) want to let any gringos from Mexico into the Country Club, which is what people called the American Board of Surgery. Are the words on my certificate just words? Does faithfully and successfully mean nothing?

Did they purposefully, no matter how I answered, fail me? I don't think so, but it was a time not of inclusion, but exclusion. To wit, in the fall of 2020 the American College of Surgeons (ACS), not the American Board of Surgery, but they're the same people, just different hats, came out with an edict. It basically said that the ACS would revamp their policy of race to include more blacks. I applauded that effort.

I think they said something like, "If we're not perfect on race, we're not perfect." By inference, then there was apparently an unspoken exclusion of Blacks (and other minorities and who knows who else, FMG gringos) before the edict of 2020. Otherwise, they wouldn't have had to change anything. If you push the clock back to the early 1980s when I took the Boards, what was in place then (their mindset unspoken), about foreign medical graduates, especially from Mexico?

We were the first class to show up. Would they keep us out of the country club? Of course, I have no proof of anything. You get no feedback so that you could do it better next time, just your denial letter. I didn't/couldn't study since I was covering the ER three weeks out of the month then helping Dr. Kopp the last week. I passed the written (qualifying) exam but not the oral (certifying). I was, in fact, the field liaison officer for the American College of Surgeons at Eisenhower.

Certificate of Appointment

PHILIP BRETZ MD

is a Member of the Field Liaison Program of the Commission on Cancer and is appointed Field Liaison Physician at

EISENHOWER MEDICAL CENTER

RANCHO MIRAGE, CA

CHAIRMAN, COMMITTEE ON FIELD LIAISON

DIRECTOR, CANCER DEPARTMENT

While my friends in family practice got umpteen times to pass their written, we got three in my day. And again, it's not like I could take time off so I could answer some guy's favorite journal club article.

No excuses, but this proved to be very devastating throughout my entire career. It was the second big blow in my life; the first was losing my father. While the American Board of Surgery is careful not to say the certification exam bestows competency, again they know damn well that hospitals, insurance companies, HMOs, and the general public use the designation for admission or exclusion from hospital staffs, etc., and whether or not a surgeon is competent. There won't be any complications if you chose a Board-certified surgeon over one who isn't, really? The list of unreachable opportunities in one's career without Board certification is almost inexhaustible. One will never be designated Chief of Surgery; you are forever looked down on as inferior. Publication becomes nearly impossible. The internal humiliation is almost unbearable for the rest of your life. Behind your back, you are treated like a leper, that's what it feels like for the rest of your life, no matter your success.

The following is directly from the General Surgery News, July 2018 Volume 45, Number 7, page 22. It is in the 'Letter to the Editor' section. It is written by Daniel J Weinberg, MD. It says, and I quote, "To the Editor - I feel a need to respond to Dr. JoBuyske's opinion article, "Meaningful Certification," in General Surgery News (May 2018, Page 1). Several points need to be made. First, I am commenting from a background of certification and two recertifications. I also trained and practiced 15 years at Presbyterian Medical Center, in Philadelphia (Dr. Buyske's institution), so I can appreciate her reference to clinical care. I disagree with a fundamental assertion made in this opinion, which is simply this: I do not believe board certification has any relevance when it comes to a surgeon's; competence. I have had 30 years to observe those who are board certified and those who are not. I've proctored people who were double-boarded. I have found, and many readers will likely agree, that this is not a measure of surgery competence or quality. It is a test of test taking. It is a publicity stunt, as the public has been led to believe that it is a measure of skill and competence.

Are lifelong learning and continuing medical education (CME) important? Of course, they are. But exams that have no relevance to my clinical practice are no measure of my competence. In fact, the certification on those grounds is misleading to the public. My exams have focused on "zebras," and not the things I do every day.

I must also disagree about the reference to proctoring, that it requires many people and many operations to assess skill. In all my years I've been doing this, I have found that it is easy and quick—a couple of cases, that'll tell me if a person can "operate" and whether or not they have any "judgment." Finally, as a professional pilot, I will also disagree with the analogy of the safe pilot and the surgeon. In flying, our skills are tested exhaustively every year in a simulator, along with judgment. It is not comparable [to the surgeon] because of the lack of performance assessment in surgery.

We are asked knowledge questions that mostly (to date) have not been related to our actual practice. So, they are very different, indeed. The solution? I would suggest really relevant, intensive CME offerings, they should be mandatory. They should be practice type-specific to the degree possible. If the public persona of a board-certified surgeon is believed to be so important, do it on the basis of those CMEs. Do away with the testing process. Even initial certification with written and oral exams has no connection to ability to do surgery. Again, it relates to an ability to take tests. Certify based on recommendations of program directors who graduate residents, and make them accountable for graduating unqualified people.

Adjust the length of surgical residencies to give trainees adequate exposure to cases so they will become competent, (as we did in the 1980s). Then perhaps, we will be closer to label "board certified" meaning something."

Ok folks, you see it's not just me.

The American Board of Surgery (a private enterprise) has never been forthcoming to the public of explaining exactly what that certification implies. I have a letter from the past president stating that the certification doesn't equate to competence, that there are many surgeons not Board-certified who are highly competent, but the Board chooses to hide that fact. There is a recent journal article from *General Surgery News* dated July 2020 authored by Ben Gerber, MD. The title is, "Fellowship or No, How Do We Ensure Quality?" The article deals with the question of how to decide which surgeons provide high-quality service. What? This article ignores all the training, and it begs the question, just what kind of surgeons are we churning out these days? One position put forward is that if a surgeon completes a fellowship (after completing their residency), it is reasonable to assume that they provide better quality service. By extension, the service provided by "non-fellowship trained surgeons" is possibly not high quality. What hogwash.

There are already multiple layers of quality assurance in the hospital monitoring every physician, including surgeons, like the Mortality and Morbidity Committee, the Quality Assurance Committee, and a number of lawsuits. These people have all served residencies faithfully and successfully. So again, just what kind of surgeons are we churning out that are so inept? Ultimately, each surgeon must know his/her limitations and act accordingly. Finally, the patients themselves can complain to the Medical Board, the hospital, and the surgeon if they are not satisfied with the care.

But superseding all this is the individual surgeon's integrity to know his/her craft like no other and provide unparalleled care. Dr. Gerber goes on. "My experience as a member of multiple local quality assurance committees has shown me that fellowship training does not automatically ensure quality care in all instances. Undoubtedly, I'm not the only person who has made this observation. I'm sure that all of us can think of some colleagues who are fellowship-trained and also have quality concerns. If the true aim is to ensure universal quality standards, then quality should be the focus rather than training or experience as surrogates to presume quality."

In the article, there is no mention of Board certification as a surrogate for quality. I think the same argument about all this training and certification to ensure quality can be made that we all know colleagues who are Board-Certified who end up in the Mortality and Morbidity committee with lawsuits trailing them. What does this all mean? It goes back to the integrity of each surgeon to know his/her limitations. It's as simple as that. A surgeon must hone their skills each and every case.

Members of the certifying team at the American Board of Surgery should observe the surgeon doing actual surgery, his/her indications, and outcomes, instead of asking questions on some topic the surgeon will never approach. An example is a thyroid or pancreatic surgery. If you have decided you won't approach a pancreas for a Whipple procedure, then you won't and shouldn't be held to be knowledgeable for every detail about pancreatic surgery.

Still, you are if, during your exam, that's your examiner's forte, just like Bernie Fisher asked me about breast cancer. Almost 70% of general surgeons are Board-certified. That means most of the complications and visits to the Mortality and Mobidity Committee are Board-certified surgeons.

But wait, isn't Board certification saying (as everyone thinks it is) that if you're certified, you're the best of the best, and therefore, there should be no need for Mortality and Mobidity committees as far as Board-certified surgeons are concerned? But we all know it is necessary.

Not being Board-certified (although by ABS's own admission, certification doesn't equate to competence) severely impacts a surgeon's entire career on several fronts. The humiliation factor for your entire career, even though you may be a great surgeon with great results and have accomplished much, makes you a second-class citizen. A non-certified surgeon cannot join and is never asked to join the American College of Surgeons to become a coveted "Fellow." The ACS is another country club after certification. Again, you're dog meat no matter how many lives you saved. Admission to any hospital is restricted to only Board-certified surgeons. For those surgeons who are part of HMOs, the same process holds true.

As my particular case unfolds, I can't help but think that my not being Board-certified helped grease the skids toward their sanction of me by the Medical Board. You see, this bum isn't even Board-certified;

he must be incompetent and guilty of doing "experimental procedures." How can it not impact everyone, creating a totally negative picture that may be (you will be the judge) totally wrong?

Apropos to this discussion is the experience of Scott Kelly, an American astronaut who not only flew missions aboard the Space Shuttle but he, along with a couple of other Russian cosmonauts, spent a year in the International Space Station. This paved the way for needed knowledge about the effect of space on the human body during prolonged periods. I recommend the book highly; it is called *Endurance*. But the reason for my mentioning him is twofold. First, he points out what a lousy student he was all throughout his formative days including high school. He graduated in the bottom half of his high school class. He somehow got into a college and tried pre-med but failed the courses. If we relied on his grades, he wouldn't have become a hero astronaut. Second, and again apropos to my childhood going down that hill no hands with burning candles in each hand, it seems I one-upped him. He also found it necessary to careen down hills on his bike. It must be a genetic thing in guys who are not content with the status quo.

One solution to the quality of surgery or family practice, for that matter, is to have open access to the public for Mortality and Mobidity conferences. But you can bet that won't happen. You see, while the practice of medicine is one of integrity, it's not like golf, where you are required to penalize yourself if you break the rules, but no one sees.

An example is a surgeon who treats a post-operative infection in the office, or brings the patient to another facility to operate on it; the original facility will just record no complication. When, in fact, there is one complication or maybe a lot, but no one is any the wiser since the surgeon decides not to report.

To defend our profession of surgery, 100 things impact whether a particular surgery will end up with a complication. To name a few, age, does the patient have co-morbidities (diabetes, COPD, heart disease, etc.), length of surgery, whether or not an organ was accidentally injured like the colon, is it a clean operation like a breast biopsy or a dirty one like a colon resection. I've always said it's so easy to criticize from the peanut gallery, but if you think you could do it better, then please step up to the plate and become a surgeon. What, no takers?

I hope those people at the American Board of Surgery have the guts and transparency to declare publicly just what their president wrote in his letter to me. Namely, the certification exam does not equate to competency. And by extension, institutions like hospitals and the like should not use Board Certification as a criterion for admission. But that won't happen either. It only means you passed that particular exam and has nothing to do with your outcomes in treating patients within your scope of expertise. Now with ivy league colleges dropping the SAT (college entrance exam) and paying more attention to recommendations, how long will it take for the same re-evaluation to hit the American Board of Surgery? The prolonged and complicated processes one goes through to sit at the certifying exam should amount to something. That would include exhaustive efforts, i.e., college, MCATs, medical school, five years of a surgical residency watched over and scrutinized daily. And finally, on completing their residency must be recommended by their program directors to apply to the Board because they completed their residency faithfully and successfully period. Then the Board decides if the applicant has met the criteria like the number of major cases, etc.

Further, thousands of non-certified surgeons provide outstanding care on par with Board-certified surgeons. The vast majority of surgeons are Board-certified, so that should mean the vast majority of complications or less than perfect surgical outcomes or things like operating on the wrong patient, wrong site, etc., are due to Board-certified surgeons. There is a published article by Tyson K. Cobb entitled "Wrong Site Surgery – Where Are We and What is the Next Step?" The article estimates there about forty wrong site surgeries that take place every week in the US. That means over 1,300 per year. It neglects to say who is responsible. Someone should go back to that article and find out the Board certification or not of all those surgeons and whether or not they were all FMGs? That would put the nail in the coffin one way or the other. The PMID number of that article is 23730251. But wait, the picture presented to the public is that it is preferable that your surgeon is Board-certified. There are other entities that look into this like The Sullivan Group, and papers by Dorothy A. Andriole, MD, FACS. Of course, any public statement by the American Board of Surgery that would in the least way tarnish them will not be forthcoming. Perhaps in the future, there may be a lifetime achievement certification by the ABS, without admitting they made a mistake years ago that cost the surgeon untold misery. They could do what's right. But don't look for that anytime soon.

An example is the letter I received from Dr. Bernard Fisher. It pertained to my groundbreaking efforts at initiating the country's first large-scale breast cancer prevention clinical trial and that I should be commended for what I had done. That effort was conceived and executed by me, a non-board-certified surgeon, while *every other researcher* in the country from the NCI, NIH, to any major cancer center didn't have the vision necessary, otherwise they would have done it much earlier. Apparently, it took my out-of-the-box thinking. My effort finally got this country to look at breast cancer prevention, with the government spending $68 million on my idea that, by the way, was usurped. This story is in *Sacrificing America's Women II*.

Interestingly, Bernie probably failed me on my certifying exam. I try not to be self-aggrandizing as I look back on my surgical career, but sometimes it's difficult not to. That is, these setbacks are catastrophic and there is a limit to what one can endure with all these one-sided attacks without being able to defend one's self. To end this sidebar on certification, in my letter from the President of the American Board of Surgery, he stated that now the Board allows five chances to pass the certification exam. So technically, he said I was still Board-eligible. This doesn't do me any good now as I'm seventy-five and not on any hospital staff.

Sometimes, though, I take great pride in what I've accomplished. I just want those examiners to know they need to find a different path rather than the totally subjective path they have been on for decades. The current path disavows all prior work upon entering that room for your exam. This is unjust since the very people who give the exam were your mentors for five grueling years of direct daily supervision, and they know your capability like a book. I also want them to know that their decision dramatically affects a surgeon's entire career. Of course, they know all this but are unwilling to change. Perhaps during the exam, they could just say to the candidate, your answers need work, and you have the option to withdraw, and this session will not count on your five tries.

That would at least show some respect for previous hard work. Or, as I said before, perhaps a lifetime achievement certification would be in order. That would go a long way to saying they made a mistake years ago, without them having to admit anything. But, of course, none of that will happen to this country club of theirs. Not only that, but to obfuscate from the public the false notion that when a patient scouts out a surgeon and selects one who is certified over one that isn't, that person thinks all will be well and no complications. But we know that isn't the case, and no one publicly lists all the complications certified surgeons make daily. Or finally, a statement by the Board so the public could learn the nuances here that Board-certification doesn't equate to competence as it says in my letter, would help. I would be content for the American Board of Surgery to go to Eisenhower and evaluate all my surgeries (they have them on microfilm) and interview whatever patients they want over forty years to see what's what. I can stand next to any Board-certified surgeon on this planet and hold my head up. Enough of this, it's very difficult for me, but it has cut deep. I'm sorry to belabor this Board thing. I'll tell you they don't let stumblebums operate on the First Lady or Secret Service. On to the next chapter in my life, EMC.

CHAPTER 5

ON THE SURGICAL STAFF AT EISENHOWER MEDICAL CENTER, RANCHO MIRAGE, CALIFORNIA

M Y REPUTATION AT Eisenhower grew because I made rounds twice daily, refined my surgery every case, and had no serious ongoing complications. See the recommendation of 100% of third-floor oncology nurses.

The reason that 100% thing is so important is those girls saw all the surgeon's care and complications. I took care of many sick patients, and I became known to the Jehovah's Witnesses as the bloodless surgeon at Eisenhower and operated on many of them. One day the cardiac surgeon approached me and asked if I wanted to try and assist on the open-heart team. Remember, I almost stayed at Loyola to do a cardiac surgical residency. I was good at it, and yes, the thought appealed to me. So, I signed up. Well, I didn't actually sign up, just started. It seemed right off the bat we could operate together with very few, if any, miscues. As a little time passed, Dr. L. (general surgeon) was dismissed unceremoniously. A little further and Dr. B. (thoracic surgeon) was also dismissed. I should have taken the cue from them. In those days, the knife dropped at 7 a.m., and we did on average two to three hearts a day, three or more days a week.

Sometimes we operated every day during the season. Before 7 a.m., we always looked at the patient's angiogram one last time. We didn't have any residents to open or close, so that meant we did everything. Sometimes they didn't clot for long periods coming off the heart-lung machine. We ended our days around 5 p.m. or 6 p.m., almost ten hours in the OR, then do it all over again the next day.

Dr. S. would crack the chest, and I would harvest the veins through as small an incision as I could. It became a game to see how small an incision I could get away with. A lot of patients had an incision all along their leg from groin to ankle (from other surgeons). Then I would move up to the first assistant position across from the surgeon, and we would put the patient on bypass. We would clean the schmutz off the vein and begin the bypasses using an instrument called a "punch" to make a hole in the aorta for the proximal anastomotic site, then find in the heart the distal anastomotic site in the coronary artery. Sometimes the artery was only a millimeter or so, which called for no f—-ups.

As far as I remember, we never had any miscues through about 3,000-plus hearts. We sometimes had to do an endarterectomy on the coronary artery as it was so involved in plaque, we couldn't sew the vein to it. Years later, we got a call from a reporter from the *Washington Post*. Under the FOIA act, he found that Medicare, unbeknownst to anyone, kept track of mortality of all heart programs in the country, doing 100 hearts or more a year. As it turned out, we weren't just the best in the West, with a mortality rate of 0.6%, but it was the best in the entire country. This was two years running around 1983-84.

KNIGHT-RIDDER NEWSPAPERS

WASHINGTON BUREAU
700 National Press Building
529 14th Street, NW
Washington, DC 20045
(202) 383-6000

OCT 2 7 1986

October 22, 1986

Heart Institute of the Desert
Eisenhower Medical Center
39000 Bob Hope Drive
Rancho Mirage, CA 92270

    I'm pleased to send you a copy of the series on bypass surgery, which I wrote along with my colleague, Michael York.
    You might be interested to know that among institutions performing 150 bypass operations or more on Medicare patients, the Eisenhower Medical Center had the lowest mortality rate in the country. Here's how the federal data looked for the top four.

Hospital	Cases	Rate
Eisenhower Medical Center	161	0.6
Deaconess Medical Center	150	1.3
Brookwood Medical Center	217	1.4
Jewish Hospital of St Louis	257	1.6

    Hope you find the series of interest, and I'd appreciate hearing any comments you might have.

Sincerely,

Thomas J. Moore
National Correspondent

It wasn't just our surgery; it was the way he developed the program. For instance, the nurse you saw on your first visit was assigned to you. She would then be at your surgery, assisting, making it easier for her to recover you in the recovery room. She knew the entire surgery result and any potential problems and headed them off. Years later, when I opened the Desert Breast Institute, I took a cue from the heart team. That is, the same doctor you saw first (me), was the same doctor you would see for decades, and was also the one who would help plan and execute treatment, if necessary, together with the oncologist and radiation therapist.

We went full tilt for the nine years I was the sole first assistant. We went for six years without a vacation. Years passed, and gradually I had given up all my general surgery. During this time, laparoscopy surgery came into vogue. I missed out on becoming proficient in that realm. While at times I forgot who I was, my bank account did well enough to buy Lot W at Thunderbird Country Club about 300 yards from President Ford. It was an acre-and-a-half on the sixth green, seventh tee, a par three. That lot cost me $275,000. At the time, that was a lot of money for sand and tamarisk trees. It was the time of Jimmy Carter in the White House, and interest rates were over 20% prohibiting me from building. However, with the election of Ronald Reagan, interest rates plummeted to 9%. In today's market, 9% seems like highway robbery, but back then, it meant Joan and I could build. We engaged an architect, and we settled on what is referred to as French pavilion (see photo).

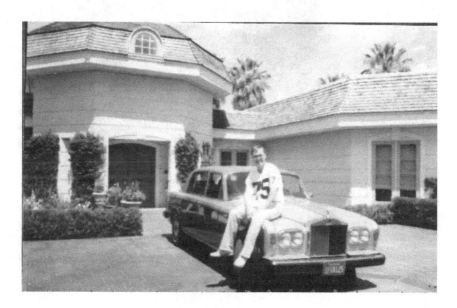

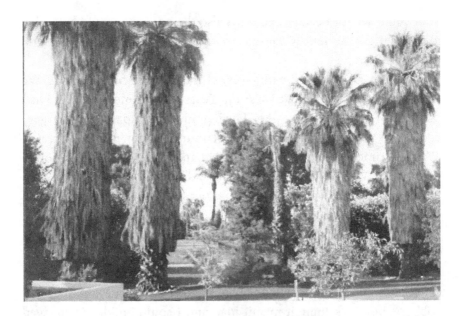

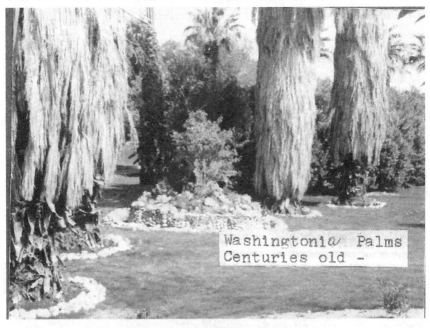

Washingtonia Palms
Centuries old -

It was 6,000 square feet. About $30,000 later, we had plans. I remember telling Tony (our architect) that I wanted at least one foot on either side of the hallway with my arms outstretched. My cousin Stan had started Phillips Construction up in Lake Arrowhead. He and his sons, Stan Jr., Jimmy, and John, would build my home. One night after the Bob Hope Classic Ball, we walked the property on the newly poured foundation. I walked the living room and decided I wanted it about five more feet totaling more than 30 feet long.

There was a vacant lot next to ours, and I inquired as to the owner. He turned out to be Fred Wilson, who was a member at Thunderbird and owned Transworld Insurance Brokers in Beverly Hills. Fred was really something.

I wrote him a letter, and he called and invited me up to his house in Thunderbird Heights. In my letter I said I recently purchased Lot W and would like to purchase his lot if he wanted to sell.

I also said I didn't have the money but could afford a $5,000 initial good faith down payment and the rest in a balloon in three years. He called, and I drove up. This is the extra land I acquired with Fred's lot. It was good to be a surgeon at EMC.

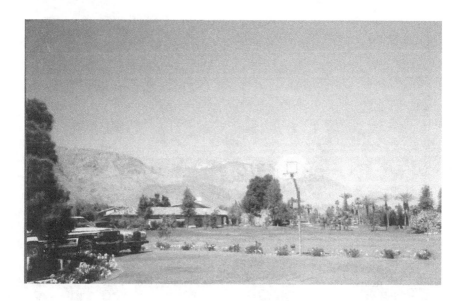

Upon entering his driveway, I noted two Rolls-Royces ("Rollers") and a koi pond that started out front and continued into the house. He turned out to be very engaging and was friends with the President, among others. He was a true high roller. He agreed to sell me the lot on my terms, and I commented on the two Rollers out front. He said one was his, and the yellow Corniche convertible belonged to Alan Paulson (founder of Gulfstream jets). He was buying it from Alan.

I sensed an opportunity and said, "I'll buy yours." He took me out and we drove around, and I bought myself a 1979 Silver Wraith II with $5,000 down. Not a bad investment. I've had all kinds of cars from the 57 Olds, to 63 split-window Vette, to a Bricklin to 928 Porsche, to a Jaguar XJ12, to Cadillac Seville, but nothing felt like that Roller. My youngest son Christian at age two would stand on my lap and steer going down the street to our house. That Roller was the only one I ever saw with a velvet interior. Now with that acquisition of Fred's lot, I had over 2.6 acres plus directly on Thunderbird Country Club.

I planted wild flowers in the form of a "B" on the lot.

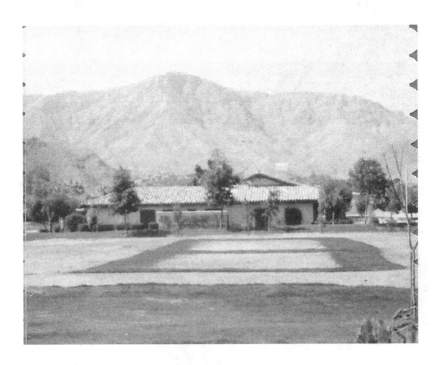

Fred would invite me to his daughter's wedding, and Joan sat next to the original Oscar Mayer and danced with Buddy Rogers. Fred also had high roller parties, and it was at one of those where I met Robert Michel, then the House Minority Leader. My encounter with Michel is detailed in *Sacrificing America's Women II* (coming soon). But let me tell you a sneak preview of that meeting. I had come up with the idea to do a large-scale clinical trial for breast cancer prevention using the drug Tamoxifen. I knew I would need support on Capitol Hill and that Fred would probably have a senator or the like at his yearly Bob Hope Classic party at the house.

I went up to Fred's house and detailed my plan for the prevention trial. He invited me up when Michel was there and introduced me. I told Congressman Michel about it and my association with the Soviet Union to work together instead of trying to kill each other.

He took me into the den, picked up the phone, called Jim Baker, the Secretary of State, and told him. This would lead to further trips to Washington and eventually to the White House. This encounter and the rest of the Tamoxifen story will be detailed in *Sacrificing America's Women II*. But that meeting with Michel taught me something. It taught me that a person in power who likes a story could act on it immediately without undue delay. Below is the response I received from Secretary Baker that the project should be pursued. What began as an idea in my brain was taking on a life of its own. The Tamoxifen trial really gets involved and convoluted and that's why I felt like James Bond and Huck Finn.

It was a true adventure story of a kid from Chicago.

United States Department of State

Washington, D.C. 20520

Dear Mr. Michel:

The Secretary has asked me to respond to your letter of February 12 informing him of Dr. Phillip Bretz's proposed joint study on breast cancer with the Soviet Union.

The Department appreciates your interest in this study and applauds the efforts of Dr. Bretz and his colleagues to find a cure for this widespread and often terminal disease. We also appreciate the significance of joint U.S.-Soviet studies not only in conquering common medical problems, but also in forging stronger relations generally.

Although we did not have an opportunity to speak with Dr. Bretz prior to his departure for the Soviet Union, a member of my staff has since contacted him and will render every assistance possible.

As you are aware, the United States and the Soviet Union have signed the Agreement on Cooperation in the Field of Medical Science and Public Health, which includes cancer research as an area of cooperation. While we welcome private initiatives to further cancer research, we cannot officially endorse proposals for joint programs made by U.S. or Soviet citizens which fall outside our government to government agreements.

Nonetheless, in light of the magnitude and potential benefit of this study, we believe the proposal should be pursued. We have advised Dr. Bretz to consult with and seek guidance from the National Cancer Institute. Dr. Federico Welsch and Dr. Wesley Simmons of the Institute are also conducting a breast cancer study with the All Union Cancer Research Institute in Moscow. They will undoubtedly welcome the opportunity to share experiences and medical data with Dr. Bretz.

Again, thank you for keeping us apprised of these events. If I can be of any further assistance to you in this or any other matter, please do not hesitate to contact me.

Sincerely,

Janet G. Mullins
Assistant Secretary
Legislative Affairs

The Honorable
   Robert H. Michel,
     House of Representatives

When I did have a little time off, we would drive to Coronado to stay at the Del. During one visit, the Los Angeles Olympics were on, and we watched the opening ceremonies. I noted one sequence was several pianos playing George Gershwin's music. I don't recall how I found out, but I could buy one of those pianos, a Kimball. It would sit in the far end of the living room at Thunderbird by the French doors.

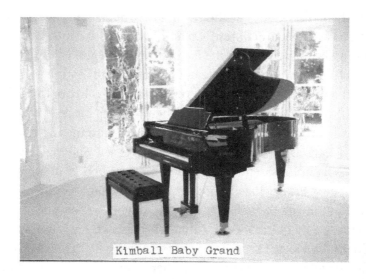

Kimball Baby Grand

At the time the house at Thunderbird went up, we lived at Sunrise Country Club. There was one street at Sunrise you could walk along, and there was a wall that separated Thunderbird from Sunrise. Joan and I used to walk by, and you could see part of our house as it was built. One day some ladies were looking over the wall and one of them said, "Look, is that the new clubhouse going up?" referring to our house. That made me feel good. Below is a night time photo of the entrance.

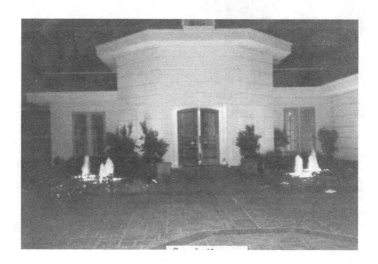

I had hit my stride (without anyone's help) and was living the American dream. Sometimes Joan and I would drive into Los Angeles to shop at the "Blue Whale," the Pacific Design Center where you could have custom furniture done. We bought all kinds of antiques, from two huge French chandeliers to big French antique mirrors to a Chinese lacquer table and a hand-carved wooden hunting piece. It was a good time. As I say in my letter to the presidential nominating committee of North Park University, I was saving lives left and right, we lived 300 yards from President Ford, and you might find us at a party with Bob Hope or Frank. It felt good to be on my game and live out my destiny. But most of all, after years of hard work to be respected in my community as a go-to surgeon, that felt the best. Back in those days, the Coachella Valley reminded me of the town in *Doc Hollywood* where the doctor was very respected, and there weren't hundreds of doctor wannabees in the hospital. It was just you and the nurse who knew exactly what she could do before calling you and when to call you.

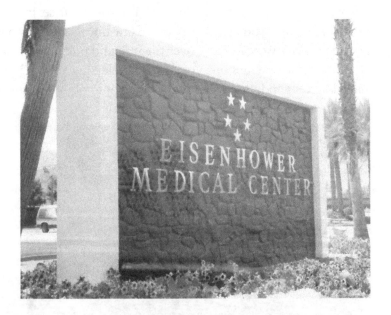

When I arrived at Eisenhower in the summer of 1979, no surgeon knew how to make a fistula for long-term dialysis. Since I was on the transplant team at Loyola, making fistulas was almost a daily event. In fact, I helped pioneer the "reverse fistula" that Dr. Peter Geis taught us.

Eisenhower enjoys a very good reputation. It all started with the generation that was there with me, and I'd like to mention those that worked with me on almost a daily basis. These guys were always there, no matter what time. It was like a band of brothers. When I arrived at EMC there were only forty-two doctors on staff. When I pulled into the doctor's parking in front, I knew exactly who was there. If I leave anyone out, I'll owe it to a senior moment. This is in no particular order; these were all good docs without regard to religion or race. We all worked together to help the patient. Dr. Phil Dreisbach, my oncologist, and fellow researcher, worked with me daily when I opened up my breast center. He would go with me to the Soviet Union.

We had adjoining offices so we could walk back and forth to see patients together, and the patients loved it. We helped pioneer neoadjuvant chemotherapy with the National Surgical Adjuvant Breast Project (NSABP) protocol B-18.

I was their Principal Investigator at Eisenhower. We first went outside the box with what we called the "Compass Treatment." That is, after making the diagnosis with a core needle biopsy, we would (in the cases that needed it) begin neoadjuvant chemotherapy (chemotherapy before surgery). But instead of the protocol of the NSABP, which called only for four rounds of chemo, we kept giving the patient chemo assuming the tumor was shrinking until the tumor was no longer detectable. It's called a complete response (CR), and we called the patients "responders." If a patient receives primary chemotherapy or neoadjuvant chemotherapy, about 80% of the time there will be a 50% reduction in tumor size. The significance of this is it would down stage a patient from mastectomy to lumpectomy.

In fact, during the clinical trial NSABP B-18, there were patients Dreisbach had given chemotherapy to, and when he returned them to me for surgery, I couldn't find the tumor. That happened to other surgeons across the country. One patient treated in 1997 is still alive in 2021. She had large breasts, and we couldn't document any active tumor on repeat core biopsy after the chemo. We discussed it, and I felt

I might be going on a fishing expedition and excavate her breast in an attempt to find an active tumor that wasn't there. On that patient and 7% of our patients back then, we treated them only with chemotherapy and external beam radiation, no surgery of any kind. That was back in 1997 and published as an abstract in the American Society of Clinical Oncology proceedings.

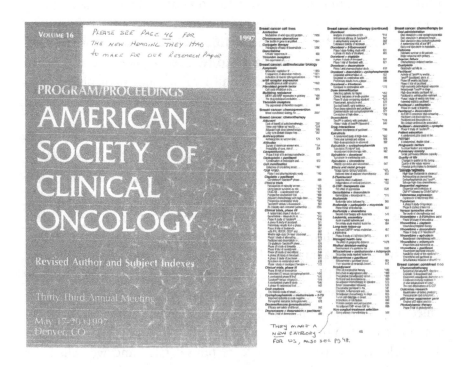

THE COMPASS TREATMENT, A NEW ERA OF TREATMENT IN BREAST CANCER NEOADJUVANT THERAPY AND RADIATION WITHOUT SURGERY

Bretz* P., Dreisbach, P., Desert Breast Institute, Palm Desert, CA, 92260
Bacus, S., Advanced Cellular Diagnostics, Inc, Elmhurst, IL, 60126

Key Words: core biopsy, strategic analysis, neoadjuvant chemotherapy, no surgery

An understanding of the natural history of invasive breast cancer coupled with effective chemotherapy opened the door for vast improvements in the care of breast cancer patients. Often, axillary node dissection was used as the major guide in recommending adjuvant chemotherapy. Over the past decade for the purpose of neoadjuvant chemotherapy, lymph node status has been supplanted by strategic analysis. This is based on core sample, tumor grade, size, lymphatic invasion, mammographic appearance, clinical exam, family history and extensive tumor analysis. This has identified aggressive invasive tumors that are likely to have already metastasized long before the patient is diagnosed. Since 1989 we have treated 96 patients ranging in age from 28 to 83 with neoadjuvant chemotheapy based on strategic analysis following core biopsy. Tumor size ranged from 1.2 cm to over 8cm. All patients have received at least four courses of CAF. Neoadjuvant therapy has identified "responders" who showed consistent tumor ablation to the point of total tumor dissolution based on clinical exam, mammogaphy and repeat core sampling. In the past five years we have continued chemotherapy including at times Taxol well past four courses, if mammographic evidence pointed to total tumor eradication.
Compass Treatment Results
5/96 (5.2%) had modified radical mastectomy
84/96 (87%) had lumpectomy and radiation
7/96 (7.3%) had no surgery, only chemotherapy and radiation
32/96 (33%) had no node dissection
18/96 (18%) had sentinel node biopsy
18/96 (18%) had no tumor removed
3/96 (3.1%) local/regional recurrence, none of the above eighteen patients
89/96 (92%)* have survived, followed from 2 to 10 years**
one patient died of myocardial infarction free of cancer*

Individualized treatment at a dedicated comprehensive breast institute following strategic analysis guidelines and response evaluation accounts for the above results. Our comprehensive team is active and in place before the diagnosis is made. These results point to patients doing better at a dedicated comprehensive center. We conclude implementation of Nationwide Networked Comprehensive Breast Centers is in order to achieve optimal patient care including lowering mortality and mastectomy rates. For those patients with no tumor found at surgery or for those with no tumor on repeat core biopsy and having no surgery, the classic paradigm of "clear margins for radiation" comes into question. We also conclude that it is possible to effectively treat some invasive breast cancer patients without surgery.

Those cases marked another time I was outside the box in breast cancer treatment, including the Tamoxifen trial and developing Desert Breast Institute. I was outside the first time when I was the first one to do a lumpectomy at Eisenhower. This all led to an invitation from UICC (a European cancer group) to present The Compass Treatment in Vienna. We called it the Compass Treatment because it was about 180 degrees from what my mentors said was the only way to treat breast cancer. That marked the first time countries outside my own would reach out to find out what I was doing and how I did it. We proved you really could manipulate breast cancer in some cases.

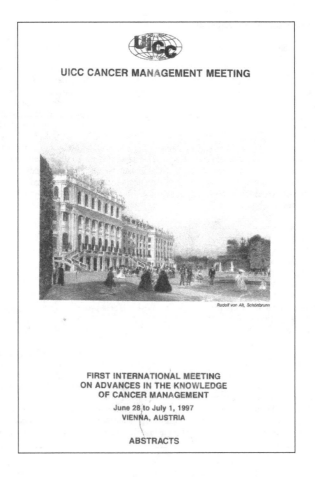

Dr. Ron Sneider was my go-to guy for pulmonary work in the trauma cases. It seems like I'd always be calling him at 5 a.m. when I usually finished a trauma case. Dr. Stuart Barton and Dr. Robert Gebhardt were my thyroid and neck guys. They were always there, no questions, whatever time it happened to be. Drs. Noel Curry, Mark Sonnenshein, and Tony Torney again were always there if I needed GI help. Dr. Phil Shaver was invaluable in assisting me with cardiology cases, in particular the "Bird Lady."

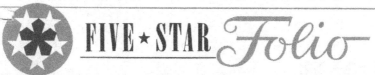

EISENHOWER MEDICAL CENTER

FIVE ★ STAR *Folio*

A CONTINUING REPORT ON THE ACTIVITIES AT EMC ★   JANUARY-FEBRUARY 1981

"If I'm ever going to see a miracle, this is the one."
EMC patient survives critical injuries

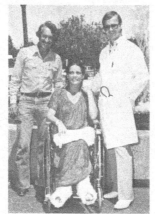

This is a story about a slender, 42 year-old woman with a fondness for breeding cattle at her Santa Rosa Mountains ranch, who was obliged to go on a 3000-calorie daily diet --the hard way. On a damp evening several months ago, she was deliberately run over by a car of "joyriders" as she jogged along Highway 74 near Anza. Clinically, she experienced three to four "deaths" during the next several weeks of hospitalization. Only sophisticated medical equipment, a physician skilled in trauma, other doctors and support personnel could pull her through during her 38-day ordeal.

Velva Eddy of Anza, Calif., who narrowly escaped death several times while hospitalized with major-trauma injuries, departs the hospital with her husband, Guy. Dr. Phillip Bretz, her primary physician, wishes her a speedy convalescence.

"Go home and feed your beefalo."

To Velva Eddy, housewife and mother of two, these were the sweetest words she ever heard.

For nearly two months, she lay near death as a result of severe colon injuries, shock-lung complicated by pneumonia, critical cardiac arrythmia, renal failure, fractured spine and shattered pelvis.

"If I'm ever going to see a miracle, this is the one," commented Dr. Phillip Bretz, surgeon and EMC trauma expert who was Mrs. Eddy's primary physician following her May accident. "She should have died many times," he added.

For a relatively small population, the Coachella Valley experiences an unusual incidence of trauma cases, the physician noted. A majority of trauma cases in large cities are gunshot or stab wounds, he explained. Locally, however, it's traffic accidents--truck drivers falling asleep on the interstate, vehicles careening off cliffs on tortuous Palms to Pines Highway 74, drivers "lulled" and entering desert spa cities at excessive speed, and so on.

Fortunately for Mrs. Eddy, EMC is

trauma-ready.

Mrs. Eddy had the severest type of trauma: multiple-organ failure.

Before her hospital discharge, the patient would undergo the intensive care of Dr. Bretz, surgeon; Ronald Sneider, pulmonary expert; Richard Stone, nephrologist; Jack Sternlieb, open heart surgeon; and Phil Shaver, cardiologist.

Support services including pharmacy and dietary were also deeply involved along with round-the-clock nursing care.

After arriving at the emergency room, Mrs. Eddy was rushed to surgery for the most critical trauma detected, a massive necrosis of the large bowel. Such a condition rates a 50 percent mortality factor.

The next crisis was shock-lung followed by superimposed pneumonia. Each chest cavity required a chest tube and the maximum pressure setting the respirator could generate over an extended period. Prognosis: 90 percent mortality rate (partially due to long term, high oxygen concentration through mechanical means).

The next insult to her body was

kidney failure as a result of overwhelming sepsis (spread of infection). The mortality rate here was 70-75 percent. She required extended hemodialysis (artificial kidney).

In short, Mrs. Eddy incurred "multiple-organ failure" of the most severe kind.

"In such instances, one thing leads to another; it snowballs and it almost always leads to the demise of the patient," Dr. Bretz said.

But Mrs. Eddy clung precariously to life. For the first several weeks, she maintained, "I never slept once. The doctors said my mind was alert, though I couldn't speak. I just felt that if I went to sleep, I'd never wake up."

Nutrition-wise, the patient was again in near fatal peril. Without hyper-alimentation (concentrated glucose and amino acids solution) her nutrient-starved body would have begun consuming its own muscles. The hyper-alimentation team was able to keep her alive, plus provide nutrients with which to build on, by means of a 3,000 calorie daily diet introduced through her subclavian vein.

continued on page 4

Classic Ball
January 1981

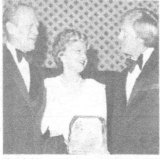

Classic Ball Master of Ceremonies Gerald Ford and EMC Trustee Betty Ford present a special tribute to golf pro Jack Nicklaus, the fourth Classic champion to receive the honor. (Arnold Palmer, Billy Casper and Bob Rosburg were honored in previous years.) The Ball drew more than 900 attendees. Proceeds of all Classic events benefit EMC and other desert charities.

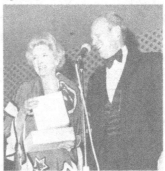

On behalf of the Ball committee, former President Ford presents Dolores Hope, chairman of the EMC Board of Trustees, with a gift to thank the Hopes for their role in the occasion.

Miracle: Velva Eddy (continued)

She faced yet another crisis: three cardiac arrests which each brought emergency physician visits from the Desert Cardiology Group. Mrs. Eddy continued to have severe abdominal infection and her white count was approaching 40,000 (as opposed to about 10,000 normal), signaling inability to fight off the sepsis, exacerbated by inability to sustain her blood pressure.

By this time, she was on multiple, maximal-dose medication for the blood pressure problem. Dr. Bretz was "more concerned than ever about her survivability."

As Dr. Bretz lay awake one night trying to think of something that could bring her back, it suddenly came to him..."Intra-aortic balloon pump." Dr. Jack Sternlieb (Heart of the Desert) who uses the pump in open heart surgery would have the key to her "second heart." To Dr. Bretz's knowledge, Dr. Sternlieb had not used the intra-aortic balloon pump in a multiple-organ failure patient.

After explaining Mrs. Eddy's case, Dr. Bretz and Dr. Sternlieb were in surgery at 3 a.m., giving her a temporary second heart. Dr. Sternlieb inserted the balloon, and one more battle in the war for patient survival was won.

"Even though we were still fighting the sepsis problem, over a period of time we were able to wean her from the blood pressure medication. Inch by inch she came back."

Still immobilized by chest, neck and abdominal tubes, Mrs. Eddy found the door to speech. Her first words: "Hi. I want to tell my husband how much I love him."

Her blood proteins improved; she no longer required kidney dialysis. And she could now talk.

"I truly believe that Dr. Bretz saved my life," Mrs. Eddy said. "I think every doctor in the hospital was here to see me. I've been treated royally, just royally."

Dr. Bretz continued: "This has

been a case where many unusual things were done. It was the only way to save this life. Multiple-organ failure on the basis of sepsis has a near 100 percent mortality factor." Hence, a miracle appeared to unfold on behalf of a steel-willed individual.

"Not only did Mrs. Eddy come back, she came back as a whole person," he added.

Mrs. Eddy is able to walk and is now home with her family. Other than the psychological "nightmares" she recalls, Mrs. Eddy's only medical exigency is recovery from surgical alteration of her abdominal wall.

"I'll be looking for steady progress in her recovery" is Mrs. Eddy's benign prognosis by her doctor.

Meanwhile, she will be able to continue raising black angus cows to buffaloes, producing "beefaloes."

That's what Dr. Bretz told me to do," Mrs. Eddy smiled. "He said, 'Go home and feed your beefalo...and put some meat on your bones.'"

Drs. Don Wasserman, Mark Kaufman, and Jeff Herz provided first-class assistance with urology cases. Dr. Steven Kopp was my surgical assistant, and I was his when each of us covered the ER, which back in the day was the entire month. Being the new kid on the block, so to speak, I took ER calls from Dr. Wayne Garrett and Dr. Joe Lesser (the man who so graciously took me in after my residency). It was always good to have another surgeon assist, one you could bounce questions or ideas off of and not just a tech handing you instruments.

But as usual, the government, with their ever-increasing army of functionaries, outlawed payment of two surgeons back years ago, so surgeons got used to operating by themselves. Drs. Robert Murphy, Robert Bush, and the rest of Desert Orthopedics were always taking excellent care of the fractures in trauma cases. Dr. Randy Blakely (RIP) was a true gentleman and excellent thoracic surgeon and was the first assistant on the heart team before my arrival. We played many rounds of golf together. BG Dr. Richard Lynch (US Army retired) taught me everything I know about reading mammography, and we have worked for over forty years. He told me once that if there was a war, he wouldn't mind being in the same foxhole serving with me. I guess as a Brigadier General, he saw my conduct as very ethical and professional. We used to trade off trying to see if one of us would miss a small cancer on mammography. I'd say, "If you can find this one, you can play with the big boys."

David Mantik, MD, PhD, (another true friend) and Dr. Ted Masek would provide excellent radiation therapy, and David and I have worked together for over forty years. David is a world authority on the Kennedy assassination and not only has written several books and articles on the subject, he is usually asked to appear on many panels and TV segments when November 22 rolls around. David is the smartest guy I've ever known. Dr. Lawrence Cone (RIP) would always be involved in some cutting-edge infectious disease clinical trial and would be there with an experimental antibiotic to help save a life. Dr. Dick Stone (RIP) would help with dialysis and renal failure patients. Since I was the only surgeon who had experience constructing fistulas for dialysis patients and had pioneered the "reverse fistula," we collaborated on many patients.

I couldn't have done any surgery without excellent anesthesia. To the following men, I owe a great debt of gratitude. Dr. Richard "Ric" Bradshaw, Dr. Jim Merson, Dr. Terry Gabrielson, Dr. John Jacobson, and Dr. Scott Levy, all these men were with me for many hours of critical surgery for decades on end. They never refused to do a case with me, so I must have been doing something right all the time. Those were the days where I might have six or seven major cases on the schedule, like constructing a new stomach out of small bowel for a patient with gastric carcinoma. One side bar about Ric Bradshaw. Now Ric was restoring a Pierce Arrow. Since this was an antique, auto parts were understandably scarce. That being said, every so often Ric would disappear for a few days on the pretense of having located a critical part. We never got to the bottom of that.

Dr. Don McEwen (RIP, a real gentleman) taught me about women's hormones. As a general surgeon, you didn't necessarily care about the difficulty a woman was having with her hormones. But as their breast doctor, it played a major role in one's understanding of what was happening to them. Dr. Joseph Lesser (RIP), who took me in right out of Loyola, thank you for having faith in me and risking your reputation.

Dr. Lesser risked his reputation because while I had attained chief resident status at a major university, I hadn't earned my bones yet. Years later, when I would lose everything, Dr. Sheryll Shearer (RIP), my radiologist at DBI, would step in and make it possible for me to continue my work. I owe him a debt of gratitude. Also, an extreme debt of gratitude to pathologists Drs. David Kaminski and Doug Bacon, both of whom traveled with me to the USSR. Their teaching me the finer points of interpreting tissue under the slide went a long way to my understanding of how breast cancer operates. Dr. Borko Djordjevic helped with any plastic surgery. At one point he owned the 007's house in *Diamonds are Forever*. Outside the medical arena I owe a debt of thanks to Steven DeLateur and Jay Ash. Steve, my de facto attorney and friend, has helped me for years, especially with the Honey Breast Implant project. Jay Ash has been not only a great friend but has helped with the billing for years. I thought I had the record of driving from the desert to Hemet every day for ten years (over 110 miles), but Jay drove for years almost daily from the desert to San Diego and back. Holy cow!

As I said, Joan and I were living the dream. I was able to buy homes for my mom and Aunt Florence and for Roy and Jan, Joan's parents. I paid for almost everything, mortgages, golf cart, etc. Roy was able to play at Ironwood on my membership and visited the clubhouse often. I was usually in the OR, unable to play. One time when I called to make a reservation for dinner, the maitre'd said they were sold out; he was sorry. Roy called a few minutes after and, "No problem, Mr. Pedersen, a reservation for six." It felt good that I was able to do that for them.

I was running on all twelve cylinders. At Christmas, we would drive out to Live Oak Canyon to the Christmas tree farm (Greg owned it) and cut our own tree. One year we cut an eighteen-footer; it was the biggest tree they had. I had bought a Toyota 4Runner from my cousin Dick, and that tree hung off the front and back, almost like the Griswolds in *Christmas Vacation.*

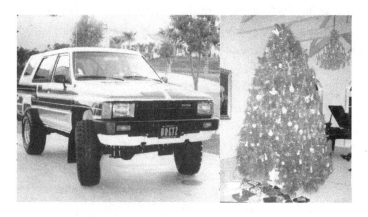

We had to tie the tree to a beam in the living room. We have hundreds of ornaments, with some being well over 100 years old. It took a couple of days to decorate it. We had real garland all over the place with poinsettias on either side of the walk to the front door, and two real big wreaths were hanging on the doors in front. I had built the big fireplace at Thunderbird so you saw it the first thing upon entering the house. It was double-sided so you could see into the living room. You had to walk up three stairs, which then led into the living room. The see-through fireplace at night looked pretty cool when you stood outside with the fountains lit on either side of the pools leading up to the front door.

We had Fior di Pesco marble throughout the entrance and down the hall on the sides. The marble was slab cut and laid down "bookend"-style, not in little squares. Ashley's room had an antique chandelier and an alcove bed. The playroom had a fire pole and a maze you had to negotiate to get down from the loft. From the entrance, you could look down the long hall to the cherub fountain by the master bedroom. We had carpet from Ireland in the living room and wood floors from Sweden in the master.

During this time, around 1984-86, we were LA Raider fans. I had six season tickets, and every game, my cousin Stan and whoever could come would drive to the Coliseum in Los Angeles. Parking was an issue until I found out about the parking lot next to the Coliseum owned by some museum. I think I paid $600.00 a year to get a pass and park there. It was hassle-free and guarded. The Raiders always had a charity event, and usually it was for cystic fibrosis. Here is the program where I am an honorary member.

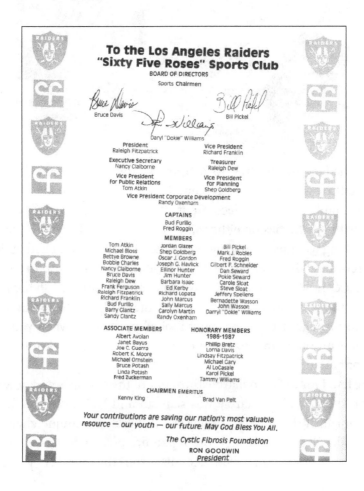

If you paid extra, you could have your player of choice sit at your table. That would be Howie Long and his wife. Jason got to sit on his lap. It was great fun, and these guys were huge in real life. OJ was there, and big John Matuszak, a real Raider. Also at that time, I had had a stretch limo made, a Lincoln. On the divider between passenger and chauffeur, I had inscribed the Raider mantra, "Commitment to Excellence."

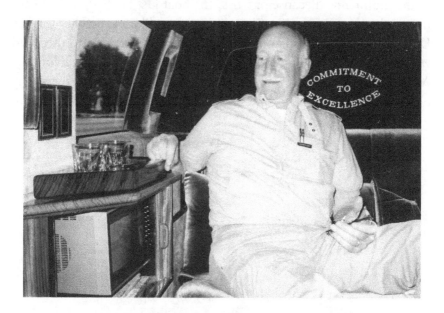

We took Stan and Darlyn (his wife and my cousin) to a Raider event. I had just gotten the limo, and I told him we would meet in the same parking lot when he came down the mountain from Lake Arrowhead. He arrived and drove around three times, looking for the 4Runner. He was stunned when we flashed our lights.

The reason for the limo was I had a partner, who was my medical student when I was Chief Resident at Loyola, and I offered him a partnership when he finished. I wanted him to work into the heart room so I could take some time off. Also, there was a small hospital up in Arrowhead, and I wanted to be there as well. It's a long drive to Arrowhead when you're tired, and the limo would fit right in. When we would drive to Las Vegas at Caesar's Palace, they would leave it right out front. In town, Ashley would stick a white glove out the window, making people think Michael Jackson was in the limo. We had fun with it.

At the same time, I had purchased a home up in Lake Arrowhead that we used on weekends, see below. I also bought a boat that we fished from on Lake Arrowhead. There's nothing like a huge snowstorm up in the mountains. Because of work, the boat just bobbed in the water mostly, but that house, like Thunderbird, was like a sanctuary for me. Up at Arrowhead, sitting out on the porch and listening to the wind whistling through the pine trees surrounding the place was hypnotic. Arrowhead was close enough so I could get back to EMC if an emergency heart came up. This happened more than not.

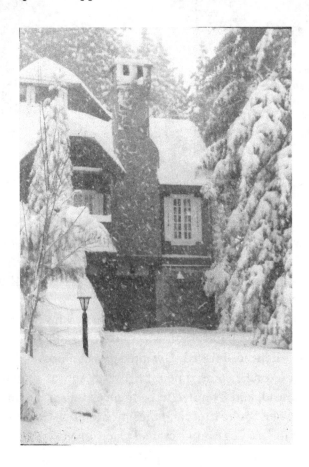

I was working very hard, and I wanted my family to have quality time together whenever I managed some time off. To make America work it's not a place of handouts and sluggards, so you just get by and let others do the innovative work. It should be a place of opportunity to exercise your G-D given talent, and use the ability you were endowed with to achieve at the highest levels. That goes for anybody period. That's what America should be, let you find your way to the top no matter who you are. It feels good the higher you go; the sense of achievement is awesome and enduring, pushing you to higher levels. You never have that satisfaction if you sit on your ass and let the world go by without helping, and you will never see that person of achievement in the mirror if you let people tell you they'll take care of you. Simple as that. It requires a lot of work, but one perk is you get to enjoy things you wouldn't otherwise. We have a lasting joke in the family that if I didn't have all these kids, I could have bought a Ferrari. But one perk with kids is you get to watch them grow and outdo you.

There are several stories during the Eisenhower era I'll detail later. However, there is one I need to touch on now. My new partner had been there for a few months. While we were operating one day, we got a call that his two-year-old daughter looked very ill. We told his wife to bring her into the ER. We ended up operating on her for appendicitis that I thought this moribund child had. Can you imagine taking on a case like that? What if I had made the wrong diagnosis, and his child would have died because I didn't send her by helicopter to the pediatric hospital at Loma Linda? You'll have to read the story but suffice it to say, a case like that is where you separate yourself from just okay surgeons. I could have just sent her by helicopter to Loma Linda, and if she had died, everyone would have thought I did the right thing.

But I was trained to deal with a situation like that. That's what surgeons do, pull off the impossible in front of everyone. In that case alone, I proved to myself I was good regardless of Board-certification. As Dr. Blakely would say, "It was a fundamental day" in coming to know yourself and what you had unwaveringly become.

As time passed, I served on various hospital committees from Mortality and Mobidity to Chairman of the Cancer Committee, and

I think the Institutional Review Board (IRB). Each of the eleven years since I joined the staff and until I reached thirty years of service on the active surgical staff, I would receive a letter from the Chairman of the Board that my privileges had been renewed without restriction. Further, it always said they took into account my ethics and professionalism (for thirty years). Again, this was always from people who worked with me on a daily basis. As letters of appreciation and endorsement began to come (see Chapter 11), I thought one said all one needs to know about me. It's the one from 100% of the oncology nurses on the third floor. There's an old saying: "You can fool all the people some of the time and some of the people all the time." Still, I can tell you; you can't fool trained nurses who work with all the doctors and know which ones they would go to if needed based on knowledge, their complication rate, surgical outcomes, bedside manner, professionalism, ethics, and patient satisfaction.

So, I value those kinds of endorsements. If it sounds like I'm building a case that some people thought I was an outstanding surgeon and a trusted ethically acting doctor at Eisenhower, you're right. Keep all this in mind when the hammer falls on me years later. I was on active staff for thirty years.

We were invited to multiple parties and intermingled with Bob Hope, President Ford, and Frank Sinatra (my mom worked for Frank). Looking back, it was like a fairy-tale life. I was saving lives left and right and we lived across the fairway from Lucille Ball and we were raising four kids, except I was in the operating room for what seemed like twelve hours a day. Sometimes I lost track of the days and myself. Ashley used to run across the two fairways and cut Lucy's yellow roses, and bring them back to Joan. Below is a photo of us at the Bob Hope Desert Classic. I took Rick and his wife, Connie, and Terry and his wife, Jackie, my mom, and Joan's mom and dad.

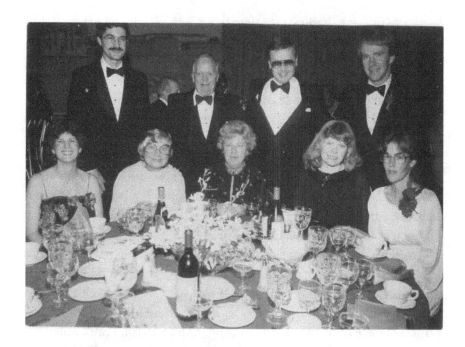

When you get married, the preacher says, "For better or worse, for richer or poorer," look out here it comes. As the heart surgeon and I were together all those hours, we often talked (during the cases) about how to grow the practice. I said one day, "Why don't you just buy the couple of acres next to Eisenhower and build our own hospital, The Heart Hospital!" He did, and probably about $5 million, and three years later, it was up. I got a call one day that, "I have to think of The Heart Hospital, and you should get up off your ass and do some general surgery."

After nine years and being the only other surgeon on the team? Of course, I hadn't done general surgery for nine years and had no referral base anymore. So, as a consequence, I lost everything. Back then, it was about $4 million. That was the last heart I did. Right after the call, I sat Joan down and told her we were going to lose everything. It was very difficult. At the time, I had used the heart money to acquire real estate in Southern California. You couldn't miss. Gold was only $400 an ounce. I suppose some might accuse me of having too much of everything.

Well, my five cars had twenty tires that I periodically had to buy, so I kept the tire guys afloat and the tune-up guy and a lot of other people. I felt I had invested wisely but mistakenly put too much trust in believing other people would always behave honorably.

I had taken a class in business at North Park College back in the 1970s. We had a guest speaker, a renowned financial wizard. He told us in the future, there will be a few of you who will be able to write a $100,000 check. The biggest check I ever wrote that cleared was for $165,000. We had a total of four homes (which various family members lived in) and multiple cars. While we didn't lose everything at once, I ultimately felt like a general being stripped of his medals. A good day for me was to come home, and one of my cars wasn't repossessed.

To take a little breather from what is difficult for me to write, there is a story involving my cousins Darlyn and Stan. Stan had built St. Louis Church in Cathedral City (known as Cat City, as Red Skelton would say on his TV show). They were very active. When Prince Rainier and Princess Grace of Monaco were visiting Frank Sinatra, Frank called the priest and asked if he could bring his guests over for a service. Then the priest called Stan and asked them to sing "Kumbaya" for Frank and the royal guests. Hard to top that. We all got a big kick out of that.

Coming up, my saga with the Medical Board was challenging for me to write as that would mark the fourth monumental disaster in my life. The first being the loss of my father, the second was not becoming Board-ertified, and now the third, losing everything I worked so hard for.

CHAPTER 6

THE DESERT BREAST INSTITUTE YEARS AND FINDING MY TRUE DESTINY

W HILE I WAS still working on the heart team, I opened the Desert Breast Institute (DBI) in 1988. Before we get into DBI, I had to insert these two photos. Legend has it that these two young ladies ignited my interest in breast work.

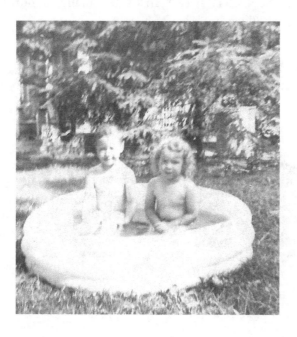

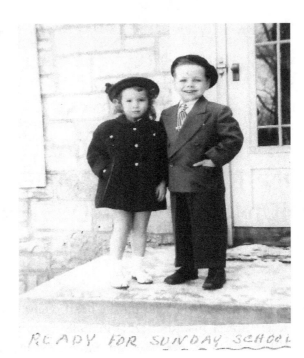

READY FOR SUNDAY SCHOOL

Below is the Desert Breast Institute; finally, a non-threatening atmosphere for all women.

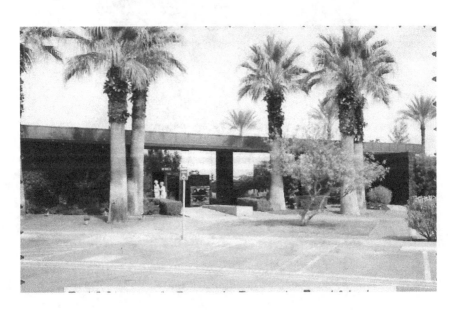

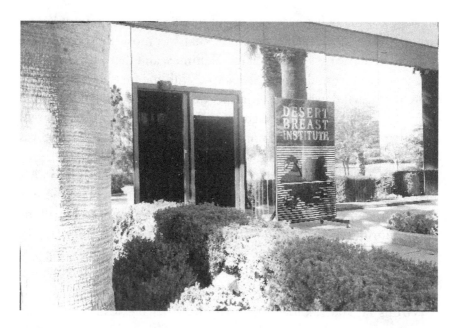

I had given a Grand Rounds in 1979 about the new breast cancer surgery, "lumpectomy." Now, so many years later, I figured all these women were living happily ever after. I had reviewed the annual death rate, and it was still at 40,000+ and continues until this day in 2021. That gave me the idea to open my own breast center, so I did, to see if I could do it better. This was in 1988 while I was still doing hearts. I figured these patients would all be outpatients, no ICU, etc., so I could see them on the days I wasn't in the heart room.

The Desert Breast Institute was the first comprehensive breast center in the Coachella Valley and one of the first in the country. The only other one I knew of was the Van Nuys Breast Center run by Dr. Mel Silverstein. Starting out, I had zero patients. I ran a two-page color ad in *Palm Springs Life* entitled, "For Women, There's Good News."

I was able to get a mammogram machine back then just because I was an MD. I did mammograms for free and only charged them the Current Procedrual Terminology (CPT) code for an office visit, needle biopsies, and more. From the first day, women were drawn to it. We would see upwards of twenty to twenty-five patients on the days we worked. I actually bet everything, my standing in the community, on Sylvia Brown doing their mammos. What was most important to me was I wanted the best girl doing my mammos, and that was Sylvia. She was great at it from day one. She stayed with me for about two years, then her husband, who was a Marine, was discharged and they moved away. I'm grateful to her; she got me off to a great start. As time went on, others took her place but none were as good as Maria Bikis. She was special with the girls. I used to include her in decision making so she would know what happens to the women she interacted with. Another mammographer that is in the same realm as Maria is Joanna Vine. She was an immense help doing not only all the mammography but all the logging for the state, FDA and American College of Radiology (ACR). She is damn good. Years later when I was performing the Lavender Procedure, Sylvia Ponder was a vital link as my ultrasound assistant in my being able to carry out Lavender.

To this day I don't know exactly why that befell me (losing the hearts), except maybe when the cardiac surgeon got the mortgage payment stubs, it was very high, so by employing another assistant, he could pocket the substantial remainder. I was never employed; I just billed insurance. It would be tough on him without me as the first assistant and my ability to not screw up and cosmetically remove the saphenous vein. Still, he could get away with only paying about $100,000 or less to the next man up saving the rest toward the hospital. As I said, I felt like a general having his medals stripped. Can you imagine the guilt and humiliation I felt having to leave the home I built and Joan's parents having to move to Arizona? Everything gone. All this happened just after I opened the breast institute.

But I just kept preserving, didn't go postal and didn't leave my family under such pressure that many men would have. It was because of my foundational upbringing and training I received at NPA, NPC, Mexico, and Loyola that made me so. To look such adversity in the face and come out on top, I don't wish that experience on anyone. One has to be prepared for what life dishes out.

During this tumultuous time, I was awarded the Carnegie Medal for an outstanding act of heroism. You can Google "CarnegieHeroFund.org" and type in my name and Bermuda Dunes, California, 1992. I was prepared for that act also.

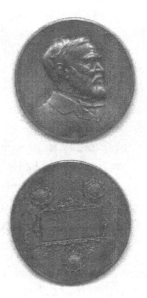

People often tell me I didn't know what I was doing, risking my life to save another person I didn't know (or know anything about). However, I knew exactly what I was doing when we came upon the accident and the occupant inside yelled out to the California Highway Patrol (CHP) officer that he was on fire. I turned to Joan and said I had to go.

My father would have turned over in his grave if I hadn't acted, considering the station in life I had achieved. When I realized in a heartbeat he was going to burn to death, I decided to act when others around, including a CHP officer, just stood there. I took a deep breath and went in, but as I did, it came to me Jesus wasn't going to let me die that day. Say what you will; that's what went through my mind. We looked evil in the eye that day and evil lost. Below is some of the letter I wrote to North Park University (NPU) Presidential Search Committee when I threw my hat in the ring to become their president.

In my career, I had been privileged to care for Mitchell Page's family, a MOH awardee for valor at Guadalcanal. You didn't need to ask any questions about what kind of man he was; it was self-evident. He was awarded the MOH for extraordinary heroism and conspicuous gallantry manning a machine-gun as the enemy broke through the lines moving from gun to gun and finally by himself until reinforcements arrived, he led a bayonet charge. You didn't question his ethics, professionalism, or conduct as it was all proven on that day in October 1942. He didn't need to take an ethics course or a course in professionalism. When the chips were down, he performed period. Some things are worth dying for if need be. The question today is, does the current generation hold anything sacred that they would be willing to die for? Didn't Jesus say, "Greater love hath no man than to lay down his life for another?" On that fateful day (and my mother died two years later on the anniversary), I was willing to do it because some things are worth dying for if we call ourselves men.

I don't want the kids at NPU (North Park University) to have to sacrifice their lives for anything but to have in the tank the ultimate commitment to mankind to do so if necessary. It all goes unsaid, of course. I don't talk about this, only to you (speaking in the letter to the Presidential Selection Committee at NPU). Sometimes, I want to go back to that moment in time as I was looking eternity in the face, and I was allowed to move in and around those flames. After I felt as though if you had cancer and touched me, you would be cured, that's how deep it ran. It was a fundamental day, as Dr. Blakely used to say.

Also, during that time of recovery (as it were), I joined (as a civilian physician) the emergency room at the Marine Air Ground Combat Center in Twentynine Palms, California. I felt guilty not going to Vietnam, so this partially made up for it. I was there for three years. I would put in a full day's work at DBI, then all night at Twentynine Palms, and then back for another full day at DBI about twelve times a month. I remember a few stories related to my experience at Twentynine Palms. There was the rattlesnake incident; a soldier brought in without a brain (having walked into the spinning propeller); the soldier brought in without a head from a helicopter accident; and a grenade destroyed a soldier's arm. We will visit those in the "Short Stories" chapter.

During that time, I ran for Congress against Sonny Bono (in the 1994 primary). I received over 6,000 votes (he sprinkled stardust on everyone), but my mother said she voted for me.

I certainly don't want to leave out two very important moments in my life. Those would be the birth of my second son Christian in 1982, and my second daughter Alexandra in 1989. Those are cherished moments that a husband and wife share. I remember Christian's birth. When Joan's water broke (he was the third child), we got into the car, and about halfway to the hospital, I thought I was going to have to pull over and deliver him. Joan kept saying he's coming, and I kept saying don't push (big help). When we got to the hospital, I jumped out and ran inside to the delivery people and said, " My wife's outside, and she is going to have the baby now." The nurses said, "Ok, sir, we'll just get the wheelchair." But when they examined her, they called Dr. Bedner (who was jogging) to jog right into the hospital. He got there just in time, and I accompanied Joan into the delivery room. As I remember, he came out fairly quickly, and all was well. When Alexandra was born, it wasn't as dramatic as Christian's birth. But again, I was in the delivery room, and when she came out, Dr. Demersseman let me grab her, and I remember saying to her, "Don't worry, your Daddy's got you." With that, the nurses took her and stabbed her in the heel to get blood. Oh well, I tried.

There are more stories of my surgical experience at Eisenhower. But now we finally come to my destiny. That is, dedicating my life to women to prevent breast cancer and trying to find a way to treat it without destroying them, which I think I have done. After residency, it takes some time in the real world to figure out just what a doctor is really good at. As I stated before, I abhorred the radical breast surgery I was taught at Loyola. But again, to be fair, back then the surgeon was the only one standing between you and the grave as chemotherapy and radiation were in their infancy. Remember, it was the "Did you get all the cancer doc" generation. But something happened when I first got to Eisenhower, which was a game-changer. That something in 1979 was the seminal article by Umberto Veronesi, MD from the Tumor Institute of Milan, Italy. He had dared to perform less than a radical mastectomy, preferring instead to do a "lumpectomy."

That is, instead of removing a woman's breast and muscles of the chest wall, disfiguring (and in some cases incapacitating her forever with nerve damage), he had a clinical trial of just taking cancer out and doing external beam radiation. Guess what? The results were the same, recurrence and survival.

So, in my book, mastectomy had become tantamount to legalized assault, just feeding a system of what Dr. Azra Raza calls in her book *The First Cell*, the "slash,-poison-burn" approach to cancer treatment in the US. Anything to perpetuate the juggernaut of the seemed necessity of major surgery, of giving toxic drugs and women needing major radiation treatment. And as Dr. Raza also notes, this is all done under "the assumed righteousness of how things are done." How could all this evidence-based medicine be wrong? And G-D help the individual who proposes anything less than what the party line dictates.

Shortly before my untimely end to the heart team occurred, I had reviewed the literature now about nine years out from Umberto's paper. As I hadn't done general surgery for almost nine years, I thought, since his paper of 1979, that women were living happily ever after. Much to my dismay, a lumpectomy was still for most on the back burner, and the mortality rate around 40,000 hadn't budged. Knowing how the other assistants on the heart team were unceremoniously terminated, I decided to open the Desert Breast Institute in 1988.

Let's get a couple of things straight that I would bet my soul on. First, my mantra from day one was to preserve mind, body, and spirit, and I didn't and don't take that pledge lightly. Second, and equally, I promised to be a voice for those that didn't have one. As time went on, there were three courageous ladies I couldn't save, and I promised each of them I would not give up the fight against breast cancer until I had an answer. Further, and let's get this straight; I never, ever acted in an unethical or unprofessional manner, period. You can come into the office and choose any chart and call any patient to verify that statement.

In the thirty-two years since 1988 and seeing over 13,000 women from all over the world (including a First Lady of the United States, a Secret Service agent, a Saudi Princess and an Olympic gold medalist from USSR), I have never, ever received a letter of complaint. I have hundreds of letters profusely thanking me, Lastly, I coined a phrase; "You're not providing cutting-edge treatment; you're making the edge," a big difference. Remember, I said that there are two types of doctors, those that do their job and go home, not letting anything get under their skin (and I applaud that effort). Then there are guys like me that opened the book that says, "Don't open this book unless you want to change the world." One of the main reasons for writing this book is that the reader can decide if I accomplished my goal, at least as far as the powers that be will let me.

I went to the people at *Palm Springs Life Magazine,* and they helped design an ad and logo. The logo would be a swan (powerful but graceful) with an image of itself being reflected.

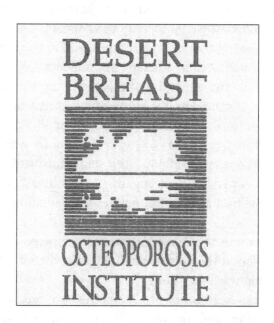

I moved off the EMC campus and got a great office right next to the hospital. It was away from the hubbub and traffic of the hospital and then in a more tranquil setting. I furnished the office (institute) with antiques and an aquarium to soften the thought of having to come in for a mammogram. As stated before, I hired Sylvia Brown to do my mammography, and I purchased a new mammogram machine from Lorad. Those were the days of big processing vats filled with developing fluid (before digital). I was proud that DBI was the first comprehensive breast center in the Coachella Valley and one of the first in the nation. Not being a radiologist, I was theoretically encroaching on their turf. Back then, as long as you had an MD degree, you could buy a mammogram machine.

On the first day of opening DBI, and the second patient to undergo mammography, I found cancer. The idea behind a comprehensive center (to my thinking) is that before the surgeon acts (who would usually get the patient from the general practitioner), every member of the team would get a chance to interview and examine the patient and let the patient get those different perspectives. Then, a consensus would arise before the surgeon dropped the knife or maybe didn't drop the knife in lieu of neoadjuvant chemotherapy or radiation. This is important, and here is an example as to why. In the age of neoadjuvant (primary chemotherapy), that is chemotherapy given before surgery to possibly shrink the tumor and downsize the patient's tumor, hopefully the patient becomes a candidate for lumpectomy versus mastectomy. It's vitally important for the oncologist and radiation therapist to examine the patient (before any surgery), so everyone knows what they are up against. In days gone by (even now), this step is too often omitted.

In the days when mastectomy ruled, the breast was sacrificed right off the bat by the surgeon, neither the radiation therapist nor the oncologist saw the tumor in the intact breast. They never got the chance. This reminds me, in my forty years of surgery, I never had one oncologist, radiation therapist, or radiologist come into the operating room to see what was being done.

While the sine qua non of my comprehensive breast center (DBI) was the inclusion and interdisciplinary consultations with other members of the team before the surgeon acted, there are a few other sine qua non's.

One being that DBI was to be thought of, not just as a doctor's office to go to yearly for mammography, but a true sanctuary where women knew our mantra to preserve, mind, body, and spirit. Further, that if a woman called with a lump and was the least bit anxious about it, she was seen that day no matter the day or time (weekends if needed). At DBI the patient would have an opportunity to discuss with each team member their opinion and obtain any second opinions before any treatment was undertaken. I knew I was on the right track when I got a call from Shelter From the Storm asking if I could help shelter an abused woman, as they were full. Of course, I did. They didn't call the hospital or any other place, they called me. I was pleased that my community recognized DBI as a place of caring and compassion. DBI and members of the team were members of the largest breast cancer research group in the world, the NSABP, and I was the Principal Investigator at Eisenhower. In fact, it marked the first time breast cancer clinical trials were brought to the Valley. Taking on such responsibility would put our research team under some scrutiny (not something you would do if you had something to hide or you were in fact, unethical).

Further, laying the foundation of trust (as all these women, over 13,000 of them, come to bet their lives on my ability to save them) matters. This is worth repeating. Remember that company out my way (Granite) in SoCal that has a bumper sticker on each of their vehicles, and it says, "CHARACTER MATTERS." You bet it does. Further, the patient is seen each visit by the same doctor year after year and decade after decade. Hence, a true knowing, caring relationship develops, and the doctor has at his fingertips everything the patients have had done and the outcome. That is, the breast center is staffed by people who want to make a career out of it. Patients are not seeing a different disinterested doctor just putting in their time.

Each doctor on staff is trained to be multi-disciplinary, and they must have knowledge across usually sacred turf. This enables a DBI doctor to act that same day. For instance, if the patient has a cyst that hurts, the doctor can immediately perform a needle aspiration, instead of the usual sending a requisition for a surgical consult that may take a week or more, then another week or more before the patient gets in. Then the surgeon may not have the skill to perform an ultrasound-guided biopsy which means more waiting and another requisition to a doctor who can. No, being able to act that same day is of tremendous importance in relieving anxiety and pain. When the patient leaves, she is fully informed about what is going on and understands what has been done to solve the issue instead of waiting weeks (with all the agony and anxiety it portends). There is literature available for the patient if she wants more information and videos of procedures. Really important is there is a host of patients who are more than willing to speak to a new patient about their experience at DBI. If new patients desire, they have access to them directly for questions they might have.

You'd be surprised how graciously women, who have gone through any procedure, are more than willing to talk to another woman who is set to undergo a procedure, comforting them and allaying their fears. This kind of caring thought process won't happen at a hospital. I think a favorite saying of mine bears repeating as it's the reason why women have come from all over the world; *we don't just provide cutting-edge treatment; we make the edge.* There is a big difference between providing what a doctor thinks is cutting edge and always (that is every day) pushing the envelope until we find what we are after, an answer to the devastation of breast cancer. That is, a minimally invasive therapy where surgery, chemotherapy, and radiation can be avoided. All the while, we are preserving a woman's body the way G-D made it, a tall order.

I can't tell you how many times my patients have come in and commented, "You're always doing something extraordinary for us." My mission is kind of like that of Star Trek, "To boldly go where no man has gone before." There are consequences to such an approach I would find out years later at the height of my career, hopefully defeating breast cancer. I just read in the latest *Photonics Focus Journal* in November 2020 that Siemens Healthineers are to acquire Varian Medical Systems for $16.4 billion dollars. Varian makes the linear accelerator to provide state-of-the-art radiation for cancer patients. How interested are giants like Siemens and Varian in developing/exploring a diagnostic and treatment regimen that can be done for pennies on the dollar, patients aren't hospitalized (can actually stay well away from the hospital setting), and they resume normal activity immediately with (for breast cancer), no surgery, chemotherapy, or radiation? And the hospitals that buy their equipment for millions of dollars, how interested are they to explore other options?

And likewise, how interested is the federal government to change how we have done things for decades which learned men profess is the only answer. Or, more likely, they profess that the answer to cancer is right around the corner. They just need continued government funding of all this research. There have been over four million papers published on cancer and just who reads all of these to determine what should be instituted?

As I said on the first day DBI opened, on the second patient's mammogram, I picked up a cancer. We were seeing about twenty-five patients a day. How is it that my small entity next to a 30-million-dollar hospital saw all those patients who formally had gone to the hospital? To start, I cut out the middle man (general practitioner) who typically orders the mammogram. Generally, family practice docs never go to actually see their patient's mammogram. They rely on the radiologist's interpretation. Therefore, the family doc never becomes fluent enough to engage a radiologist about certain mammography findings to change management. I have a list of breast cancer cases missed by, of course, Board-certified radiologists certified to read mammography. I call it the master f——-up file. One case was seven years that cancer was visible on mammography, and it just grew. That ended up in a lawsuit.

In another case, the radiologist said that in order to tell if a focus on mammography was breast cancer, he would order films every six months for one-and-a-half years. That's why at DBI, eventually, I had a radiologist right there with me, and we discussed findings right then and there (the radiologist and surgeon) with the patient still there to be examined. That way I learned all the radiologist knew, and he learned my thoughts on the subject to perhaps alter his thinking on how to approach certain findings.

The radiologist saw long-term results of decisions I had made. Second, today's women are not stupid; they know if the technician takes more than four views, she sees something so the patient asks the tech *Did you see anything*? The tech, not being a radiologist, typically says you have to ask your doctor; otherwise, she is playing doctor. Then the prolonged wait ensues, typically more than a week, sometimes two, then you might get to talk to a secretary because the doctor is "busy" seeing patients.

At DBI patients talked to the doctor that day and know what is going on before they leave, usually with peace of mind and able to omit the anxious days of prolonged waiting for results. Typically, at the hospital, the big wheel usually doesn't stop to cater to one woman's questions. At DBI, the wheel doesn't turn unless all the questions are answered right then and there by the actual breast doctor versed in diagnosis and treatment. Does this approach (part of The Lavender Way) sound better than the treatment patients usually get? If you say yes, you're getting the drift.

But the culmination of the Lavender Way/Lavender Procedure took about thirty-five years for technology to catch up to breast cancer. If one doesn't bother to look at these technologies, they never see the light of day or their potential.

I got deeper into breast cancer research and refining my lumpectomy skills (into a cosmetic lumpectomy versus a regular lumpectomy), see below. You will see the progression of my thoughts on how less invasive procedures produced the same results, arguably then better than mastectomy. In about thirty-two years, I would change the name from DBI to Visionary Breast Center. The State of California issued me the certificate to change the name. Below is what I call a cosmetic lumpectomy. That is, instead of making an incision directly over the tumor, 99% of the time I make a circumareolar incision. I cut down about 1 centimeter or so, then tunnel over to the tumor. The tunneling provides a supportive wall so no indentation takes place. This was self-taught and I was after this patient to get the incision tattooed as then you literally couldn't tell I was there. She said she didn't want to as it reminded her of me. How many men have that for a compliment?

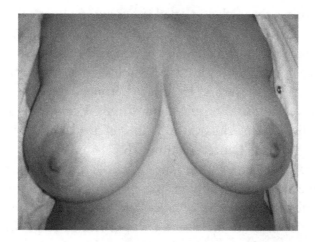

Alternatively, here is an example of a surgeon who didn't give a damn. The patient told me she asked him to do a circumareaolar incision (around the nipple), but he said he didn't have time. This guy shouldn't be doing any breast surgery in my opinion. Please realize that I also only see a small fraction of patients out there.

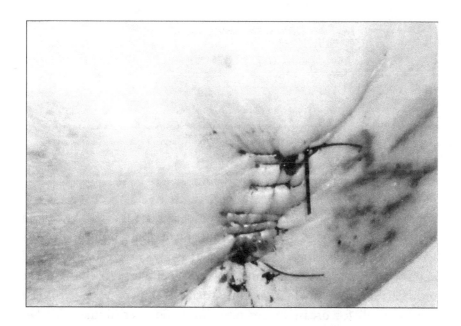

While this is chronicled in detail in *Sacrificing America's Women II*, I will relay enough now to get the picture of my personal commitment to the women of the United States of America and the world. If I was going to call myself an institute and not just be on the cutting edge of breast cancer diagnosis and treatment but make the edge, I figured I needed to get DBI into formal clinical trials. I contacted the NSABP and was able to join. This was in late 1989 or in 1990. It marked the first time National Cancer Institute (NCI)-supported breast cancer clinical trials were brought into the Coachella Valley. I was the first to do a lumpectomy at Eisenhower, the first to develop a comprehensive breast center in the Coachella Valley, and now the first to bring breast cancer clinical trials to the desert. I was named Principal Investigator (after some interviews and vetting) at Eisenhower and was probably the first surgeon in the Coachella Valley to obtain an NCI Principal Investigator number 17790, which is still active in 2021. Years hence, the medical board's expert would disavow that my number was active, see below for proof and where does the prejudging stop? Note the date! Somebody was wrong.

Subject **NCI RCR Registration Approved for Dr. Phillip D. Bretz (IVR-17790) Request R000148410**
From   <RCRNS@nih.gov>
To   <drbretz@visionarybreastcenter.com>
Bcc   <RCRNS@nih.gov>
Date   2021-02-05 16:35

Dear Dr. Phillip D. Bretz (IVR-17790),

The Cancer Therapy Evaluation Program, NCI has approved your registration packet for request **R000148410**.

You are currently registered as an **INVESTIGATOR** with an **ACTIVE** registration status. Your registration expiration date is **21-Feb-2022.**

Comments:

After joining the NSABP, we were invited to Vancouver, British Columbia for their annual meeting at which about a thousand research doctors attend. I was so nervous I forgot any identification (no driver's license, etc). When we got to our Canadian destination, they just waved us through (it was a different time, folks). When we perused the active and available protocols, I was stunned to discover there was no protocol (clinical trial) for breast cancer prevention. So over dinner with Dr.

Dreisbach, my team oncologist, (it just popped into my head), that the US should be doing a breast cancer prevention trial with the drug Tamoxifen. He said, you're probably right, but who is going to listen to you? When we got home without telling anyone, I buried myself in the library, and Barbara Potts (EMC's head librarian) got me every article ever written on Tamoxifen. I wrote my protocol in twenty-four hours and sent it into the FDA and the rest as you'll read is history.

One of the first trials we helped pioneer was N.S.A.B.P. B-18. This was a clinical trial to test the difference between neoadjuvant chemotherapy (meaning chemotherapy before surgery based on core needle biopsy) to postoperative chemotherapy. Until this trial was done, doctors had never seen the impact of chemotherapy on the tumor left in situ (in place, not excised). This trial, probably more than any other except maybe the OncoVue genetics risk, helped open my eyes to what we could do to manipulate breast cancer and help the patients.

To wit, we found out (and others confirmed B-18's findings) that 80% of the time, there will be a 50% reduction in tumor size, and about 30% of the time, there will be a complete response. As we enrolled more patients into B-18, something very interesting came to light (before any analysis of the entire trial). This observation that I had would start me on my path to not just step outside the box but never go inside again. It was probably the start of me being called the "Lone Ranger." What was this epiphany?

I was sending patients to Dr. Dreisbach, and he began the protocol for chemotherapy, which lasted four months. All during that time, I didn't see the patient until they returned for surgery. To my astonishment, in some of these patients, I couldn't find the tumor on physical exam, nor repeat mammography or ultrasound or repeat core biopsy. I didn't know it at the time, but those patients were part of the 30% group with a complete response. Toward the end of the trial, I sat down with Dr. Dreisbach. I said if we encountered any of these complete response patients off the trial, wouldn't it be possible just to do radiation and no surgery? Otherwise, it would amount to a fishing expedition or excavation to try and find cancer that probably wasn't there, or at least small enough now that radiation would kill it off. I would just destroy the breast, something I vowed not to do. We talked to our radiation therapist (Dr. Mantik), and it was decided we would offer that option to patients who had a complete response.

It wasn't a helter-skelter decision on my part and the result, not of any clinical trial to date, but the experience of a group of researchers who cared for breast cancer on a daily basis for decades. We would try and identify any residual tumor via mammography, ultrasound, and biopsy. If we couldn't, the patient would be good to go with just radiation and, if appropriate, an anti-estrogen, if that's what the patient decided on after reviewing all options with all of her doctors.

As luck would have it, a patient with large breasts (who is still alive in 2021) had a complete response of a tumor over 2 centimeters. Before offering her the option to avoid surgery and just do radiation, I did all I could to find that tumor but was unsuccessful. Knowing the options and knowing she would probably be one of the first women in the world to opt for such a treatment, we went ahead only doing radiation. That was no breast surgery and no axillary lymph nodes dissection.

As I said, she is still alive in 2021 and her treatment was back in 1997. Certainly her treatment was well outside the standard of care (no evidence-based medicine), yet we did it, and she is still alive. That's because decades of specific experience count. Three experienced cancer doctors believed this was feasible, and the patient had the right to decide her treatment regardless of "standard of care" when she had a chance to consider all options.

Back then, in the early 1990s, this option of avoiding surgery after neoadjuvant chemotherapy was exercised by 7% of our patients. All lived out their lives except one, who had a local recurrence eighteen years after and then underwent The Lavender Procedure (I will explain later), again after full disclosure of options like mastectomy. I ended up calling this treatment (of just radiation, no surgery after neoadjuvant chemotherapy resulting in a complete response), the Compass Treatment.

It was 180 degrees from how I was taught was the only way to treat breast cancer, yet they did really well. How was that? The Medical Board said nothing to me about this and the Compass Treatment was way outside the box. I waited until 1997 to try and publish this. It was successfully published as an abstract in the *American Society of Clinical Oncology* (the country's largest oncology peer-reviewed medical journal).

If you read the abstract, you'll see we successfully treated invasive breast cancer with no surgery (in the late 1990s), just chemo, and radiation. I think that marked the first time something like that was published in such a journal. In the past, aggressive surgery was the sine qua non, part of the holy trinity, surgery, chemotherapy, and radiation. Don't you think someone, anybody, would have read that and said, "What the hell is going on here? How can this be? You have to do surgery because that's the way it has always been done." This marked the second time (the Tamoxifen trial was the first) I looked outside the box. Eventually, I would end up so far outside the box I couldn't see the box anymore, and I would be by myself, the Lone Ranger.

This compass idea marked the second time I knew (under the right conditions) that you could manipulate breast cancer to a better outcome using less invasive means. I wondered just what other things I could bring to the fight to defeat this plague? I loved my work and found the research very exciting. By this time, I probably had (if memory serves) about seven physicians who had me operate on them or a member of their family. One doctor told me another respected surgeon on staff said I was the best breast surgeon in the country. I never said that or professed anything like it, but learned people recognize somebody pushing the envelope that no one is pushing, and were grateful.

I can tell you, when any doctor has the honor of being asked to operate on another doctor or their family, they do not ask you out of chance. They have seen the playing field and who gets the best results. They know you are skilled, ethical and professional. There is no other way to say it. Those kinds of accolades make one feel like all the work has paid off, and as Joan says, "I was serving my purpose."

After the "Bird Lady" in about 1981, Dr. Kopp and I were called into the administrator's office. We wondered what grievous act we had committed? It turns out the EMC Board had decided EMC should try to be the trauma center of the desert, which had yet to be decided which hospital would be chosen.

They would use the experience of the "Bird Lady" to justify EMC as the designated trauma center in Coachella Valley. Dr. Kopp and I were the chosen ones to be EMC's trauma surgeons. That felt good as there were other surgeons on staff. Desert Hospital (now Desert Regional) hired a fellowship-trained trauma surgeon and they got it. Every so often though, we would get a Marine helicoptered in from Twentynine Palms. It was an honor to care for those men.

After I was no longer doing hearts, my income dropped precipitously. That's when I lost everything. To supplement my income, I worked in the ER (as a civilian physician) at the Twentynine Palms Marine Air Ground Combat Center. I did this for three years. Working a full day at DBI, then an hour twenty-minute drive to Twentynine Palms and start a twelve-hour shift from 7 p.m. to 7 a.m. and drive home with just enough time to shower and eat. I would work between twelve to fifteen shifts a month. Like I said, there are a couple of stories of my experiences at Twentynine Palms that are interesting, which I go into in Chapter 14, "Short Stories of a Surgeon."

With the publishing of my abstract, "The Compass Treatment," I received an invitation to speak in Vienna, Austria at the UICC's First International Meeting on Advances in the Knowledge of Cancer Management. This would be the first of many invited speaking engagements outside the US. Over time I found it interesting that countries outside the US were very interested in hearing about my research while in my own country, nothing. When you read "The Compass Treatment," you must realize how revolutionary it was (especially back then) to propose any kind of treatment of breast cancer that didn't involve surgery. A knife never touched those patients. The abstract was published in the American Society of Clinical Oncology, the country's largest oncology group. Am I the only one who thinks it strange that no one ever tried to contact me about this and just say Phil, how did you do that?

Vienna was really cool. It was a city that you could just walk around and be serenaded by violin players playing Mozart. We got to visit

Mozart's home as well as Beethoven's and St. Stephen's Cathedral. I got my fill of weinersnitchel. If you ever get to Vienna (Wein), make sure you stop by the Hotel Sacher for their renowned torte. The entire experience was very uplifting and pushed me to further pursue my out-of- the-box thinking. I very much liked engaging foreign countries and people we regarded as enemies like the erstwhile USSR. I found out that they liked to fish and enjoy life the same as us: the real people, not the government, who spent more time counting their missiles than taking care of their people. I've always been treated with great respect in any country I visited to speak.

In the USSR a funny thing happened when we got together for lunch. During lunch I thought I heard someone speaking Spanish. It turned out one of the Soviet team was in Cuba during the Cuban Missile Crisis. Since I went to medical school in Mexico, I engaged this guy, and there we were communicating in Spanish in Moscow. Their genuine desire to learn (in a non-arrogant way) what I had to say was always evident and very different from any experience I had in the States.

There wasn't some self-appointed hierarchy (as Dr. Raza would say) that disregarded you out of hand because you weren't an academic surgeon and on top of it not Board-certified. .

After Vienna, I continued to try and publish something of note at least every other year. My various publications and presentations in peer-reviewed journals are detailed later. And by "something of note," I mean something no one else has done to reduce further the abominable procedures performed on women in the name of science and good medicine. An example of something no one else had done is my invention of the "Autologous Free Fat Patch to Surmount the Problem of Skin Spacing in Accelerated Partial Breast Radiation (APBR)."

This was published in the journal of the American Society for Radiation Oncology (ASTRO), the largest radiation therapy group in the country.

Supplement to

INTERNATIONAL JOURNAL OF

Radiation Oncology

BIOLOGY·PHYSICS

VOLUME 75, NUMBER 3, SUPPLEMENT   2009

PROCEEDINGS
OF THE
AMERICAN SOCIETY
FOR
RADIATION ONCOLOGY
31ST ANNUAL MEETING

ASTRO

TARGETING CANCER CARE

McCormick Place West
November 1–5, 2009
Chicago, Illinois

Official Journal of

ASTRO AMERICAN SOCIETY FOR RADIATION ONCOLOGY

PAEDIATRIC RADIATION ONCOLOGY SOCIETY

Affiliated with
LATIN AMERICAN ASSOCIATION OF THERAPEUTIC RADIATION AND ONCOLOGY

0360-3016(20091101)75:3S;1-2

ELSEVIER
ISSN 0360-3016

Visit www.redjournal.org for the IJROBP's online submission and peer review system

2091 An Autologous Abdominal Free-fat Patch Surmounts the Problem of Skin Spacing during Accelerated Partial Breast Radiation (APBR)

P. Bretz[1], D. Mantik[2], T. Mesek[2], S. Ling[2], P. Dreisbach[3]

[1]Desert Breast and Osteoporosis Institute, La Quinta, CA, [2]21st Century Oncology, Palm Desert, CA, [3]Eisenhower Medical Center, Rancho Mirage, CA

Purpose/Objective(s): A problem in dosimetry planning using a partial breast radiation device is lack of skin spacing. As a consequence of this lack of skin spacing many after-loading catheters must be extracted without treatment. Each member of the comprehensive team must be aware of the surgical and radiation techniques that optimize individualized treatment. In order to solve this problem of skin overdosing, we have developed two techniques.
Material/Methods: APBR is used to treat the area most likely to develop a local recurrence, i.e., that centimeter around the original lumpectomy margin. If successful, high dose rate brachytherapy using Iridium-192 is administered in two sessions per day over five days for a total dose of 34 Gy. Instead of elliptically excising the tumor, often leaving little skin spacing and frequent skin indentation, the surgeon enters the breast through the areola. The initial incision is carried down for at least a centimeter and then cautery is used to divide the tissue until the tumor is reached. The tumor is excised (with clear margins) preferably in the shape

of the balloon. This technique allows for a supportive wall of tissue. For cases that still have skin spacing problems an autologous abdominal free-fat patch transfer has been devised. The patch is removed through an appendectomy-like incision just medial to the left anterior superior iliac crest. The size varies and the thickness of the patch removed generally is at least 1 cm thick. The patch is trimmed and two stay sutures are used to tack the patch to the roof of the defect.
Results: Since having to abandon our very first attempt at balloon placement we have successfully implanted and radiated 35 patients using the above two techniques including the fat patch in 15 cases. Patients have been followed for 10 months up to seven years without any local recurrences. Three patients developed spider-like vein prominence and some firmness over the lumpectomy site but no long term severe effects have been encountered. In some cases the fat patch is visible on ultrasound and mammography. In our last patient we used a new type of multi-lumen catheter/balloon but could still not safely protect the skin. We, therefore, placed a patch the same day and used it that same day, a dramatic result visible on CT.
Conclusions: APBR remains an evolving art, especially with new devices steadily emerging. The art includes shaping the lumpectomy cavity to conform to the balloon options, as well as advances in radiation planning. All must dovetail harmoniously to achieve a superior outcome. Wherever this may lead, though, we conclude that the two techniques cited here can be employed immediately to reduce skin doses. If employed, these techniques will promptly permit more frequent use of after loading catheters.
Author Disclosure: P. Bretz, None; D. Mantik, None; T. Mesek, None; S. Ling, None; P. Dreisbach, None.

You can go right down the list from founding the first comprehensive breast center in the Coachella Valley, the Desert Breast Institute, to bringing into the Valley National Cancer Institute-funded clinical breast trials, to the Tamoxifen clinical trial, to the cosmetic lumpectomy, to pioneering accelerated partial breast radiation, to the fat patch, to the Compass Treatment, to pioneering a vaccine clinical trial, to engaging the erstwhile Soviet Union, China, Mexico, Honduras, Brazil, Canada, Africa, and Vietnam to bring freedom from the curse of breast cancer to those women and make the world safer, all this now via the Lavender Way and Procedure.

Again, I point all this out, not to be self-aggrandizing, but to drive home the point that I didn't have to do any of this. I could have just done my work for the day and gone home as so many others do for decades. But I felt I had a calling, and I made that promise to those three ladies that I wouldn't quit until I had an answer. Notice I didn't say "CURE" or "THE," but "AN" answer. They can throw all the insults and sling arrows but they can't do away with or cover up my cancer-free patients.

All this (I think) adds up to someone who had done the due diligence and what could be done without red tape to free women from this curse, versus some unscrupulous unethical, unprofessional, negligent doctor. That's not me, it's the seven-and-a-half year out cancer-free patients from the Lavender Procedure that are the point.

I might add here that if and when you read a medical journal article, they usually have a list of authors. You'll find the last name at the end of that list is usually the department chair or the like.

That way, even though the department chair didn't contribute a lick to the article, they get to have their name on it and can list it in their publications. All mine (except the last one on the Lavender Way/Procedure) are in abstract form because there are only so many hours in the day to devote to an article without help.

Now each one of those items listed, like the Compass Treatment, has a story all its own on how I came up with the idea, which in turn has led me to refine my non-invasive approach further, a journey that has taken decades of commitment to reach the goal.

With publications and presentations, that led to an invitation to speak in China. It was December 2017 in Beijing. So now I've been to the two biggest Communist countries in the world. China was a real experience. Not only did they pay me a stipend, but they flew me first-class on Air China. In LAX when I checked in, they directed me to the first-class lounge. I couldn't believe my eyes. They had a huge bar with whatever liquor and about ten items on the buffet. I called Joan and described the place, and she said, did you intend to leave your credit cards at home? *What?* It reminded me of when I went to Vancouver for the NSABP meeting and forgot my identification. What no credit cards? I had about $500 in cash, but it was too late to go back home. If anything went wrong, I couldn't get back.

I just had to go with the flow and hope for the best. However, it wouldn't have made any difference. They never let me pay for anything while there. First-class (only two people there) was very enjoyable, to say the least. The stewardesses hovered over me with hot towels what seemed like every ten minutes. You had your choice of Western or Eastern meals. I chose Eastern on the way over. As a pilot, I was a little familiar with how a big plane like that should behave, and the pilots were pretty damn good, a very gentle ride on Air China.

I was expecting us to be flying over the ocean the entire plane ride, but that wasn't the case. It's actually pretty easy to hit Beijing from the US. We just followed the US coast until we hit Alaska, then made a left and followed the Aleutian Islands, which stretch out like an arrow pointing to China. So, it seemed there was always a little land under us.

Upon landing in Beijing, I didn't want to get off the plane. Immigration was a little edgy, just like Moscow, but no problem. The Beijing airport is very well appointed. I was driven to the City Wall Marriott. It turned out the sponsor of the event (whose first name was Tiger) billed it as a "high-end" medical conference. He occupied the top two floors (like our Howard Hughes at the Desert Inn in Las Vegas).

The next morning, I made it to the elevator and a couple entered with me. I know a little Chinese and said good morning, and they said they were from Ohio. When I walked into the restaurant, I couldn't believe my eyes. There in grand display were Santa Claus and Mickey Mouse. Although I didn't say it, I thought, hey, wait, you guys can't do this, you're commies. The buffet was first class.

Tiger's people got to me and escorted me to a room. The entrance to the room was guarded by two women dressed in traditional attire. On the doors on either side hung two large flower arrangements that were three feet long. The door was opened for me like I was royalty.

I hadn't spoken one word of my lecture. How did they know I wasn't going to bomb (as in being disappointing)? I guess my meager reputation preceded me. In the room there were again large flower arrangements in all corners and a bigger one in the middle of the table.

Then they proceeded to pin a corsage on me. That took all of about five minutes, and then it was off, apparently to the lecture hall or a gulag, I didn't know which. I couldn't believe the next thing that happened. While I stood with Tiger at the entrance, they began to play blaring music reminiscent of "Rocky." It wasn't only that; there were a couple hundred lights on the ceiling going back and forth. I did feel like a prizefighter entering the ring. Back home, no one would receive an entrance and ovation like that. I didn't know how to react. Next, I was escorted by a beautiful Chinese movie star to the stage. I had given my computer to a stagehand and never had the opportunity to see how the PowerPoint would look. It turned out the slides were about ten feet tall, so all 2,000 people in the audience could see. I guess they really liked my presentation. They didn't allow for any questions, though. After, in the lobby, I was asked to pose for pictures and sign autographs of about fifty people who had lined up to get a picture with me. This kind of treatment can really go to your head.

Throughout my trip, I had access to two (I assume Tiger's) brand new Mercedes 600s complete with driver and interpreter. They took me to the Great Wall and shopping. When we entered one large store, each floor was devoted to one thing like shoes or jewelry. I couldn't believe they had huge angels hanging from the ceiling, complete with trumpets and "Silent Night Holy Night" blaring in English. What the hell was going on here? All the women were dressed to the nines with Gucci bags or the like, knock-offs or not. Out on the streets were hundreds of Mercedes, and I never saw a junk car. I figured the genie was out of the bottle and never going back, the capitalist genie, that is. They liked their individualism too much.

They took me to Tiananmen Square. I never saw so many surveillance cameras. About twenty military men came marching by. It was like a non-event. I don't think the average Chinese is that into the military scene. The Forbidden City seemed to go on forever. I saw a kid with "Dream Big" on the back of his jacket. That's not the communism I know. There was a separate place where all the concubines stayed, apparently hundreds of them. It was probably good to be the emperor. We all went to a restaurant where Peking duck was the specialty. Dinner at Tiger's was something else. Besides being surrounded by Ming Dynasty furniture, the table we all sat at was round, and I think I counted fifteen place settings. There were about three people with towels on their forearms who observed you drinking wine. When you took a sip, they were immediately there to fill your glass. Then there were the toasts, almost like in Moscow, one after another. The toasting was another glass of some special liqueur. It seemed the food just kept coming, from crabs that came from his private lake to ribs, etc. Tiger showed us around his office. He apparently had a couple of satellites that monitored all maritime movement around China. He had a screen that took up the entire wall, and he could change screens with just his hand movements. It was all quite impressive.

To show you that the Chinese have a sense of humor, here's what happened at the end. I was dressed in my jeans to fly home and got a call that Tiger wanted me to come down and say goodbye to the audience, still over 2,000. So back in my suit I go with my Commie pin on and retake the stage with the music and lights.

During the course of the finale, Tiger's partner came over to shake my hand. As he did, he said and translated to me that I had a really strong hand grip. I have been told that many times. I took the microphone from him and said, "It's because I'm feeling breasts all day."

Nothing happened with the audience. Then when the translator told the audience in Chinese, there was great laughter. They got it, and I waved. After, I felt like a celebrity with many people again lining up to get a picture with me. I never had any reaction anywhere else like that.

During one of our dinners, Tiger said he wanted to do 1,000 Lavender Breast Centers, and I was feeling pretty good about that. Ultimately that never happened, which was very disappointingly enigmatic. The other thing I really wanted to taste was authentic chow mein, and that never happened; it's mostly American food over there. That's probably why their cancer rates are climbing.

Some may remember President Nixon's visit to China to "open it up." China's President at the time, Chou En-Lai, had ordered the first every tally of cancer in China. It turned out then there were provinces in China that had basically no cancer or heart disease. But as one moved toward Beijing, the graph lit up. Now decades later it's another story about cancer and its rise in China. Is it Western diet creeping in? A book called *The China Study* by Dr. Campbell tells the entire story.

At the airport I went through their version of TSA, which was no big deal. Then I waited in the first-class lounge at which there was no shortage of good eats. Upon hearing my plane called, I proceeded to the gate. There was only one plane. There were people lined up to check in, and I went a little further where it said "first class." There was no one there, and I was ushered in. As I walked down the jetway, I could see a table on the side with uniformed men behind it. As I approached, I could see the stewardess standing by the plane, and they stopped me and said, "open." What the hell, I just opened my case for the TSA people, and now again? No problem, I think they just wanted to see what the gringo had in his suitcase. So now I'm about twenty feet from the stewardess, and there is one more guy (not friendly-looking) checking everyone out before they got onto the plane. I didn't look at him twice.

When I passed him, the stewardess came out a few steps and grabbed me and brought me inside. Once inside, she directed me to my unit and provided me with silk pajamas and slippers and, of course, a drink and a hot towel. As the plane taxied out, I felt like I had done really well but was glad to be heading home. The thought crossed my mind of that scene in *Midnight Express* where actor Billy Hayes is heading out and just before the plane takes off, it is called back to the gate and he gets arrested. I crossed my fingers.

As the new Boeing 777 lifted off, I had music playing in my ear and watched the lights of Beijing fade in the distance. The ride home was very gentle, and the stewardess made sure I lacked for nothing. When dinner came, she made sure the utensils were placed just so. I watched our progress on my private screen, and I hoped we wouldn't get shot down flying over just north of Incheon, South Korea. Once we came into US territory, the words United States of America came on the screen, which made me feel good.

On landing at LAX, I wondered if any of the crew ever just walked out and asked for asylum because there were no Chinese guards, just the stars and stripes looking at you as you deplane. I have to say (and as you will read in *Sacrificing America's Women II*), I was treated so very well by both the real people of the Soviet Union and the real people in China. As far as I could tell, the real people of both countries really liked gringos. As I said, Tiger wanted to do the 1,000 Lavender Breast

Centers but to this day, I don't know what happened. I never heard from China after my visit.

Back home when all the patients I would see were the result of word of mouth and with doing fewer surgeries, I looked for other opportunities. One such opportunity was afforded me in Hemet or more specifically San Jacinto, California. Dr. Vidhya Koka and her husband interviewed me and hired me on. I had to learn what EMR (electronic medical records) meant and how laborious it would turn out to be, taking time away from actually knowing the patient. The issue with EMR is, if you don't click the right buttons (of which there are hundreds of options) and it's not recorded for the HMO quality assurance committee, then you didn't do it, even though you did.

I could have folded my breast practice but I didn't, remembering the promise I made to those three girls years before. I owe the Kokas a generous measure of gratitude for taking me on when I wasn't a family physician, but my ability as a surgeon would come to prominence suturing the many lacerations that came into urgent care. I spent ten years there driving back and forth from La Quinta each day (except the one day I was at my breast center). It was about 112 miles back and forth on I-10. Generally, I would see at least one bad accident a week as I navigated the freeway. One day while driving, I spotted a car parked on the freeway in the right-hand lane with no one inside. As I called 911, I was looking through the rearview mirror and sure enough, a car just plowed right into it. Situational awareness, people.

I can recount a couple of patients I had come to know well. Incidentally, my record of seeing patients in SJ was eighty-two in one day, and you want to know why medical care is suffering and patients are suffering as a result of mismanagement by HMOs? Guess. There was one little guy about six years old who was a trisomy (mongoloid). Even with a room full of people, when he saw me down the hall he would yell, "There's my doctor," and run into my arms. Whatever I was doing instantly came to a halt to catch him when he jumped. For many patients, I doled out medication samples given to us by the drug reps. For many, they didn't know where their next meal was coming from let alone buy medication. I always made sure I did what I could to help out. One thing that disturbed me was many of the patients didn't know there was a World War II or how that came to be. I don't know how the country will survive without everyone knowing its courageous history. Our country doesn't run automatically, it takes all of us contributing to the extent each can. We all have to care about the country and do our part to uphold its virtues.

One has to understand that all the activity and growth of economy doesn't just happen. If one just keeps picking fruit from the tree and doesn't tend to the tree, soon there will be no more fruit. But that's another story. At Thanksgiving at the annual dinner at SJ, everyone would gather around to watch me (the surgeon) carve the turkey (no pressure). There are a few people I worked with that made my job much easier and I owe them a great thank you. In no particular order, Dr. Koka, Mr. Koka, Andrew Pulumati, Nina Kumar, Miguel, Desi, Elma, Carla, Gil, Lucy, Leslie and Jeff. Everyone answered the call for our patients many times under difficult circumstances. If Perez is reading this, "How many were there?" Just an inside joke. Adela Amaya at Radnet made sure my MRIs were scheduled promptly.

As soon as the Medical Board edict came down, each HMO in turn told Dr. Koka I could no longer see their patients so I had to withdraw from their practice and that was my principal source of income. Again, just like the American Board of Surgery washes their hands saying it's not us that prevents a surgeon from not being let on staff of a hospital, it's the hospital. The Medical Board, but silently, says we didn't take away his principal source of income, he still has his license. They, in effect, absolve themselves. So, too, do the HMOs.

Once you've been branded, everyone assumes they found something very bad and instead of the HMO calling you in to get your version (two sides to every story), you are summarily dismissed. They say, look, it's not us. If the Medical Board found enough wrongdoing, then it must be true, right?

It's not just losing your main source of employment; it's losing every opportunity to do any business outside of medicine. In my case, that involves losing opportunities to develop Lavender Breast Centers and developing Honey Breast Implants among many other ideas I have.

I lost count of the number of letters to CEOs of organizations that I know could joint venture in these projects as some proport to want, "a world without cancer." I believe what happens (although I take great pains in assailing myself discussing the Medical Board issue in those letters), is the people then Google me and there it is, a confirmation of how negligent I was. Who the hell would want to do business with that guy? While I understand that, the Medical Board's edicts cut deep, it's not just a slap on the wrist as the *LA Times* intimated in an article published July 14, 2021. Probably the only job I can get now is at a gas station convenience store instead of what I was cut out for, saving lives and preserving bodies.

But I must say that just yesterday, I saw two patients who typify the problem in this country and really pisses me off. I am disquieted that women like these are being wasted because of some arrogant people who think they know all the answers. And I'll be the first to say I sure as hell don't know all the answers but I think I can offer one after seven-and-a-half years of following up on the Lavender Procedure and cancer-free patients. If the powers that be knew the answers, I wouldn't be seeing women like these two coming into the office in desperation. These are probably the same arrogant people who thought they knew all the answers back when I initiated the Tamoxifen prevention trial (see *Sacrificing America's Women II,* coming soon) and caught them with their pants down. Let me clarify, I never initiated anything to catch anybody with their pants down, anything I came up with was to help women period. Eventually, when I got going with the prevention trial, I wanted the NSABP to run the American side and I would run the Soviet side. I never wanted to exclude anyone. This entire saga is detailed in *Sacrificing America's Women II.* Let's just say with my foray into developing a clinical trial, there was blowback from the get go. But years later when the Tamoxifen trial was completed, I was right all along as Tamoxifen lowers the risk of breast cancer by about 50% in high-risk women.

It isn't just the NSABP; it's all of them that have swallowed the slash-poison-burn Kool-Aid that refuse to look outside their money-making juggernaut. Don't misunderstand me here. I'm not saying of all these cancer doctors their primary focus is to make money. It's just how it works out that there is a lot of money to be made. Why rock the boat? How do you get the system to look at alternative less expensive treatments? Again, it was not my intention to catch anyone with their pants down. But it just shows what one person (again White, Black, Hispanic, Yellow or Red) with an idea, unhampered by a suffocating bureaucracy staffed with functionaries, can do and very quickly.

My sole purpose was to help the women of my country and the world by putting an end to the misery breast cancer causes. I believe the Lavender Way and Lavender Procedure accomplish this. It needs to be national, and only the President of the United States can do it. As Dr. Raza calls them, the self-appointed opinion-makers are so entrenched and won't let anyone displace them.

Indeed, probably all of them are Board-certified ACS fellows or a like entity in their own specialty like oncology. You will come to understand very clearly (I hope) just how disruptive the Lavender Way/ Lavender Procedure is and how much of a threat it is to bring down the inner circle and make things right for EVERY woman period. If the women knew the results of Lavender, I think the house of cards might just come tumbling down.

Getting back now to the two ladies, one had never had a mammogram and the other had a mammogram a long eight years ago. I explained there is a burgeoning number of women who are forgoing mammography for whatever reason like the fear of repeated radiation or pain. I see a constant flow of these women, and I'm out of the loop. How many women like these two are out there? The first lady (in her fifties) said she noticed a lump in June, then had an ultrasound ordered in August (by someone other than an MD), who had an ultrasound nearby. Situations like this with people not knowing what to do or how to go about it (dabbling), have caused a real delay in this patient's care. Her tumor is the size of your fist now with palpable lymph nodes and metastatic disease. In August, they told her she had fibrocystic disease with a few small cysts. She has a slim chance of survival. Could the Lavender Way have helped her?

I am angry with the system having created an environment where women are afraid of mammography and not coming to see any doctor. Then they resort to some type of this alternative nonsense. The surprising thing is their denial is so strong that they continue to incorporate alternative chance remedies even with the tumor growing through the skin.

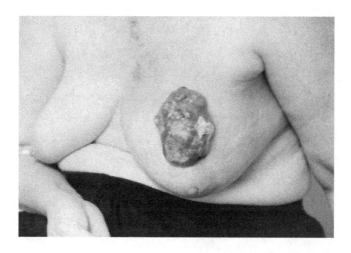

There is no doubt in my mind that if the Lavender Way was up and running across this country, patients like these wouldn't be in the mess they are in. Likewise, the other patient who never had a mammogram, noticed a lump in her breast that was causing redness and skin wrinkling and was rubbing iodine on it. I'm beside myself seeing patients like these who will be robbed of a long prosperous life because of the system, which no one wants to change. Scenarios like these two patients are totally preventable.

From the movie *Cool Hand Luke,* in which Paul Newman played Luke, "What we got here is a lack of communication."

That was said just before they shot him.

From the movie *The Accountant*: "You're different and sooner or later different scares people."

CHAPTER 7

THE LAVENDER WAY AND LAVENDER PROCEDURE; HOW I GOT THERE

H ow did I come up with those names, Lavender Way and Lavender Procedure? Let's go back a few years and review my continual quest to do less invasive procedures with better results. I started a new phase with Accelerated Partial Breast Radiation (APBR) around 2004. Up until that time, I was still on the chemo, surgery, and radiation train, but when the makers of MammoSite contacted me to learn APBR, I jumped at the chance.

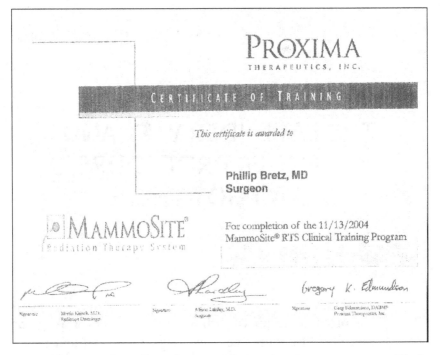

APBR seemed to fit right in with my less invasive quest. Heck, who wouldn't want twice daily targeted radiation via the MammoSite catheter for just five days versus five days a week for six weeks with a booster at the end? That's called "external beam radiation," which radiates the entire breast. External beam had carried complications in the past like pericarditis, pneumonitis, rib fractures, and well-known peau d'orange and global breast shrinkage.

I remember a case at EMC when another doctor went on vacation and asked me to see a couple of his patients. A lady came in who had a lumpectomy done, and her entire breast was black from radiation burn. APBR allowed obviating all that with truly targeted radiation.

The rationale for APBR is that about 90% of the local recurrences after lumpectomy occur within 1 centimeter of the original lumpectomy wall. The catheter has a balloon at the end which is blown up with saline and, upon proper insertion into the lumpectomy cavity, abuts the surrounding margins 360 degrees. The image below has the "fat patch" as well and is a pretty good placement.

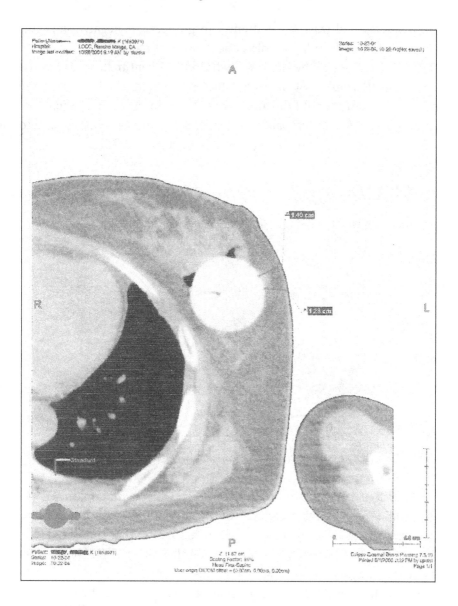

Thus, when the radiation therapist inserts the focus of radiation, it effectively kills any cancer within that 1 centimeter. It was a pretty cool technology to come up with, and if it worked, would eliminate the need for external beam radiation. I did about forty-five or so APBR cases and have yet to have a local recurrence or re-recurrence. One of the things

I quickly learned was, in an attempt to get clear or negative margins (where there is no identifiable cancer), one sometimes gets close to the under-surface of the skin, well within the 1 centimeter. So in those cases, APBR would not be acceptable as it would totally destroy the skin. This was a patient I did and burned the skin. After this patient was when I invented the "fat patch," to prevent any further burning and to expand the pool of women who could benefit from APBR.

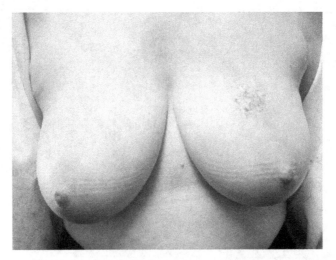

Left breast partial breast radiation with skin burn
secondary to lack of skin spacing

After that case, it popped into my head that why couldn't I just excise an Oreo-sized fat patch out of the abdominal wall and use it as a buttress to provide that 1 centimeter cushion. I did that and called it an "autologous free fat patch." I had that published in ASTRO. I hope other surgeons saw that and were able to utilize it. It makes a big difference to the patient. Thus, APBR was a great advance I was able to help pioneer. Again, I didn't have to do any of that. I could have just said, "Well, we can't do APBR," instead of coming up with a new surgical procedure. At Hines VA, we had done a research trial with veterans coming back from Vietnam to see if they were exposed to dioxin (agent orange). We took an Oreo-sized piece of fat from the abdominal wall to analyze; that's how I came up with the idea of the fat patch for APBR. It worked like a charm with no evidence-based medicine, just experience and ingenuity.

Then a world-renowned breast cancer surgeon, Dr. Mel Silverstein, was pioneering Intraoperative Radiation Therapy (IORT) and again, from the Tumor Institute of Milan in Italy. IORT goes like this: the surgeon performs the lumpectomy, and then a machine (about the size of a large suitcase) is wheeled up to the table, and an arm with a ball attached (which is the radiation source) is lowered into the lumpectomy cavity. Radiation is then applied for twenty minutes while the patient is asleep. The big deal is, when the patient awakes in the recovery room, she is done with her surgery and radiation. For me this effectively put a fork in APBR, and I sent Mel a number of cases.

Again, I didn't know if IORT would perform as advertised? After a couple of cases, I couldn't ethically give the option of APBR to patients knowing that IORT was available at Hoag Hospital in Newport Beach. APBR was great and had great results, but IORT trumped it.

It would be interesting to know (but we will never know) exactly how many surgeons in the Coachella Valley sent cases to Mel for IORT? Knowing what a quantum leap it was to benefit patients, did any surgeons search IORT instead of the same old radiation offered at the hospitals in the Valley? I say if a surgeon wanted to be included as a "breast surgeon," then they should have sought out IORT.

Again, I didn't have to do it, and the patients would have been none the wiser. But ethically, it was impossible for me not to include IORT as an option. In following these IORT cases, a thought struck me. I had met Dr. Ken Ramming (RIP), who was pioneering cryoablation surgery in the early 1990s. He was at John Wayne Cancer Center and his focus was metastatic colon cancer to the liver. Resecting the liver for one or multiple foci of cancer is fraught with potential complications from bleeding to poor prolonged recovery to death on the OR table from uncontrolled hemorrhage. While Dr. Ramming's cryoablation (just freezing the tumor) didn't do anything for survival, it did arguably give patients a better quality of life. He had let me watch a case of a patient I referred to him, and I felt it was the right decision on the patient's part to choose cryoablation.

Then the light bulb went off, all because of my results with APBR and seeing IORT results. That is, if we were essentially betting patients' lives on the ability of these two FDA-approved modalities (although relatively new and no widespread use) to cure patients (as best we could), why couldn't I just freeze the breast cancer? If one uses the gun analogy, what difference does it make if you get fatally shot with a 45 caliber or a shotgun? Either way, you will be dead. So, in using cryo, if cryo could kill the cancer using the theory of "targeted kill," then it would open a whole new chapter for women. Why? Because it could be done not only outside the OR but outside the system altogether for not much money. Further, any trained doctor could do it. Cryo would be of tremendous help in countries with limited resources where there isn't an oncologist on every block. Because cryo is so mobile, it could be done in any trained doctor's office or an eighteen-wheeler, instead of a threatening hospital.

It would have the capacity (coupled with the Lavender Way) to level the playing field almost overnight for the underserved, and especially African American women. Breast cancer is the biggest killer of Hispanic women, and that would end too, if I could get our country to embrace a new path to the diagnosis and treatment of breast cancer. I could see a revolution coming. Consider the following:

1. I had been down this path before with the Tamoxifen prevention trial, and it turns out I was right with my assumption that Tamoxifen could be used for active prevention (without my having any "evidence-based medicine"). I had the ability then to know in a heartbeat that Tamoxifen could save untold thousands of women from breast cancer. I could see it as plain as day when no other researcher could. Now, armed with almost forty years of experience fighting this disease, I could also see the contribution of cryo to change the landscape for ALL women everywhere dramatically. Remember, all this technology is FDA-approved and, therefore, has gone through clinical trials with positive results. It's just that no one is using it for several reasons. I'll name a few so you get

the drift of how difficult it is to bring technology to a level where all surgeons are doing it. I'll list them in no particular order. One of the biggest reasons is the fear by surgeons of being sued. Why? Because in cryo, a surgeon doesn't remove the tumor. Excising the tumor, let alone the entire breast, has been the mainstay for decades to "get it all." Now we are asking them to forget all that and just freeze the tumor. You see how that causes consternation.

2. There is no one to teach you, and since the patient is awake, you can't screw up during the procedure like saying "Oh crap." You have to have a certain level of expertise to pull it off. There was no one to teach me.

3. The representatives of the companies just set up their machines, they weren't doctors. In my case, I always let the significant other enter the room to hold the patient's hand or look at the tumor being killed on the ultrasound monitor. Having the significant other in the room accounted for the dramatic change from grief to almost joy. It changed the whole psychological foundation of the family. To do that, you have to be good.

4. A lot of surgeons' practices are being bought up by hospitals, and if, for instance, a breast surgeon then works for the hospital, few months might go by when the surgeon receives a call from the CEO. And the CEO says, "Doctor, we bought your busy breast practice as we thought you would feed the pipeline of chemotherapy and radiation and, of course, your surgeries, where we make our money. To date, we haven't seen a case. Is there a problem?" Now the surgeon says, "Well, I'm just killing the cancer in the office. No need for surgery or the rest." You can see how that would not go over well.

5. Cost is another factor. The surgeon gets to use all the hospital's equipment without charge. Neither does the surgeon pay for the staff or their malpractice insurance, etc. This isn't

the roaring 80s now where specialists were revered, and seemingly everyone bought all kinds of equipment. The glory days are over, so a $100,000 price tag for cryo equipment is beyond the reach of the majority. The surgeon has to pay for each probe, and you have to buy two in case one fails during the procedure. Probes can only be used once, and they cost roughly $1,300 each, probably more now.

6. Fear of failure is another problem being faced by the surgeon. While a monkey can't operate, any butcher can carve out a tumor in the breast. Cryo is very precise, and there is no stumbling, especially with the patient and family watching.

7. But mostly, it's having to let go of nearly everything you learned for years of how to treat breast cancer. That is hard to do to potentially face severe ridicule and action of governing bodies if things go south. Remember, cryo is apparently not "standard of care" according to some people. It takes a surgeon with some guts to start doing something out-of-the-box. Most surgeons are inside the box where it's a safe haven.

8. While a surgeon wouldn't think that a fellow surgeon would write a complaint to the Medical Board without first having the guts to confront him/her, that's exactly what happened to me, when all that surgeon had to do was pick up the phone and ask me what I was doing. I would have invited that surgeon to come, learn and watch a case. I had several doctors who inquired do just that, come and learn. I have included that letter written about me by that surgeon to the Board, see Chapter 8. Incidentally, the Medical Board has never told me about that letter. I found it in a chance encounter (my lawyer never told me either) in the discovery material from the Board.

9. Lastly, there are turf battles in the hospital as to who exactly is going to do this, surgeons or radiologist or any doctor interested, since it's not really surgery? A typical scenario

would be where the surgeon sees a patient and is sure it's a
breast cancer and sends the patient for a mammogram and
schedules the case. Then the patient calls to cancel a few days
later because the radiologist "just froze it." Bingo, turf war.
While there are other reasons a surgeon might not want to
venture into cryo, you get the idea of what's going through
their heads.

Just like it was meant to be, when I got the cryo equipment, three
patients showed up, two with local recurrences and one with breast
implants who had retained cancer at the margins by another surgeon
and didn't want her breasts butchered again. The two local recurrences
were both my patients, and each was about twelve years out from her
original surgery. The surgeries years ago consisted of lumpectomy and
external beam radiation. Now the standard-of-care and the "book" say,
if a patient has a local recurrence following lumpectomy and external
beam radiation, the only option is mastectomy.

Both recurrence cases were well into their eighties. Some surgeons
faced with a patient in that age group wouldn't recommend any
treatment. But with cryo, it makes a huge difference. The one patient
had developed Alzheimer's, and she couldn't remember my name. She
was on a blood thinner as well. The other recurrence patient wanted her
breast saved and was thrilled with the new possibility of cryo. Another
thing cryo offers is probably no real "loss of time." Meaning, I always
followed up with all the cryo patients two months after the Lavender
Procedure with mammography, ultrasound, and core biopsy. I had an
independent radiologist do the core sampling as I didn't want it said that
I "missed" the cancer (all done by a third party). This held true for first-
timers also, and because a lot of the patient's tumors were discovered at
very small sizes (less than 1 centimeter), most were hormone positive.
All that time then, they were on an anti-estrogen depending on their
age and hormone positivity of the tumor. That's why there was really
nothing to lose attempting cryo.

If it worked, great, if not, the patient could opt for another attempt
or move to a more conventional procedure. In addition, some people

have criticized me for not doing a lymph node dissection. First, increasingly there is a move to omit lymph node dissection even with micrometastasis in the sentinel node. Why? Because there is no difference in survival in those cases, nor is there an enormous burden of cancer developing in those nodes over time.

Lymph nodes are part of the lymphatic system in the body. They are responsible for making antibodies against things like bacteria or viruses. There are thousands of nodes all over, and some you can feel. If you ever felt the neck of a child that has recurrent sore throats or ear infections, when you felt their necks (on either side), you could feel what feels like little lumps that are mobile (they move when you push on them or palpate them). Your tonsils are part of your lymphatic system. Lymph nodes vary in size.

Usually, they are the size of a lima bean but can get larger normally. In some parts of the body, they are clustered like in either axilla. The other part of the lymphatic system is they are connected by lymphatic vessels, just like arteries or veins. They generally run alongside. The real damage with cancer-infected lymph nodes is when they empty into the bloodstream and seed the body with cancer.

The big deal (historically) with lymph nodes is in cancer; the more lymph nodes that are removed at surgery that contain cancer, the worse is your prognosis. In my personal effort to rid a woman of breast cancer, the greatest number of lymph nodes I ever removed is fifty-eight. I believe the average number nationwide is about fifteen. No question, I left that woman very damaged.

That's how I was taught like thousands of surgeons coming of age in the 1970s. I have spent my entire career trying to rectify that situation. I hope I succeeded. Someone with no lymph nodes with cancer is much better off than someone with five or more nodes involved with cancer. Historically, lymph node involvement indicated the need for chemotherapy.

This was before the onset of neoadjuvant chemotherapy, where we gave chemotherapy before any surgery for invasive breast cancers 1 centimeter or larger without regard to lymph node status.

Why? Because invasive cancers do what they do, given time (spread).

In the 1800s, it was thought breast cancer just got bigger and bigger and then went to the first lymph node, the second, and so forth in a very orderly manner. That's what gave rise to the concept of "getting it all." The rationale was if you have three lymph nodes involved with tumor and the surgeon could get to the fifth one with a normal one in between, the surgeon had gotten it all. Dr. Bernard Fisher (RIP), Director of the NSABP from its inception in the late 1950s until a few years ago, as a result of the clinical trials they did, put forth the concept of breast cancer being a systemic disease.

Given an invasive tumor's size and genetic make-up, even though we couldn't demonstrate cancer that had spread, the concept of micrometastasis or occult metastasis came to be. That accounted for women who died of breast cancer in the past with negative nodes. Then we thought we had gotten it all because the surgeon removed fifteen negative lymph nodes, which should have said she was cured, but somehow, the cancer can spread. We now know that had to be micrometastasis. That was the rationale for neoadjuvant chemotherapy. How did the cancer spread if not through the lymphatic system? President Truman had a sign on his desk that read, "The buck stops here." President Clinton, I'm told, had a sign on his desk that said, "It's the economy stupid." All cancer-treating doctors should have a sign on their desks that reads, "It's the bloodstream stupid."

What if we could find cancers before they hit the bloodstream? But back then, if we knew the patient probably had metastasis, even though we couldn't demonstrate it on any scan, there was a better chance of killing every last cell. That edict by the NSABP probably accounted in large measure for the juggernaut of what is now the slash-poison-burn approach to try and kill every last cell. If we could do that, then 40,000 plus women would not be dying of breast cancer yearly despite being given a ton of chemo. That's why Dr. Raza points out that we should set our sights on finding and treating the first cancer cell, not the last. That's what I think I have done with Lavender Way, starting with the genetics risk test followed by non-radiation modalities to find ultra-small cancers. The smallest cancer I've found is 4 millimeters, less than and size of an eraser head on a pencil. I'm convinced that's what makes the difference in how you should manage breast cancer the Lavender Way.

If you read the *Divine Comedy* by Dante Alighieri (1320), there is a part where Dante is led into hell by Virgil. When they come to the entrance, there is a sign that reads something like, "All ye who enter here abandon all hope." I am convinced that to understand the potential of cryo and the Lavender Way, the sign should read, "All ye who enter here abandon all previous dogma you have learned about diagnosing and treating breast cancer."

If you don't and hold Lavender to the standards of decades-old dogma, then you will come to the wrong conclusion about Lavender's merits and me. I think that's what happened to me. It is so unbelievable that anyone (meaning me) who dares to execute this diagnostic and treatment regimen would be labeled negligent or incompetent or any other adjective you can put in there.

I did three patients the first time I tried cryo. I did the easiest first, which was Corinne. She had a less than 1 centimeter local recurrence more than ten years out and now eighty-three years of age with advanced Alzheimer's. Her cancer was clearly seen on ultrasound and I could feel it. Next would come Doreen. She had a local recurrence after about twelve years out from lumpectomy and external beam radiation.

Lastly would come the most difficult, and that was Rosie, who had breast implants and a retained cancer from another surgeon. I told Rosie that I or anyone else probably should not tackle a case like hers without doing about fifty cases, but she had faith in my ability. Rosie in 2021 is pushing eight years out with no evidence of any local recurrence nor any lymph node involvement. So, I either guessed right on these patients or perhaps I did/do know something that eludes others.

We would see how the other two cases went that day and then judge whether or not to do Rosie. You see, surgery is like NASA firing off a rocket. If you don't push the launch button, then nothing happens. No harm, no foul. But once you drop the knife or push the launch button, then it's game on, and you better be prepared. You know, all throughout my surgical career, I never laid awake at night sweating out if I was up to doing a difficult case the next morning. Loyola and Drs. Freeark, Pickleman, Warpeha, MD, PhD, DDS, Greenlee, Raffensperger, and Folk saw to it that they trained me well. By the time one finished their surgical residence at Loyola, you were an extension of each of those surgeons. At some point, a surgeon has to know if he/she has what it takes to do a difficult case even though they may have never done a case like that before.

When I had the probe placed on Corinne's cancer and pushed the button (it lit up a nice shade of blue), I thought, as I saw the iceball engulf the tumor and killing it, that this would be a real game-changer, a miracle. And seven years hence now I'm sure of it. Am I the only one to see the light here? Look, I'm aware of at least two clinical trials, FROST and IceSense3. At least one of those trials continues to use post-procedure radiation. That being the case, we don't know if the patient is cured, if it was the cryo or radiation? Did I push the envelope extirpating my patients from the system to see if cryo could stand on its own? You bet I did and guilty as charged. But I made that decision based on forty years of experience diagnosing and treating breast cancer. I hope you come to the same conclusion I have and that is the Lavender Way potentially finds cancers before they can spread. Then we can use cryo to kill it and come full circle to "getting it all." Otherwise, years and years go by with seeing if radiation is necessary involving more clinical trials. Then, as always, who or what entity can declare finally that cryo can stand on its own? When does cryo cross the finish line?

As I said, when we finished, both Corinne and Doreen, and Rosie went off without a hitch. That is, I was able to insinuate the probe into the cancer between the skin and the implant wall, some feat if I do say so myself. Immediately after I finished Rosie, she said she was hungry and wanted to go over to Lavender Bistro (in La Quinta, California) for something to eat.

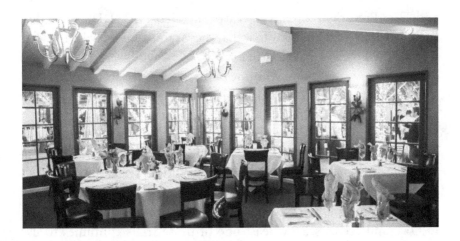

Lavender Bistro is right across the street (a one-minute walk). I had put the finishing touches (a dab of antibiotic ointment) at the probe entrance site and a 2x2 gauze. I never had to use a single stitch on any patient. Immediately we walked over, and within fifteen minutes, Rosie was enjoying a lobster salad and, as I said, toasting with a sip of chardonnay. She didn't get drunk and had a significant other with her. She toasted with the wine because none of the forebodings of another botched surgery ever happened. For that, she was very happy. It bears repeating, she is seven-and-a-half years out cancer-free.

Wilma, a patient from Texas, flew to us because even though she could feel the tumor, at age eighty-three and with a history of three strokes and on blood thinners, she said her doctors in Texas wouldn't operate on her. She kept feeling it every day and worrying. She didn't tell me about the strokes until after her procedure. But it points out that the Lavender Procedure is well suited for this type of high-risk patient. Why? Because it's a twenty-minute procedure, and the patient is fully awake. Right after Wilma's procedure, Nick (the owner of Lavender Bistro) opened up just for us to serve a spectacular lunch and, yes, toasting with a little champagne. I can't tell you how different it was to see the radically changed scenario from sorrow and dread of disfiguring surgery and dread of chemotherapy and radiation to the utterly uplifting psychologic (almost euphoric) state of the Lavender Procedure. You can get a sense of it in the videos.

This might be a good time to let you read my informed consent. Pretend you're a breast cancer patient and trying to decide on what procedure you are going to opt for. Since cryo has not been around for decades like lumpectomy, and since there aren't thousands of cases to know its secrets, I called it "experimental." Mind you it wasn't experimental since it is FDA-cleared. It was just that no one, especially back eight years ago, was venturing into cryo for reasons already elucidated. In addition, I made sure each patient knew exactly how many patients I had done and what their number was. Some of them memorized it to say, "I'm number twelve."

So, let's discuss "informed consent."

To me, informed consent should relay to the patient what reasonably the patient should expect in terms of the procedure itself and potential complications. It has to stop somewhere though. For instance, while the Coachella Valley is on the San Andreas earthquake fault, you wouldn't put in the informed consent that the surgical light might fall on the patient if an earthquake came.

In my informed consent, I trace my path to finding and embracing cryoablation. That is, how I came to believe in cryo, that it wasn't something I dreamed up in my garage. There was a sequential step approach taking years from radical mastectomy to modified radical mastectomy to lumpectomy to APBR to IORT to cryo. All that took decades to perform the procedures and see the results and change the approach accordingly. The overriding idea was to initiate ever less invasive procedures and achieving as good a result or, ideally, a better result. I think I've done it, but you be the judge.

During my first case (Corinne), I said to myself, *if this works, this is a real game-changer,* and it has been. What I've espoused for years, I began to see in real life. That is, there is a burgeoning number of women who are not only refusing mammography but refusing any traditional treatment. They opt instead for alternative treatments like ozone.

There are quite a number of these. I had one patient from Wisconsin who stood naked for an hour surrounded by multi-colored fluorescent lights. What happens to these patients? As years go by, as we have seen, the tumor grows until eventually it grows right through the skin. It's the damnedest thing. I've asked myself a hundred times why anyone would not seek medical help if they felt a lump or for sure, if they realized a mass was growing despite any alternative care? I never really got an answer from any of them about this conundrum, except they didn't want the effects of radiation or chemotherapy to injure their bodies. What? Apparently every one of these women didn't ponder what cancer would eventually do. I understood their reluctance to undergo surgery, chemotherapy, and radiation but never understood that they would be in such denial that eventually cost them their lives.

So yes, I had women come in with 3-centimeter tumors that had refused any treatment, and the tumor was about to break through the skin (not the patient below). I did perform the Lavender Procedure on them just in an effort to prevent the tumor from becoming a local nightmare. The following image is one of those I warned you about. If you don't want to see it skip ahead two pages. My guess is, though, you'll want to see what kind of suffering is inflicted on women which I say could be almost totally avoided.

This page intentionally left blank. The image has its own page.
Skip ahead two pages if you don't want to see it.

This page intentionally left blank.

This page intentionally left blank.

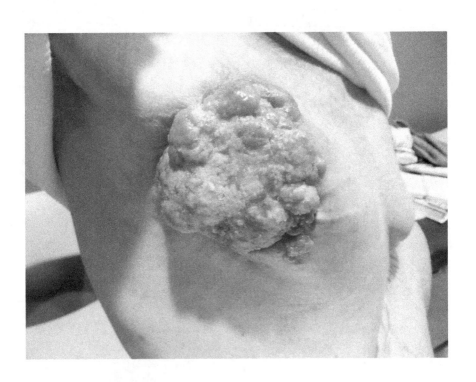

This page intentionally left blank.

This page intentionally left blank.

This page intentionally left blank.

The patient pictured had tumor growing for seven years out of the skin. Now she wakes up every morning, and parts of it fall on the floor. It stinks to high heaven and bleeds. Yet, she still refused any treatment. So out of sheer concern for your fellow man (woman in this case), you offer help because you're a doctor trained to help relieve suffering.

Then you're soundly criticized for doing Lavender as it's not indicated. I obviously didn't perform Lavender on the above patient, it was too far gone. But what are we to do as cancer doctors when they knock on our door? For me, I helped them as, in many cases, I was their last resort. I'll take any criticism but that's what I took the Hippocratic Oath for.

Perhaps others have forgotten that or if they never took the oath, they have no idea. What I mean by that is functionaries put in place by a system that increasingly erodes the position of doctors (notice I didn't say "providers"). These functionaries can, at will, wield power over the defenseless doctors. These functionaries know this, and that emboldens them to screw us more. It's almost as if they have unlimited power with no one to answer to, no checks or balances. I talked to a person who should know. That person (male or female) said that the Board's mantra is to "revoke" that physician's license as investigators of the Medical Board. Of course, just like the American Board of Surgery says, they are not responsible (unsaid) for non-certified surgeons not getting on a hospital staff or other employment; the Medical Board will at all times espouse fairness in every aspect of their conduct.

Though in this day and age of fairness to all (supposedly), if I were in charge, there would be enough people at any meeting with the accused to make it appear at least that there was fairness involved, perhaps just like a jury and at least someone of the accused own race to remove any inkling of racism which we are all concerned with today. For instance, in a general military court martial there are usually eight members hearing from witnesses. There were no witnesses like Mrs. Smith, who supposedly originally wrote about my doing an "experimental" procedure or the lady with PTSD, where the Board's expert said I performed a procedure that was not indicated. In my case those patients could have probably helped resolve the issue, and there would be simple answers to simple questions like was the equipment all FDA-approved or not? There would be someone on the Board charged to look into that matter, i.e., the company's 510(k), and resolve it openly. That would have resolved the implication in the competitor surgeon's letter that I had somehow cooked up some hairbrained procedure in my garage.

Also, a question to follow, how are the patients doing in the case of a doctor trying to treat cancer patients? And it would be mandatory to disclose any complaints to the accused at the meeting. Like in my case, I think to be fair to me, they should have shown me the surgeon's letter and let me refute it sentence by sentence or not. I was never told of the existence of that original complaint by that surgeon. My own lawyer never told me about it. I only became aware of it in going through the "discovery" material the Board sent to my attorney. As it was, it was well over a year into the Board's action against me.

Because the nuances of medical decisions are so foreign to people like the governor of the state, who maybe ultimately the Board answers to, it's hard for outsiders not to just go with whatever finding the Board makes. Guilty or not, the process should be totally revamped.

As time went on, I had both cryo machines by the two companies in my office. They both worked well. The Sanarus system looked a little sexier and was more streamlined than IceCure at the time. I understand IceCure has a new machine, perhaps emulating the Sanarus product more. Sanarus, since they didn't listen to me about how to attract doctors to use their equipment, went down the tubes and was recently bought out by Hologic. These big companies don't get it and won't listen to someone who has been on the front lines for decades, oh well.

Again, neither company offered any actual surgeon or another type of doctor versed in the management of the machine to oversee and assist me at any time. I learned from the first case, like Abraham Lincoln teaching himself in his log cabin.

As I said, my first case was Corrine, and I could feel the tumor, so that was the easy case that day and gave me valuable insight on how to manipulate the probe and how the machine functioned. For instance, I learned from Corrine that the operator should have five 20cc syringes filled with sterile saline at the ready in case the iceball came too close to the under-surface of the skin.

By the time I hit my fifth case, I had pretty much mastered the technique necessary to carry out successful cryoablation (a.k.a. the Lavender Procedure). I harkened back to Dr. Pickleman at Loyola with his cards, asking the medical students, "How many ways are there to get screwed?" In my paper, I detail pretty much everything I came to know that was important to carry out the procedure. Remember, I did these with the patient awake and family members present to ask questions during the procedure. That's why Lavender reverses all the dread and unhappiness associated with breast cancer, past and present. I'm equally sure that I would be roundly criticized for allowing family members into the operating theater, as it were. But that's how I did it and learned how to reverse all the negative aspects of breast cancer treatment.

I can hear the critics now: "Letting those people into the close operating environment will increase infection rate." Let's look at that statement probably justified under the old operation techniques. The fact is, infections are dictated by how long a procedure lasts (allowing more time for bacteria to invade tissue) and if the case is classified "dirty" or "clean." For instance, a colon resection where potentially harmful bacteria are present that could possibly contaminate the operative field would be classified as a "dirty" case. On the other hand, breast surgery would be a "clean" case. Further, and more apropos to the Lavender setting, is the only place bacteria could invade the patient's body is through that tiny 3-millimeter poke to allow entrance of the sterile probe. Further, if the operator takes the time, he or she can apply antibiotic ointment around that entrance site to prevent any possible infection.

I never had any infections, nor will anyone else who performs Lavender prudently. Can you picture tiny bacteria sensing the entrance site of the probe and scurrying to insulate themselves between that potential space of skin and the probe, squeezing through? As they say in the NFL, "Come on, man." I realize my shortcomings like no "evidence-based" medicine for me to make the no infection rate statement, but that's the real world. You don't have to do ten clinical trials and have debates by self-appointed opinion leaders to dictate to the underlings what to do. That's why progress in cancer treatment is so slow. Surgeons or any cancer doctors are no longer allowed to use their brains.

Decades of experience are nullified and the doctor must toe the line until a "consensus" is in place and the G-d almighty insurance companies approve it. I'm not called the Lone Ranger for nothing and proud of it. Although at times I feel more like Don Quixote like the song says, "He strove with his last ounce of courage to reach the unreachable star." For me, though, the windmills are real. But just look at the results!

Speaking of results, I've kept you in suspense long enough. Let's take time now to look at my paper. After that, take time to look at the video on my website of the eighty-six-year-old patient talking on her cell phone to her son in Seattle while her cancer was being killed. Since her original surgeon insisted on a mastectomy, and she went out to eat right after the Lavender Procedure, maybe I did something good. As well, her cancer was in the right breast, and she uses a cane in that hand to walk and steady herself. Suppose the original surgeon had proceeded with a mastectomy and injured one of the many nerves or caused lymphedema with an axillary lymph node dissection that would possibly have spelled disaster for her?

She is now ninety-two in 2021 and cancer-free, but that won't count to the system. Or does it? How outrageous my conduct was (unethical, unprofessional, and an extreme departure from standard-of-care) to let the eighty-six-year-old talk to her son on her cell phone while her cancer was being killed. Or was it outrageous after all?

How about a breath of fresh air from eons of horrific disfigurement and death? Remember the promise I gave to those three girls I couldn't save decades ago, not to give up until I had an answer? Someone has to show the way to get us all out of this stagnation of destroying women's bodies and a continued climbing death toll. I would also point out that due to the very negative dialogue in my paper toward the system, I found it very difficult to get it published. However, two journals have now published it. You can go to *RAS Oncology and Therapy Journal* and click on Oncology and Therapy Journal or scr@sciencerepository.org and click on Surgical Case Reports. Both are probably in the archives now.

I will let the American public decide if I was so far out of line that my medical license should be revoked. I will also ask them to ponder if there was perhaps something else afoot? The derogatory dialogue in my paper was never meant to be trash-talking or just ridicule. But I did find a way to prevent disfigurement and death and turned this thing around so I thought people would take note. That never happened despite multiple attempts to let the Lavender Way and Procedure see daylight.

That's the reason for this book, besides giving my grandchildren something to remember me by. You see, at age twelve, upon losing my dad, I didn't have the thought beforehand to ask my dad anything about how he dealt with life or the war. Since some people have said I have accomplished something, I wanted Mr. O. and Dr. H. (maybe a doctor someday) to have something to read and fall back on when things get tough. Because let me tell you, losing your father at twelve, not getting Board-certified, losing your job (heart team) and losing your home and everyone else's you paid for, being shut out of the Tamoxifen trial (that I thought up), everything you worked for, and losing your medical license (stayed with terms and conditions, making you feel like a criminal) and being humiliated in my community is a lot to bear.

The Medical Board did a hell of a job destroying me and everything I stood and stand for. They should all get promotions for bringing me down. I came to know the four "Ds" very well. That is disillusionment, depression, despair, and death, although I never got to the last one. I try not to feel sorry for myself, or some people would say "just sour grapes," but sometimes the thought is there, and sometimes it's overwhelming. I guess some people will say now, come on, he was just too stupid to pass the oral Board exam, simple as that and he deserves what he is getting. Really? Whoever says that, let's put their record next to mine and see what is what. The important lesson is to keep going each day and use all the talent that G-D gave you. That's all we can do.

These last few sentences are not meant for the reader to feel sorry for me. It is meant for people to know that even in the worst of times, you must find the strength to keep going. Each of us is not just us but the product of generations of people who had it very tough to get us where we are today. Giving up is not on the agenda. But for anybody, including Mr. O. and Dr. H., you must know that getting through tough times requires you to have built a very strong foundation, including the Lord, to see you through. Ok, enough, I didn't mean for this to be a sermon.

The next part of this book is the most difficult to write. Before we venture into Hell's Half Acre, let me quote from a book called (and I recommend) *Everything is F-cked: A Book About Hope* by Mark Manson. It's from page 62 and it reads, "Every institution will decay and corrupt itself. Each person, given more power and fewer restraints, will predictably bend that power to suit himself. Every individual will blind herself to her own flaws while seeking out the glaring flaws on others, Welcome to Earth. Enjoy your stay." I have to say, except for my dad's death and the Medical Board issue, I have enjoyed my stay immensely. However, as you read my case with the Board, it started in 2015 and ended November 2021, about six years. This encompassed almost six years of extreme anxiety, dread, despair, losing my principal source of income and forever wondering if all I had accomplished would not see the light of day? Six years? Some people would call that cruel and unusual punishment. All that time I felt I was being treated as a criminal with a probation officer, quarterly forms to fill out and relentless edicts like an ethics course. The only thing I didn't have were ankle bracelets. In my opinion this entire episode should have been handled different, like in-depth interviews with all parties to know what was what. Of course, I want the reader to make up their own mind once they read all of this. Should there be repercussions to others or more on me?

CHAPTER 8

MY SAGA WITH THE MEDICAL BOARD

I WILL TRY MY best to present only the facts, and as I have wanted all along, I want the reader to decide if there was always fair play involved or something nefarious and seemingly clandestine. The phrase "cancel culture" has only come about in the last few months of 2020. Just keep that in mind. I'd like the reader to think of the consequences of the Board's actions have been not only on me but my family with the humiliation, embarrassment, ridicule, job loss, and worst of all, my being prohibited from doing the Lavender Procedure, saving breasts and lives. I had been receiving about three to four emails a week (before Board action) from women worldwide who had been diagnosed with breast cancer and wanted to fly here for me to perform the Lavender Procedure. Now with the Board action and saying I was negligent at every turn, women see that first and assume I'm an unscrupulous shyster, and any chance I had to help them is gone.

They all had seen my TEDx Talk ("dr. bretz ted talk" on YouTube). The video you'll see as a link on my new website of the eighty-six-year-old was meant to be played after my TEDx Talk. However, since I was emotional for the first couple of minutes (oh hell, call it like it was, I cried), and only being allowed eighteen minutes for the talk, they didn't run the video. Therefore, the talk was kind of disjointed, not allowing the audience to see the frosting on the cake, as it were. Even so, almost 40,000 people, probably mostly women, have seen it. It's like it has a life of its own, which is good. That means the powers that be haven't been able to snuff out Lavender totally. You might see my talk was quoted and downloaded by a Dr. Sircus. It just points out how others interested in less invasive techniques value pioneering work.

I will start and end with the same thought. There are three things in play here: (1) is that after forty years, the Board finally caught up with me before I did more damage or (2) that somehow at the end of what some people have called an illustrious career, I turned into Mr. Hyde or (3) there was something else afoot. I'll never know about (3) as it's all in the shadows and unsaid.

First, let's look at my history with the Board. They have renewed my medical license for forty years without incident up until 2020. When I first thought about becoming a doctor, I said to myself, if in becoming a doctor I could save one life, it would have been worth it. But over the course of those forty years (like every surgeon), one saves thousands of lives. Should that count for anything? Obviously, it shouldn't count against an illegal act or the like. How any entity would go about dispensing any judgment without knowing my past (or just summarily dismissing it) and without ever asking just how my patients were doing with all FDA-approved equipment remains a mystery.

So, let's start. By the time I came to Mrs. Smith (named changed), who was the one who filed the complaint, I had done five Lavender Procedures and was pretty confident in my ability to perform the procedure. About that time was when the TV spot came out. Apparently now the TV station has taken it down to avoid any relationship with me. I waited over a year after performing the first cases to go public with my results.

I didn't do one case and go public to say that I have cured breast cancer in a twenty-minute in-office procedure, as some have intimated. I initially was unsure of the ability of this cryoablation to treat breast cancer. I didn't know if they would all have complications, lymph node spread, or skin involvement, but none of that occurred as I waited. Those in Group 1 & 2 were all doing well breast cancer wise except for the lady with Alzheimer's who fell and one patient who developed a primary lung cancer about three years out. The Alzheimer's patient expired by the time the paramedics arrived.

That means that all in Groups 1 and 2 were/are cancer-free, and I either guessed right on having no lymph node involvement, or I really knew what I was doing based on forty years of experience and that I spared all those women the ravages of breast cancer, including disfigurement, bankrupting cost, and escape from death. But again, that doesn't count. It seems to me that if you are found guilty by their "expert" for not performing lymph node dissections, and then years later no lymphadenopathy shows up, who is at fault and who knew what and who didn't bother even to try to learn a new technology? Not only those technical things like nodes but to be found unethical (because I was sentenced to a course on ethics) and as well, a course in professionalism with my conduct being deemed unprofessional, added to the distress. When the edict from the Board's "expert" came down on my birthday, yeah on my birthday, was it a coincidence? With the verdict apparently in, I was never called in to confront the "expert" on each of his verdicts. I was told to just sign the verdict and I said I wanted to add "under duress," but the Board wouldn't let me do it.

You can fool some of the women all the time and all the women some of the time, but you can't fool all the women all the time. Women are smart now and can ferret out a caring, competent physician that they are willing to bet their lives on. A term I heard is "authenticity of caring."

Take time now to review the sampling of letters from women all over the world, so you see what they think of me and the treatment they received, many are handmade cards (Chapter 11).

Because of the Tamoxifen prevention trial and other things like Carnegie and running for Congress, I was kind of a grade B celebrity in a town of straight A list celebrities (the Coachella Valley). I think I've been on the front page of *The Desert Sun* for something or other (all good) about seven times or so over the past forty years.

I called my contact at the TV station, and because of my history, they did a very nice segment back in 2015. It aired and a lot of people saw it, including a competitor surgeon in town who took offense for some reason. Instead of just calling me and asking if that surgeon could come out and see what I was doing or see an actual case (which is what would have happened years ago just out of camaraderie), that surgeon just fired off a letter to the Board. We can start this convoluted tale by your reading it below.

11/5/15 3:43 PM	Page 1 of 2
Board:	**Medical Board of California**
License Type:	**Physician's and Surgeon's**
Complaint Number:	8002015017972
Incident Date:	10/29/2015
Description:	On 10/29/2015, Dr. Phillip Bretz presented a procedure on the local news which stated that breast cancer can be treated without surgery. He called it the Lavendar Procedure since he went to the Lavendar Bistro across the street from his office with a patient who had been "disease free" for 2 years from his procedure to drink chardonney and celebrate. The procedure involves placing a cryoprobe into a tumor. There was no mention of type of tumor, grade of tumor, features of the tumor, sentinel node status, or use of radiation. He teared up during his interview stating that he had been developing this for several years in order to keep women whole. He had used it on 5 patients. He stated that surgeons in the community use "cookbook" treatment for cancer. He did not mention that the patient is left with a permanent hard ball-- we know this since cryoprobes have been used for benign fibroadenomas-- but not for cancer. I have a patient who was scheduled for surgery next week for a 1.4cm grade 2 infiltrating duct cancer. Her breast MRI shows that the tumor invades the skin and nipple of the breast. Dr. Bretz saw this patient and is scheduling her for the cryoprobe procedure (for cash of course). He will not know margins or nodal status, and will undoubtedly have to destroy the nipple. It is not in the patient's best interest to undergo treatment that is not based on proven therapies. I would appreciate it if you could look into this situation since many patients are now inquiring about this. I think you should also be aware that Dr. Bretz has lost hospital privileges, trained in Guadalajara, and does not mention ever being board certified. His office is at 78034 Calle Barcelona Ste B, La Quinta, California 92253.
License Type:	**Physician's and Surgeon's**

I had never met this surgeon, although I would have welcomed that surgeon to see everything and actually start doing Lavender on that surgeon's own patients. I didn't need to do another case to prove to anybody how good I was like any surgeon has to (unspoken, of course) when they go on staff at a new hospital. I came to know Lavender because it was a lifelong professional quest to defeat breast cancer. I have a track record and history, no dabbling, just total commitment to women. I was never apprised that the first contact with the Board was via that surgeon. In fact, the Board never disclosed that letter to me, and I only found out about it almost two years into this mess when I went through my attorney's documents.

So, getting back to Lavender, I was feeling pretty good about things and feeling really good about Lavender. I had done Mrs. Smith (name changed) days before, and she was scheduled to come in for a post-procedure check on the nineteenth of the month. On the sixteenth of the month, I get *the* letter from the Medical Board (investigation unit) that Mrs. Smith had filed a complaint, see below.

BUSINESS, CONSUMER SERVICES, AND HOUSING AGENCY - *Department of Consumer Affairs*   EDMUND G. BROWN JR., *Governor*

MEDICAL BOARD OF CALIFORNIA
Central Complaint Unit

Phillip Bretz, M.D.

La Quinta, CA 92253

Patient:
Control Number:
Dates of Service:

Dear Dr. Bretz:

The Medical Board of California is in receipt of a complaint regarding the care and treatment provided to the above named patient. Pursuant to the provisions of Section 800(e) of the Business and Professions Code, we are providing a comprehensive summary of the complaint filed against you.

The complaint alleges the following: Dr. Bretz is performing experimental cancer treatments called "the Lavendar Procedure", which is not the standard of care nor an approved treatment for cancer. The treatments are being performed in the office of Dr. Bretz as he has lost his hospital privileges. The procedure involves placing a cryoprobe into a tumor.

Pursuant to Section 2220.08(a)(2)(B) of the Business and Professions Code, the Medical Board of California is required to provide you with an opportunity to respond to the allegations noted above. As such, in accordance with the enclosed Authorization for Release of Medical Records form, please provide a written summary of the care and treatment rendered to this patient and a copy of your curriculum vitae. You may also provide any additional expert testimony or literature which you feel would be pertinent to the Board in evaluating this complaint.

In addition to the above, please forward a CERTIFIED copy of the patient's medical records, including diagnostic images if applicable, to the Medical Board of California. Please complete the enclosed Certification of Records/Declaration of Custodian of Records to certify that the records are a "true copy" and a complete set and return it with the records to the address shown below. It would be appreciated if you would also include a copy of this letter with your response. Pursuant to Business and Professions Code Section 2225(e) and 2225.5 (copy enclosed), failure to produce the records by the date requested may result in citation and fine or assessment of civil penalties of $1,000 per day.

The records, summary and copy of your curriculum vitae are to be provided by 2/15/2016. Please send this material to the attention of:

2005 Evergreen Street, Suite 1200, Sacramento, CA 95815-3831 • (916) 263-2528 • FAX: (916) 263-2435 • www.mbc.ca.gov

When I read the letter from Mrs. Smith, what struck me most was the word "experimental." I totally forgot the AD HOMINEM attacks elucidated within the second paragraph. It says, "Dr. Bretz is performing experimental cancer treatments called the 'Lavender Procedure,' which is not standard-of-care nor approved treatment for cancer. The treatments are performed in the office of Dr. Bretz as he has lost his hospital privileges. The procedure involves placing a cryoprobe into a tumor."

Let's look at this a little closer.

Both companies (Sanarus and IceCure) have 510(k) approval from the United States FDA. That means the companies have the right to market their cryoablation systems to treat whatever the FDA says they can treat. In the interest of space, I'll just insert the 510(k) from IceCure so you can read it yourself and draw your own conclusions. Both 510(k)s are on the internet. First note the date. This is four years before I performed my first case. Then see page two.

NOV 2 9 2010

5. 510(K) SUMMARY

IceCure's IceSense3 device

K 102360

Name and Address of Applicant:

IceCure Medical LTD.

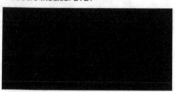

Contact Person and Phone Number:

Date Prepared: November 21, 2010

Name of Device

Trade/Proprietary Name: IceCure Medical, IceSense3 device

Common Name: Cryosurgical unit and accessories

Classification Name: Cryosurgical unit and accessories (21 C.F.R. § 878.4350).

Manufacturing Facility

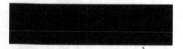

Predicate Devices

The IceSense3 System is substantially equivalent to the cleared IceSense™ System (K072883), the cleared Galil Medical Seednet family (K052530) and Sanarus Medical's V2 Treatment System (K062896).

Intended Use / Indications for Use

The IceSense3 is intended for cryogenic destruction of tissue during surgical procedures. The IceSense3 is indicated for use as a cryosurgical tool in the fields of general surgery, dermatology, thoracic surgery, gynecology, oncology, proctology, and urology. The IceSense3 may be used with an ultrasound device to provide real-time visualization of the cryosurgical procedure.

Urology

- _The system may be used to ablate prostatic tissue._
- _The system may be used for the ablation of prostate tissue in cases of prostate cancer and benign prostatic hyperplasia_

Oncology

- _The system may be used for ablation of cancerous or malignant tissue._
- _The system may be used for ablation of benign tumors._
- _The system may be used for palliative intervention._

Dermatology

- _The system may be used for the ablation or freezing of skin cancers and other coetaneous disorders._

Gynecology

- _The system may be used for the ablation of malignant neoplasia or benign dysplasia of the female genitalia._

General Surgery

- _The system may be used for the ablation of leukoplakia of mouth, angiomas, sebaceous hyperplasia, basal cell tumors of the eyelid or canthus area, ulcerated basal cell tumors, dermatofibromas, small hemangiomas, mucocele cysts, multiple warts, plantar warts, hemorrhoids, anal fissures, perianal condylomata, pilonidal cysts actinic and seborrheic keratoses, cavernous hemangiomas, recurrent cancerous lesions._
- _The system may be used for the destruction of warts or lesions._

IceCure Medical LTD.   Section 5   Page 2 of 4
IceCure IceSense™ 3   510(k) Summary
510(k) Submission

Looking at the second page under "Oncology," you'll see, and I quote, "The system may be used for ablation of cancerous or malignant tissue." Now if we go back to Mrs. Smith's initial letter to the Board, you will see the totally incorrect/false statement just after, "not standard of care NOR AN APPROVED TREATMENT FOR CANCER." Unless I'm totally wrong or can't read English, doesn't the 510(k) from the FDA issued in 2010 under Oncology say, "The system may be used for ablation of cancerous or malignant tissue."? Without making any of my own accusations, it sure looks like to me at least someone took false statements as true and used them against me. And dare I say unjustly?

Now whether or not it is standard-of-care, I will readily admit it is not. That's one of the reasons in my informed consent I said I considered it experimental not because it was unapproved by the FDA, but because we didn't have many years of follow-up as we do for lumpectomy. In fact, as you'll see, I intentionally let the patients know and wrote it in each of their informed consents, just what number they were that I was doing. Mrs. Smith was number 6 and that's what it said on her informed consent. Would you feel comfortable with a commercial pilot if you were his sixth passenger? I just had a lot of experience that patients were totally comfortable with me and they were so displeased with the other doctors, they put their faith in me to do what I did/do best.

Once a device is approved by the FDA and marketed, then anyone who is appropriately trained can use the device or not. Elsewhere in this book I list a lot of the reasons doctors were/are reluctant to venture into the cryo arena. It's like a car manufacturer. Once their vehicles are approved safety-wise, etc., and they market the vehicle to the public, maybe no one buys their car or very few, like the Ford Edsel. But that doesn't mean the vehicle is not road-worthy. Likewise, in cryo, just because the vast majority of surgeons, radiologists, or the like are not venturing into cryo doesn't mean it's not very good, indeed I, among others, have proved it is. And as far as my calling the procedure The Lavender Procedure, the historical surgical literature is replete with surgeons (having invented a procedure), naming the procedure after them, like the Janeway gastrostomy named after Henry Harrington

Janeway, or the McVay hernia repair named after surgeon Chester McVay, or the Halstead radical mastectomy named after William Halstead. I could go on and on here. But I didn't name the procedure the Bretz Cryoablation Procedure, I named it after something that would bring peace of mind and some grace to this situation of having been diagnosed with breast cancer. By the way, I have a letter off to the FDA asking them flat out if cryoablation of cancer is "experimental or not." I hoped their reply would come before the printing of this book. Their declaration will weigh heavily. It did come and it follows; I liked that they're not beating around the bush.

The negative inuendo and ad hominem attacks continue in the letter by Mrs. Smith and again I quote, "The procedures are performed in the office of Dr. Bretz as he has lost his hospital privileges." While it's true the procedures were performed in my office, I did so to rid the patients of the totally frightening experience of a cold sterile hospital setting.

In addition, the cryoablation systems by both companies were/ are meant to be used in exactly that fashion. But the fact that it says I performed the Lavender Procedure in the office "as" he has lost his hospital privileges is again another falsehood. Elsewhere in the book I deal with this issue in a more thorough manner. Her letter makes it sound like I was kicked out of the hospital for some grievous act or the like which again is false. I let my staff privileges lapse because I no longer required the hospital setting for the surgery I was doing. My surgery could be carried out in any outpatient surgical setting or as it came to be in the office.

I hope the preceding explanations help the reader understand what I was/am up against. If you took Mrs. Smith's complaint at face value, then yeah, you would go after me. But in your going after me, for G-D's sake, endeavor to find the truth.

As I read her letter I thought, what the hell is this? Everything had been explained to Mrs. Smith and her family on multiple occasions. Oh yes, another thing the Medical Board got me on was Mrs. Smith signed her informed consent on her first visit. Yes, that's true; however, she and her daughter were so fed up with the conduct and pronouncements of the surgeon who filed the complaint that she knew what she wanted, that was to come to me and Lavender. Now, what went unsaid and never mentioned by the Board was while she signed her consent on her first visit, she didn't have her procedure until seventeen days later. She signed her informed consent on November 3, 2015, but didn't actually have her Lavender Procedure until November 20, 2015. Is that enough time to give a patient? During those days, I met with Mrs. Smith and her family (even on one weekend) to answer all their questions.

What happened was, I gave her the informed consent to begin reviewing and went to talk to Joan (my wife and Office Manager), and when I came back, she had already signed it. It was made out that I somehow forced her or insisted she sign right then and there. Nothing could be further from the truth. The truth was she had been so badly treated and frightened by the surgeon who wrote to the Board, she wanted out of there at all costs. In fact, that surgeon told Mrs. Smith and her family if she came to me, I would destroy her breast and nipple, she would have a large lump there forever, and she would die. Can you imagine the gall of this surgeon not really knowing anything about me, just shooting from the hip? Because why?

No, Mrs. Smith had plenty of time to reconsider, and/or get another opinion. Notice that in my informed consent, that even though cryoablation is FDA-approved for cancer treatment as per the 510(k)s of each company (therefore, by definition, NOT experimental), I considered it (as I said) experimental and told Mrs. Smith and all the other Lavender girls. Meaning, we don't have decades of experience as we do with lumpectomy. In fact, no surgeon in the world has decades of experience. Dr. Fukuma in Japan probably has the most experience. Then, even though I didn't have to mention in the informed consent, I told each patient just how many cases I had done and listed their own number in that informed consent. Some of the Lavender Girls just referred to themselves as number 15 or the like. As I said, Mrs. Smith was number 6.

I counseled Mrs. Smith and her family that yes, her tumor was close to the skin, and there was a chance of damage. However, this procedure is not like launching a rocket. When you push the launch button of a rocket, you hope it doesn't explode as there is nothing you can do once that launch button is pushed. No, on the contrary. With Lavender, if at any time during the case I felt the skin was in danger or anything was wrong, I could just push the "stop" button to avoid any untoward effects. That fact was also ignored. It was presented that I rushed her into a bad decision to proceed with Lavender. I also came up with a new way to not injure the skin which I would have employed in Mrs. Smith's case if necessary. You'll read about it in the paper. That idea came from Corrine's case where I needed the 20cc syringes filled with saline to act as a buffer. I ended up having to fill those as we went along. After that first case, I learned to have them at the ready. I'm a fast learner.

Mrs. Smith's procedure went very well, and we actually went over to Lavender Bistro to eat and toast. Her family was with her. As I said, I was feeling good about my ability and how cryo performed.

Her case was indeed difficult, but with the saline skillfully injected (as the iceball grew) between the tumor and skin and around the nipple in a timely fashion, all was well. She is now going on four years out cancer-free without lymph node involvement.

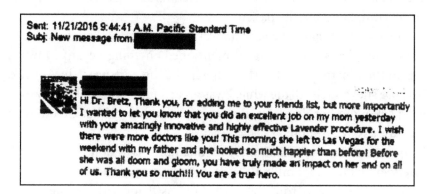

Sent: 11/21/2015 9:44:41 A.M. Pacific Standard Time
Subj: New message from

Hi Dr. Bretz, Thank you, for adding me to your friends list, but more importantly I wanted to let you know that you did an excellent job on my mom yesterday with your amazingly innovative and highly effective Lavender procedure. I wish there were more doctors like you! This morning she left to Las Vegas for the weekend with my father and she looked so much happier than before! Before she was all doom and gloom, you have truly made an impact on her and on all of us. Thank you so much!!! You are a true hero.

Who was right and who was wrong? She was scheduled to come in on the nineteenth after her procedure was flawlessly carried out and we even went to Lavender Bistro after her case with her entire family. Again the "Lavender Experience" was strictly voluntary. But I received the letter from the Board on the sixteenth. I thought, what the heck is going on here? I had heard nothing about any difficulties whatsoever.

Also, see the email I received from her son, where he states his mother basically looked and acted like a new woman. Sounds to me like I really turned this entire family around with Lavender.

She and her husband drove to Las Vegas that weekend. What was she trying to do, entrap me with something coming in on the nineteenth when I received the Board's letter on the sixteenth? But I told Joan we would see her. She came in and acted normal as can be. Nothing was wrong on physical exam, and her breast looked great. Everything had gone well. I didn't say anything (perhaps a mistake), and she never mentioned any problem with me or the fact that she had signed a complaint to the Board. The whole thing was very strange. Not as strange as what I'm about to tell you.

Here is something never disclosed to me, but at this point, I would endure about one-and-a-half years of distress and disillusionment in trying to figure out this whole tragedy.

You see, Mrs. Smith didn't understand what she was signing (according to her daughter) and signed that complaint under duress and threat of a lawsuit (by that surgeon) if she didn't sign the complaint against me. As you'll see, I believe the competitor surgeon wrote the entire complaint, not the patient.

Once I found that out a year-and-a-half later, it made all the sense in the world. That's why she never mentioned anything negative toward me on the nineteenth when she came in for the post-procedure check, because she thought all the while I was great. I found this out on my own by speaking to her daughter a year-and-a-half later. That encounter I will discuss in a minute.

In my opinion, perhaps the Board should have done an in-depth interview with Mrs. Smith and family members to determine exactly what occurred here from the start. Or was it too late for me in the Board's eyes based on that surgeon's letter? To my way of thinking, the Board should have turned their sights away from me and onto the surgeon who started all this by threatening the patient and telling Mrs. Smith she would die if she came to me, let alone the false statements the surgeon made to the Board in the original letter.

As you will come to find out, nothing ever happened to that surgeon.

Exactly how this came about, you will have to read later so as to fully understand. I found out the truth, though, and that was Mrs. Smith had no clue what she was signing beyond it looked official and never wished anything bad to happen to me. In fact, once Mrs. Smith became aware of the trouble I was in that she helped cause, I was told by her daughter she cried and together they wrote a letter of retraction to the Board. That's what they told me they wanted to do. As such, I gave them a copy of the Board member's cards and told them to send it to them certified return receipt requested. I never heard anything if the Board ever got that letter of retraction/exoneration or cared to do anything about that new information. You can read her letter on the next page.

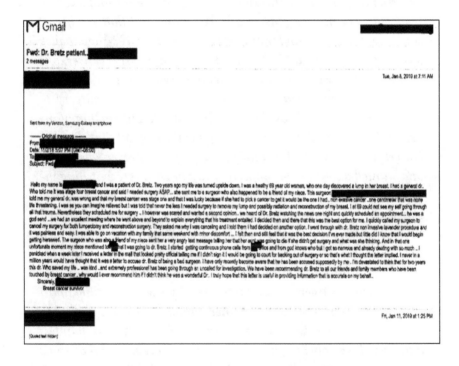

This is a typed copy of the email (for easier reading) I received from Mrs. Smith, with grammar uncorrected. I also noted that as I had given her daughter all three of the Medical Board people's addresses present at my face-to-face, this particular email was only directed to the Board's surgeon, not the Principal Investigator nor the Attorney

General. I don't know if the other two ever received this letter or what difference it ever made, apparently none. The target was set. They had put too much time on me not to ferret out a wrongdoing somewhere. If one looks at every doctor's charts, you will find something wrong somewhere.

Hello my name is Mrs. Smith and I was a patient of Dr. Bretz. Two years ago my life was turned upside down. I was a healthy 69 year old woman, who one day discovered a lump in her breast. I had a dr. who told me it was stage four breast cancer and said I needed surgery ASAP . . . she sent me to a surgeon who also happened to be a friend of my niece. This surgeon (surgeon's name and location redacted) told me my general dr. was wrong and that my breast cancer was stage one and that I was lucky because if ▉ had to pick a cancer to get it would be the one I had..non invasive cancer..one centimeter that was none life threatening. I was as you can imagine relieved but I was told that never the less I needed surgery to remove my lump and possibly radiation and reconstruction of my breast. I at 69 could not see my self going through all that trauma. Nevertheless they scheduled me for surgery.. I however was scared and wanted a second opinion.. we heard of Dr. Bretz watching the news one night and quickly scheduled an appointment.. he was a god send..we had an excellent meeting where he went above and beyond to explain everything that his treatment entailed. I decided then and there that this was the best option for me. I quickly called my surgeon to cancel my surgery for both lumpectomy and reconstruction surgery. They asked me why I was canceling and I told them I had decided on another option. I went through with dr.Bretz non invasive lavender procedure and it was painless and easy. I was able to go on vacation with my family that same weekend with minor discomfort..I felt then and still feel that it was the best decision I've ever made.but little did I know that I would begin getting harassed. The surgeon who was also a friend of my niece sent here a very angry text message telling her that her aunt was going to die if she didn't get surgery and what was she thinking.

And in that one unfortunate moment my niece mentioned to ███
that I was going to dr.bretz I started getting continuous phone
calls from ███ *office and from god knows who but I got so nervous*
and already dealing with so much..I panicked when a week later I
received a letter in the mail that looked pretty official telling me if
I didn't sign it I would be going to court for backing our of surgery
or so that's what I thought the letter implied. I never in a million
years would have thought that it was a letter to accuse dr. Bretz
of being a bad surgeon. I have only recently become aware that he
has been accused supposedly be me. I'm devastated to think that
for two years this dr. Who saved my life ..was kind.. and extremely
professional has been going through an uncalled for investigation.
We have been recommending dr. Bretz to all our friends and family
members who have been touched by breast cancer. Why would I
ever recommend him if I didn't thing he was a wonderful Dr.. I
truly hope that this letter is useful in providing information that is
accurate on my behalf.

Sincerely, Mrs. Smith
Breast cancer survivor Fri, Jan 11, 2019 at 1:25 PM

This is all getting hard to believe, I hope. Remember, I was in the
dark with all of this for a year-and-a-half.

Let's look at that letter from the competitor surgeon now. Read it
again a couple of pages back. I make no corrections on that surgeon's
misspelled words or grammar. We'll go through it line by line so you
can understand. And I must say that if you read this letter without
knowing anything about me and assume that the person who wrote this
is not a sociopath, then yes, you would want to go after that apparent
unethical, scamming, unprofessional surgeon who is fleecing patients
left and right on unproven treatments. Here goes.

First sentence: "On 10/29/15 Dr. Bretz presented a procedure on
the local news which stated that breast cancer can be treated without
surgery."

My reply: That is what is hoped but implies that I was performing
some nefarious procedure that was my own invention and

unscrupulous. I guess I had the right vision as my patients in Group 1 (the ideal patients), including those with local recurrences, which the system calls for mastectomy, are into their seventh-year cancer-free without any lymph node involvement. Who was right and who shot from the hip ignoring, by the way, a number of studies that led to FDA-approval of 100% kill for cancers 1 centimeter or smaller? All that surgeon had to do was visit the website of Sanarus to find that out instead of lashing out. Again, if you're the spear of the Medical Board (the first person to pull the trigger), it would make sense to pull that trigger as everyone knows breast cancer has to be treated with some type of surgery. And now it was brought to their attention by an obviously knowledgeable and caring doctor that didn't want that doctor's patients leaving the practice to come to me and an unproven procedure. Yes, going after me with both barrels makes all the sense if one doesn't delve into the facts or see the results of cryoablation, a.k.a. Lavender Way/Procedure. How would one get the facts? Does one solely rely on the opinion of a doctor who probably never did a cryoablation or do you explore all the facets of a doctor who has done at least twenty-five cases and has years of follow-up experience to know the truth? Wouldn't it have made more sense to just come out to talk to me and perhaps interview multiple patients, instead of never giving me the opportunity?

Next sentence: "He called it the Lavendar Procedure since he went to the Lavendar Bistro across the street from his office with a patient who had been 'disease free' for two years from his procedure to drink chardonney and celebrate."

My reply: First, the surgeon can't correctly spell Lavender or chardonnay. That said, the negative innuendo is that I coerced the patient into going to Lavender Bistro to get drunk. That is not what happened at all. As for the patient who did the TV spot with me, it was her idea after her procedure to go to Lavender Bistro for something to eat as she had been NPO (nothing by mouth) all day. And yes, with her significant other present, she ordered a glass of chardonnay (did I spell that right?) to toast (not to get drunk or party), as none of the bad things she envisioned happened to her. That's what happened as opposed to what is implied in the letter. Going to the restaurant after the procedure was true but only to drive home the point that we had turned this disease upside down and inside out. How dare someone intimate without knowing anything of the goings-on and history (of the patient having disfiguring surgery and being scared to death) to make it sound like we got drunk or close to it. That is unacceptable to me when a phone call could have settled it or at least tried to.

How we came up with the name Lavender Procedure was, as the lobster salad was being served, Joan asked me if I knew what I had just done? I said something like, I hope I killed the tumor.

She said, "Instead of waking up in a cold threatening hospital recovery room with her breast disfigured and a tube in her throat, she is over here having lobster salad, a major turn around." That's when we decided to call it the Lavender Procedure. Before I did, I inquired with the owners, Nick and Michelle if it would be, ok? They were on board and came over to the office (as one would expect) to see the machine and videos. Later I ordered Lavender bracelets (like the yellow ones for Livestrong) and the waiters and Nick and Michelle wore them. We were seeing something that had plagued women for millennia being turned into something very positive (finally).

Next sentence: "The procedure involves placing a cryoprobe in a tumor."

My reply: Yes, it does, among other things like carefully explaining the procedure, knowing the biology of the tumor, along with tumor analysis and surgical options so you feel the patient is a proper candidate. And above all, the patient has enough time to explore second opinions and then comes to the conclusion that Lavender Procedure is right for her.

Next sentence: "There was no mention of type of tumor, sentinel node status, or use of radiation."

My reply: Of course, there was no mention of the nuances of the tumor. This was a public message (not meant for surgeons), and the spot was short. And not wanting to confuse people, we just said it was cancer. But for you the reader, let's answer the questions posed by the surgeon. It was a ductal carcinoma in-situ (DCIS) tumor in a patient with breast implants. Sentinel node status was negative clinically, and I don't know any surgeon that would insist on a sentinel node biopsy under those conditions. Yes, in the literature, there is documentation that about 5% of DCIS tumors harbor an invasive component. I suppose you could make a case for Sentinel Node biopsy if the DCIS tumor was LARGE. I felt it unnecessary, and she is cancer free going on seven plus years, see mammogram report below. Further, I had a Board-Certified radiologist I worked with through all the Lavender Procedures do a follow up ultrasound on Rosie and everything was normal. CASE CLOSED if you're thinking rationally.

As to the radiation, radiation works best on rapidly dividing tumors (like a highly aggressive invasive ductal carcinoma), and DCIS is usually slow. So, for a smaller DCIS, I would discuss radiation and, of course, send the patient to the radiation therapist for their input prior to any procedure. I wouldn't recommend radiation for her as we would burn a bridge. Say, for instance, a patient elects not to use external beam. If there is a local recurrence, I've always treated it like a new cancer and radiate it then (after surgery or repeat cryo), since it declared itself as a more aggressive tumor. I never had a problem doing it that way because my patients were followed so closely that any recurrence would be small, not golf ball size, as in a patient who hadn't been seen for three years. That is another benefit of the Lavender Way, that the patients are followed closely for the rest of their lives. This is in contradistinction to most surgeons who never see the patient again after they heal from surgery. It's someone else's problem. We are taught as surgeons to use everything upfront without regard to any prolonged observation period to see if there would be a recurrence. After a breast cancer diagnosis, each patient is followed differently. Usually, I see them every six months for two to three years, then yearly but sometimes that is altered because of various circumstances like a more aggressive tumor that may have a higher rate of recurrence.

In the case of cryo, the first reevaluation is at two months with mammogram and biopsy by a third party. If there is no evidence of retained cancer, great, we continue to watch closely. If there is retained cancer as we have said, we either go back for a second try at cryo or move to lumpectomy or the like.

Remember, the idea behind cryo is to extirpate the patient from the "system." Otherwise, the patient is still ensnared by the system. We have to cut the umbilical cord, it's a brave new world that will let us finally see the light of day. If we don't cut the umbilical cord, the system still wins and women continue to be sacrificed. What's your call?

Next sentence: "He teared up during his interview, stating that he had been developing this for several years in order to keep women whole."

My reply: "In order to keep women whole?" What's wrong with that? That's the mantra of DBI to preserve mind, body, and spirit period. Then yeah, I did tear up (just like at the beginning of my TED Talk) because I participated in what I call the Holocaust on women with the aggressive surgeries of the 1970s, and now I had finally found an answer. Notice I didn't say THE answer. But the real problem I have with this sentence is the statement that "I had been developing this for several years." What the hell? I didn't develop anything. I just used technology that was already FDA-approved that any surgeon could have done if they had the vision. I couldn't and can't help it that 99%+ of my fellow surgeons in our great country either refuse to step outside the box to achieve better less invasive treatment for women, or they're afraid they can't pull it off or afraid of lawsuits, who knows? But that sentence is way out of line, agreed? It makes it sound like I cooked this up in my garage. You can begin to see my not being Board-certified led the Medical Board to jump to a conclusion they never backed off of. It would be nice to hear under oath if the investigator had it in for me from the start, no matter what I said.

Next sentence: "He had used it on 5 patients."

My reply: So, what? You have to start somewhere if you're are going to pioneer an FDA-approved new method. Cryoablation was (back then in 2014) dismissed by nearly everyone. Mrs. Smith was number 6.

Next sentence: "He stated that surgeons in the community use "cookbook" treatment for cancer."

My reply: I don't have access to that TV segment anymore, but at the time I reviewed it, I probably said I don't use cookbook treatment or the like. Even if I did say doctors in the community use cookbook treatment, what do you call it when all you hear is what Dr. Raza calls the slash-poison-burn approach?

That's okay, I stand by it in any case. Perhaps I'm subconsciously calling my fellow surgeons out to say, what the hell are you doing now? That's why nationwide Lavender Centers would stop all this slash-poison-burn approach, as Dr. Raza so eloquently puts it. Sounds to me that is what Dr. Raza is implying of all cancer doctors everywhere that continue to drink the Kool-Aid.

Next sentence: "He did not mention that the patient is left with a permanent hard ball-we know this since cryoprobes have been used for benign fibroadenomas-but not for cancer."

My reply: What? Wow, it appears this surgeon can predict the future, saying the patient would be left with a hard ball. The surgeon says "we" know this. Does that mean the surgeon has done several cryo cases and that's the result that surgeon had or just reading in a journal? I can't believe anyone would suggest that, not knowing my skill level or the outcomes of cryoablation (a.k.a. Lavender Procedure).

I want to know under oath the experience of that surgeon with cryo and if that surgeon had actually done cases. If that surgeon had, then that sentence would never have been written, see Ruth's video on the website.

Some ice balls disappear totally after a year or are absorbed down to the size of a kernel of corn that has never bothered any of my patients versus having their breast taken off or forever being disfigured.

Next sentence: "I have a patient who was scheduled for surgery next week for a 1.4 cm grade 2 infiltrating duct cancer."

My reply: Yes, the surgeon actually means "had" a patient scheduled as Mrs. Smith left that practice to come to me because she and her family were fed up with the treatment and the yelling and irate behavior that surgeon demonstrated.

Next sentence: "Her breast MRI shows that the tumor invades the skin and nipple of the breast".

My reply: If that were true, her breast should be being devoured by retained cancer five years out and it is not. Yes, perhaps it does show possible invasion of the skin and nipple, but where then is the recurrence that was bound to happen? If there is no local recurrence, then I either miraculously killed the cancer in the skin and nipple, or it was never there in the first place which is probably the case, just overread MRI images. Mrs. Smith never had surgery (just Lavender), no chemo, and no radiation. There should be cancer all over the place. But all we have is an intact breast without scarring. Who was right again in the long run? Again, when recommending Lavender (so as to omit any disfigurement), remember, we do an exhaustive workup about two months after, including mammogram, ultrasound, and biopsy. Then if there is any demonstrable retained cancer, the patient has the option to undergo another attempt at cryo or move on to traditional procedures. Even lumpectomy has retained cancer rates approaching 40% across the country necessitating a second surgery with more disfigurement. And all the while after Lavender, the patient is on an anti-estrogen to prevent the cancer from spreading.

You have to know enough to know that sometimes MRIs, like every image generated, can be overread. In my forty years of doing breast surgery, I have never had cancer eating the nipple even when the imaging report says there is cancer extending to the nipple or extending to the chest wall.

Next sentence: "Dr. Bretz, saw this patient and is scheduling her for cryoprobe procedure (for cash of course)."

My reply: Holy cow, I can't believe the audacity of this surgeon! The correct way to phrase it is cryoablation, not cryoprobe (as an aside). This further reflects the minimal understanding of the procedure and what is involved by that surgeon. But here is another outrageous unsubstantiated shooting from the hip again accusation that I'm charging cash, of course. That surgeon is correct. I did charge cash for Lavender. Why? Simple, there were no codes back seven years ago to bill Medicare or any insurance companies.

Anyone doing cryo couldn't bill them. But you can see (again) if you start putting the puzzle pieces together, not Board-Certified, doing, alleged by Mrs. Smith, "experimental" procedures, going to destroy the skin and nipple and basically hijacking the patient from what would be correct tried and true standard of care treatment. Let's add the intimation of "fleecing" the patient by charging cash.

The fact is that when I did the first three patients (like all the cases), I had to buy the probes. These probes initially cost about $1,300.00 apiece. I never gave it much consideration as I thought there would be codes, but there weren't. So, with those first three patients, I lost $5,230.00 dollars since I had to pay for three probes, pay the ultrasound tech, and for the liquid nitrogen. I didn't go back to the patients and say, you owe me $2,500.00 (which is what I charged initially). I thought it unethical as, before the procedure, I said insurance would pay for it. That's how unethical I was. Just so you know, as time went on and the two cryo companies were losing money, they upped the charge for the probes in one case to $4,000.00 and stipulated you had to buy two probes per procedure in case one malfunctioned. Initially, I was charging $2,500.00 per case. If you subtract the cost of the probes $1,300.00 and $300.00 for the ultrasound tech and $130.00 for the liquid nitrogen, and that's not including drapes, gloves, anesthesia, I made about $700.00 per case. As has always been my conduct, if a patient couldn't pay, that was that. I was trained to save lives flawlessly period. This patient wrote the *Desert Sun* in 1990. I guess this patient didn't think I was unethical.

CANCER: Uninsured patient thanks doctor

This long-overdue letter is to publicly express my profound thanks to Dr. Phillip Bretz of the Desert Breast Institute for saving my life.

In November 1990, I became one of the rapidly growing number of women in this country to be diagnosed with breast cancer.

As a single, self-employed young woman, I carried no health insurance.

I thank God that I happened upon the Desert Breast Institute in my search for treatment.

I don't know if people fully understand how rare the following attitude is in the medical community, but Dr. Bretz was completely undaunted by the fact that I had no health insurance.

His genuine concern, from the moment I was diagnosed, was that I begin receiving immediate, aggressive medical treatment for cancer.

During my subsequent encounters with other local doctors and medical institutions, I learned with anguish and shock that there are members of the medical community who will watch you die if you have no health insurance.

I want to thank you, Dr. Bretz. Today, following nine months of chemotherapy and radiation, I am by all indications cancer-free.

It is with deep gratitude and affection that I remember your warmth, humor, encouragement, and passionate dedication to fighting and eradicating breast cancer. Thank you for my life.

Before beginning radiation treatment, I was fortunate to discover California's Major Risk Medical Insurance program.

Others interested in information

Now, as years passed and a limited number of surgeons got into cryo, the going rate they came up with was $6,800.00. I ended up at $6,000.00. This figure is still a far cry from the roughly $150,000.00 for standard care involving possibly multiple surgeries to get all the cancer, chemotherapy and follow-up visits and radiation. So, for that surgeon to intentionally infer that I was seemingly scamming patients on some "experimental" procedure is an outlandish wrong against me. You'll appreciate the next sentence as to the depths of the apparent "hatred" toward me by this surgeon and everything I stood/stand for. Again, no repercussions of any kind against these false and negative innuendoes that proved not to be true but intimated very bad unethical, unprofessional, negligent conduct on my part. Really? I had to take a break before answering the next couple of sentences as they are so egregious, awful, and appalling. Can anyone recite the nine warning signals of a sociopath?

Next sentence: "He will not know margins or nodal status, and will undubtedly have to destroy the nipple."

My reply: First, I think the surgeon meant to type undoubtedly instead of undubtedly. Oh well, I think the surgeon was in such a hurry and angry it was overlooked. "He will not know the margins." You see, in cryo, since we don't remove the tumor, we NEVER know the margins. But we know its genetic makeup and history in the family and patient and its size. From there we can determine the size of the iceball we want to develop to encompass/engulf the tumor with a margin of normal tissue around it. I call the peripheral kill zone (PKZ). Again, I must point out the problems that arise when the uninformed insist on applying the old method's standards (slash-poison-burn approach), refusing even to learn what is possible with cryo/Lavender. Remember the sign upon entering Hell that Dante saw and what the corollary is to Lavender?

This issue of the nodal status is a real stickler and will take decades (probably) to get over. The insistence to violate the patient by removing lymph nodes simply because that is the way it has always been done to my thinking borders on unethical behavior, knowing the results and potential of the Lavender Procedure. Again, I know the genetics, size, history, etc., and have done a physical exam, ultrasound, and mammogram without finding evidence of clinical nodal involvement. Four years later, I either guessed right (as there is no lymph node involvement), or perhaps I did know what I was doing not submitting Mrs. Smith to an unnecessary surgery. No one is interested in how I managed to do it.

Increasingly, there are papers in the literature that have found no need to sample the nodes even with micrometastasis since it didn't make any impact on recurrence or survival. In any case, I feel that's where four decades of experience in dealing with breast cancer should give a surgeon, not the authority to do outrageous procedures but to know that all things considered, one didn't have to do the nodes in Mrs. Smith. She is now over four years out and just about perfect. Over and over again, the proof is in the pudding. Who was right, and who deserves an apology?

To say that I will undoubtedly "have to destroy the skin and nipple" is just so outrageous. I don't know any surgeon in their right mind who would dare to predict anything close to that of a fellow surgeon's proposed surgery. One might say yeah, pancreatic surgery is fraught with a higher rate of complications, but they wouldn't use words like undoubtedly which implies it *will* happen.

Of course, none of those things came to pass, and Mrs. Smith is now over five years out from Lavender. What do you think about this kind of conduct? Perhaps the surgeon didn't know or thought the Board would just give me a slap on the wrist. But if that surgeon knew how devastating the consequences have been of losing my livelihood, being prohibited from doing cryo ever again, and suffering ongoing humiliation in my community I served well before that surgeon came into town, would that surgeon have preferred to just call me? I think we have to seriously question the mental balance of that surgeon who, by the way, is in the community without any consequences of all these half-truths and prophesized false outcomes. What have we created here? The unconscionable defamation of character is unacceptable and uncalled for. If I were to address that surgeon directly, I would say, "You killed me, my family, and my G-D-given ability to save women from the likes of you and every other person who can't look at the results and say sorry, go back to doing Lavender, we need you."

I try not to get angry, but sometimes it's just too difficult to ignore. I'm very sure nearly every surgeon in this great land would condemn the behavior of that surgeon without first having the guts to talk to me and get to know my reasoning. These are ad hominin attacks.

Back to the surgeon's letter to the Board.

Next sentence: "It is not in the patient's best interest to undergo treatment that is not based on proven therapies."

My reply: There the surgeon goes again with another untruth apparently swallowed by the Board as gospel. All this is not making me look like a great surgeon. Someone not versed in ferreting out the truth could be easily convinced that my license should be taken. So, were the results proved or what?

Before shooting off the surgeon's mouth, all that surgeon had to do is go to the websites of Sanarus or IceCure and see the plethora of data. Or better yet, call me. The FDA had all the data, that's why the FDA APPROVED cryoablation for killing cancer. What else can I say? And do I need to reiterate it's the patient's prerogative to have whatever treatment they choose once apprised of ALL the options? Or today in this country is it really the patient's prerogative? It's no one's business if something is in someone's best interest or not. Unless we are creating an environment where the patient's wishes are dismissed, and they HAVE to have whatever the Board or a consensus group says.

Then why go to medical school anymore? Just have doctors who act like robots, not deviating one iota from the rules set forth but not by them. But folks, the ability to care for women (making the edge) is the result of a researcher's decades of experience. Again, it made it sound like I'm just treating patients on a whim, a devil-may-care attitude. You know now (I hope) that is farthest from the truth.

Next sentence: "I would appreciate it if you could look into this situation since many patients are now inquiring about this."

My reply: Why ask the Board? Doesn't the surgeon have enough authority or guts to just start doing it? Or is there a reason that surgeon somehow can't and is, therefore, deeply troubled having to lash out? The key word here is "many." That's right, many patients were leaving that surgeon's practice (coming to me) like rats off a sinking ship once they found out the truth about avoiding surgery, chemotherapy, and radiation or the cookie-cutter approach, if you like. And many were just appalled and tired of that surgeon's yelling outbursts. Was there something holding that surgeon back? Was it lack of skill or being prohibited by some organization that surgeon belonged to? I hope I'm hiding the obvious enough without disclosing persons or organizations. It will just take some investigative reporter to find the truth behind all this and disclose that surgeon to the light of day. Say what you want about me, folks. Still, to me, it's hard to argue with results, especially the ones I was able to achieve against a much-dreaded disease and merits at least consideration by any knowledgeable person. It reminds me of the Star Trek movie where Captain Kirk and the entire crew violate almost every rule set forth by Star Fleet Command, but at the trial, all is forgiven because they saved the earth.

Next sentence: "I think you should also be aware that Dr. Bretz has lost hospital privileges, and trained in Guadalajara, and does not mention ever being board certified." This surgeon acted like a private investigator. My results must have really bugged that surgeon. Let's look at this half-truth.

My reply: What does this sentence make it sound like? To me, whoever reads it will think, oh boy, on top of everything else, this guy has lost his privileges at his hospital and he was trained in subpar Mexico and probably never Board-certified. What a loser! We're gonna get this guy and stop him from injuring any more patients. Right, because that's what that surgeon's letter to the Board makes it appear. But it's an unrelenting assault and character assassination stacking one untruth upon another. Why didn't the Board (when I met with them) show me the surgeon's letter and ask me straight out?

Ok, now the truth and see if it changes your mind. I have lost my hospital privileges? The truth is, after I lost my position on the heart team and having been out of general surgery for almost ten years, that I lost my referral base and the breast business, with its overhead, let me just get by. With the work at the Marine Corps base at Twentynine Palms, I was able to keep a nice roof over my family's head but I lost my houses and cars.

As a consequence of all that, I couldn't afford malpractice insurance then as I was doing very few surgical cases per year. I had become a dedicated breast surgeon (outside the hospital) and hadn't done a hernia for years and couldn't do a laparoscopic gallbladder. I just let my time at Eisenhower lapse.

Further, now with Lavender, I didn't need the hospital and I could get insurance again. I could do any surgery at an outpatient surgical center. The letter makes it sound like I had done some deeply grievous infraction of ethics or the like, and the hospital terminated me for some horrendous act. You can easily see how untrue negative innuendo successfully builds a case.

It goes on, I was trained in Guadalajara. Doctor, let's get it straight, I went to medical school in Guadalajara but I was trained at Loyola University Medical Center in Chicago. How dare anyone belittles Mexico in this day and age of tolerance and understanding. That surgeon, if not to me, owes the Mexican government, Guadalajara, and the UAG an apology.

That surgeon also should apologize to every doctor of Mexican descent on staff at all the valley hospitals and across America. The last part of the sentence is about board certification. I have dealt with this issue prior to this, and you know the score there. But remember, this was a limited TV spot, and that kind of information would not have been disclosed regardless. We're finally done with this.

The kicker is I was never told by the Board that this competitor surgeon was the first to come forward. It was about a year-and-a-half into a three-year ordeal of sleepless nights that I found this letter. It was amongst the "disclosure" information obtained by the attorney assigned to me by my malpractice company. I just stumbled onto it. The pieces began to slowly come together of what had happened to me and why. I knew Mrs. Smith hadn't conjured this up on her own and wouldn't since everything went so well.

The only thing I knew at first was Mrs. Smith had signed the complaint about "experimental" procedures I was doing. Then after a few days, four more letters of "investigation" with the badge on the front indicating you're involved in some sort of criminal action arrived. Joan went into the post office to sign for the registered letters. If she had just married the guy in the green Dodge Dart, she wouldn't have had to submit herself to this humiliation!

Two of the patients, the Board ultimately dropped. Evidently, the Board couldn't find anything wrong with my charting or treatment. In fact, I sent them back to that surgeon as that was their HMO doctor as they would have to live peaceably with that person. At the same time, another patient called us to inform us the Medical Board threatened her with legal action if she didn't come forward. She said no, she wouldn't sign, and they never did anything. I complied immediately with the Board's request for the charts. I also wrote personal letters to the "investigator" in charge detailing what action I took and why. I also invited that investigator on multiple occasions to come out to the office so he could see firsthand. He never responded to any of those letters and never came out.

I thought (if I were an investigator) that at least I would come out and interview the doctor before any action was taken. As I have said, with renewing my license for forty years without incident, you would think, just out of courtesy of knowing a doctor had cared for thousands of people under very stressful conditions, that some respect (not for me but my station in life) would be forthcoming. Nothing.

While dissecting all these cases would be another book, let's concentrate on two, Mrs. Smith and the lady from Romania. I waited months for the next step with the Board. When it finally came, I was to show up at their Riverside offices. My attorney from the malpractice company came also. She said I should under no circumstances speak my mind. She had come out to the office and knew my propensity to communicate fully. She said the Board would use anything I said against me. So just answer yes or no if possible. My attorney also said the Board was "——l." When we got there and walked in, there were three people, the principal investigator, an older Asian doctor and the

Attorney General of California. I thought, was I going to be read my Miranda Rights?

They asked several personal questions like was I taking any illegal drugs and what drugs I did take, and why. They recorded the interview and can replay it for the public as far as I'm concerned. Like I told the investigator all along, I have nothing to hide.

I think I said already that my leg took a few days to recover where my attorney kicked me to stop explaining. When we came out, I told her exactly what would happen, and I turned out to be right. This was before their "expert" looked at any of the cases. I said they are in this too deep now, and they will revoke my license, stayed with terms and conditions like I always see in their quarterly reports of doctors they have sanctioned.

We already detailed their "expert's" complaint of my treatment of Mrs. Smith. How many times do I have to say the proof's in the pudding? If someone is accused of some wrongdoing or negligence of something that has yet to take place but is predicted based on the old paradigm, like lymph node involvement, and years later there is no lymph node involvement, then only two things were responsible. (1) I was just lucky or (2) I really knew what I was doing based on forty years of personal experience, which was not passive. It included starting the first comprehensive breast center in the Coachella Valley and one of the first in the country in 1988, becoming a principal investigator with the NSABP and National Cancer Institute #17790, and, among other things, like being the author of our country's first large-scale breast cancer prevention clinical trial using Tamoxifen and inventing a new surgical procedure for APBR (fat patch) so more women could benefit. All this besides serving as Cancer Committee Chairman, etc., at Eisenhower. I was also selected to be a principal speaker on President Bush's (HW) Breast Cancer Panel.

Then, if no lymph node involvement and no damage to the patient's breast occurred at the same time her cancer was killed apparently successfully, then just perhaps we should have met face-to-face, and the "expert" (who probably never performed a cryo procedure) could have asked, "Phil, how did you do this? Because if this is true what you achieved, then we need to get the message out and let California lead the way by setting up cryoablation teaching centers." But something like that was/is only in my dreams.

The other patient (the lady and former gymnast from Romania) was where I was extremely negligent in that I performed a procedure which was not indicated. That was the lady who had had a lumpectomy with resultant retained cancer at the margins by, I believe, the same surgeon who sent the letter to the Board. The patient decided she wouldn't have another surgery. This was probably based on her PTSD from being tortured in Nicolae Ceausescu's prison when she tried to escape. After explaining all the options from mastectomy to re-lumpectomy, including radiation and anti-estrogen to cryo, she opted to try cryo even though I told her multiple times (with a friend present) that she was not an ideal case since she already had a lumpectomy and there was no real target.

But I could try and get the margins since I knew where the surgeon made the incision. That seemed reasonable since, as usual, in two months, we would obtain a mammogram and perform a core needle biopsy to determine if cryo was successful or not. Then if not, she would have to make a choice to proceed with standard treatment or do nothing.

I felt all along for forty years that once a patient was given all the options of treatment, then it was up to them what treatment, if any, they wanted and not some standard of care dictated that they had to do or else. Or has our country changed to now include care dictated by some authority instead of free choice by the individual? I'm not trying to convince the reader here, just presenting thoughts that may not be at the fore.

Now months went by with the expert having the charts and assessing my wrongdoing. One day Joan got a phone call from a new patient who said she was referred by Mrs. Smith. *What!?* Now you remember, after she had filed the complaint (about more than a year-and-a-half ago), she visited the office after her procedure, not mentioning that anything was wrong or out of the ordinary. After that, I wrote her a letter detailing why I couldn't see her anymore because of what she accused me of. Now out of the blue, we get a call that Mrs. Smith has referred a patient. What the heck was going on all this time? This episode really threw me for a loop. I hope it motivates you to ask the same question: what the heck is going on here?

Now comes the coup de grace. I call Mrs. Smith's daughter as I hadn't had contact with her mother all this time. I didn't know if she had passed away or had metastatic disease or lymph node involvement or what. Mrs. Smith's daughter came in, and I first asked her how her mom was doing. It turned out she was doing just fine and her mammograms were fine. In that instant, it felt like a massive weight was lifted from me as I had treated her right, irrespective of anyone's opinion and accusations.

I told Mrs. Smith's daughter just what had happened to me as a consequence of her mother's action. She started to cry. She had not known that her mother had done that and was wondering why I declined to follow her anymore. She wanted to write a letter to the Medical Board. You can review that letter again. I was a little shaken when I read her letter. Also, I just picked up that the email was directed to the older surgeon who was at the one and only meeting I had with the Board. I don't know if Mrs. Smith's letter was never acknowledged and if the Board's surgeon had ever relayed that letter to the principal investigator or the Attorney General. Would it have made a difference? I think it should have and at least called into question the motives behind the initial attack by the competitor surgeon. Looks to me like too little too late. To me it was everything, to them nothing.

Considering what's in the letter, whose behavior was unethical? That surgeon never had any investigation into that possible fraudulent writing. Now with that letter, I really didn't understand further pursuing of me by the Board since, as you can read, Mrs. Smith had nothing besides glowing reports for me in spite of my not following her. I made sure her daughter had the names of the three people on the Board as I copied their cards. I told her to send the letter return receipt requested. A FedEx-type letter would be best. I was sure I was going to get a call from the Board that since the person who accused me of "experimental" procedures had withdrawn that accusation that that would end things. It's like if a fight breaks out and the police are called, if no one wants to file a complaint, then nothing is done about anything, and people go their own way. Fat chance. The Board never acknowledged receiving the letter from Mrs. Smith detailing being harassed by the competitor surgeon who threatened her with legal action if she didn't sign a complaint and further, that Mrs. Smith would die if she came to me. I just couldn't believe what was happening to my family and me.

As things wound down months later, I received the certified letter (on my birthday) from the Board detailing their action against me (before I had a chance to review or comment on the "expert's" findings), including revoking my license (stayed with terms and conditions), just as I predicted months earlier when my attorney and I came out of the Board meeting. Guess they made their minds up.

Their action against me was typical of what I had seen for decades in their quarterly reports of action against doctors. As I said, the letter came on my birthday, a coincidence? I was not only required to take Ethics and Professionalism courses (approved by the Board) and about double the continuing medical education (CME) requirements, but I was assigned a probation officer (just like a criminal), and to top it off, I had to (at my own expense) obtain a proctor to review 10% of my cases for the three-year period I was to be on probation.

The entire process was meant to demoralize you to the point of just turning in your license. I think that was their hope. I have about a year-and-a-half to go now on probation. The probation cost is $4,800.00 a year. I asked if, because of COVID, I could get a reduction or make payments, but the answer was no. I had to come up with the entire amount by January 31, 2021. Even if I am able to complete my probation, I will still not be allowed to resume Lavender Procedures when I am totally able to do so to save minds, bodies, and spirit. I was told next year the fee is more than $6,200.00. In 2021, considering COVID, is that abuse?

The Board did say I could do cryoablation under the umbrella of a clinical trial. The problem there is I had already found that used correctly, that Lavender could do away with surgery, chemotherapy and radiation. Yet one trial that I knew of had the patients undergo radiation. In my opinion, if they wanted to test the limits of cryo and get a definitive answer, there should have been no radiation. As it is, yet another trial somewhere in the future will have to answer that question which I already answered. That's why if California decided to institute Lavender Centers and the Lavender Procedure *as pilot clinical trials*, that would resolve the issue the quickest. That would certainly mean the Governor would have to have enough guts to do it. But for me to become involved in a clinical trial that wasn't going to answer the critical questions was a waste of time.

I recently got a call from my probation officer that he was coming out again. I wasn't going to include this slice of the pie but I decided no, I want the public to know exactly what one has to endure. Now we all know the effects of COVID on everyone, right? The government has gone out of its way to assist people with the PPP program, loans from the SBA, states even let criminals go to prevent outbreaks in prisons. We were all basically shutdown. Still, as I write this, people are not wanting to venture out except for necessities. I'm sure you know how COVID impacted you and your family. With that backdrop in mind, out comes my probation officer to ask me the same question, if I'm taking illegal drugs, if I've been involved with the police, etc. He's a nice guy though, all things considered, just doing his job.

At the end of our meeting, he tells me that he has been told to tell me that I'm in non-compliance of my probation. What? I said, I've done everything the Board has asked, like paying the fees, filling out the quarterly reports, having my charts reviewed on time, taking and passing the ethics and professional courses (over $1,000 each) approved by the Board and last, but not least, all the CME hours. What do they want? I ask if they wanted me dead? Without answering that specific question, he said I was in violation because I wasn't seeing enough patients. I think he said he was sorry. I showed him the video of Ruth from Uganda, that she was now five years out and cancer-free. After he left, I sat down and wrote this letter to the Board.

From the Desk of Phillip Bretz

5-15-21

To the Medical Board of California

I just received an email from the Board asking patience and understanding concerning erroneous emails recently sent out. I might ask the Board for the same understanding to this letter. Since being placed on probation, I have complied as my probation officer can attest to every edict by the Board including, but not limited to, fees paid, additional CME, approved courses on Ethics and Professionalism, meetings with my probation officer, mailing charts to my monitor and he has complied also, and filling out quarterly reports and sending hard copies of everything to the Board.

On a visit on May 13th 2021, I was informed by my probation officer I may be held in non-compliance of my probation because of insufficient numbers of patients, like I'm not practicing my trade. Below are a number or reasons why my patient flow is not to be expected like it was when I was on hospital active surgical staff.

1. *As of 5-14-21 Riverside County still has posted on their website COVID as MODERATE. It still restricts any meetings of numbers of people and still social distancing and masks etc. My patients are mostly Medicare age and a lot of them are still frightened to venture out of the house for anything except food and other essentials.*

2. *Unlike a family doctor that may see say a diabetic patient several times a month to establish a routine for diet and blood sugars, I generally only see my patient yearly if all is well.*

3. *While there has been a burgeoning of 'telemedicine,' my work as a breast doctor is (forgive the pun) 'hands on.' I can't expect the patient to tell me how a lump feels or even if she has one or not.*

4. *Some of my patients have called the office to say they are very concerned about going to the hospital especially when over crowded with COVID patients and sitting with numbers of people exposed despite social distancing. They say they will come in when all this settles down, so that limits the patients I see as well.*

5. *Many of my patients come from long distances like Chicago, Washington state. Because of travel restrictions and again being exposed to people on the plane, those patients are not coming in.*

6. *I have been in practice so long that a number of my patients who I've kept out of harms way concerning breast cancer or actually saved their lives are now so old they are moving to be closer to their children. And most of the doctors that I was on staff with are either retired or dead so that referral base is gone.*

7. *Because of COVID the patients who do call for an appointment we space out so as not to have any more than one patient in the office at a time. My time with each patient approaches an hour so that also limits daily patient load.*

8. *Seeing me after they get a 'clear letter' from whatever mammography facility means that coming to see me is an 'option' which some don't exercise yearly.*

9. *Since I'm not on any staff, any referral base has been lost for years and I don't advertise and my only way of obtaining new patients is through old patient referrals.*

10. *Lastly, the Board has seen to it that I'm in a 'catch 22' situation especially with attracting new patients. Most people are internet savvy and can Google anything including doctors. Any potential new patients who Google me find straight away I'm on probation by the Board and therefore decline to engage me.*

It is for these reasons I ask the same understanding of the Board as to the numbers of patients I see. The office is open 40 hrs a week from 9 AM-5 PM. Because of the above now being known to everyone. To revoke my license (if that's the contemplated next step) after 40 years of serving the women of California (that is over 13,000) patients, no lawsuits for my breast work and having my license renewed without incident by the Board all those 40 years would seem a cruel and unusual punishment by many. And to totally take away my only livelihood would also seem to be cruel and unusual punishment.

As always, I invite anyone from the Board to pay me a visit (as I have never had anything to hide), and see what I have accomplished and know what happened to those women I did perform cryoablation on. It might interest the Board to know that all the patients in Group 1 are alive and cancer-free going on seven years with no axillary lymph node involvement that was predicted.

It takes a long time to know what I know and I do my best daily for each patient. In fact, yesterday after coming home, I received a frantic call from a patient that she had just received a text from the hospital saying they saw something on her mammogram and wanted her to come in for an ultrasound within two weeks. The patient called me crying that she was so upset with no one at the hospital to talk to late Friday.

She felt the hospital had no compassion about the fear invoked in a woman that gets that call of an abnormality found on mammography and that they left her high and dry and afraid. After my wife and I were home relaxing preparing dinner, I said we would meet her and her husband at the office in an hour.

She was so grateful. And last week a new patient referred by an old patient had an abnormal mammogram was scheduled for a biopsy at the hospital. When she underwent imaging, the doctor present at the time said he wouldn't biopsy anything and didn't know what the other doctor had seen. There was no discussion of the two doctors in front of the patient to resolve the issue and the patient was left petrified and confused as to exactly what went on. She came to me and I saw her the same day and resolved the situation. She also was very grateful as was her husband and was glad she was now in my breast practice.

And I just saw a Black woman from Blythe who came to see me for the last time as she is now 86 and with her husband passing, it is difficult for her to travel. That is typical of what is happening now with my patients. But she is almost 30 years out from an aggressive breast cancer that I apparently cured and she still has her breasts intact again like G-D made them. I guess Black Lives matter to me (as all women do) decades before it became national news.

I'm also sorry the Board chose not to follow up on the competitor surgeon that wrote the original complaint not just filled with erroneous inuendo but telling the patient that left that practice I would destroy her breast and nipple and that she would die if she came to me. Of course, none of that happened and that patient is cancer-free with her breast intact like G-D made it. That surgeon also threatened the patient with harassing phone calls and the threat of a lawsuit if she didn't sign a complaint against me. Again, the Board never told me it was a competitor surgeon in town that filed the original complaint about my performing cryoablation an FDA approved procedure and more than a year and a half into the Board review the patient found out what had happened to me and cried as she immediately wrote a retraction letter. Apparently, sadly this made no difference to the Board.

Make no mistake, I serve a great purpose in my community and have for 40 years. I've played a very pivotal role in breast cancer research having founded the first comprehensive breast center in the Coachella Valley in 1988 and being designated a Principal Investigator by the NCI for over 20 years which is still active 17790. I was first to bring National Cancer Institute clinical trials to the Valley and was asked by the State of California to testify in their investigation of the drug Tamoxifen since I am the author of our country's first large-scale breast cancer prevention clinical trial. And that trial proved that Tamoxifen lowered the risk of breast cancer by 50%. That came from me (FDA IND 34,223) not a major cancer center. While this is a spattering on my accomplishments, I will also say I was awarded the Carnegie Medal for an outstanding act of heroism.

It didn't make any difference to me if that person was Black, White, Hispanic, Yellow or Red. I was willing to sacrifice my own life to save another human being. I went into a burning SUV twice to save a man who was on fire from an accident.

To me I answered the ultimate ethical question on that day. While I will continue to comply with everything the Board asks of me until my probation period is over, there needs to be an understanding of my situation and role of caring for women by the Board.

Regards,
Phillip Bretz

Below is the response I received from the Board, or more specifically, it appears one person at the Board has the authority to wield this kind of power. As I already stated, next year the "fee" for probation is over $6,000, and if my probation is extended that would mean an additional $6,000 or more in the year 2023 when I'm supposed to have completed my probation. There is no way in hell I can achieve the desired number of patients now, especially with COVID hanging over everyone's heads. My patients are mostly Medicare age and, as a result, do have comorbidities, which we all know makes COVID more deadly. Unless a miracle happens, I won't be able to afford the continued (apparently forever) years' fees, so my ability to help people, oh hell, let's just say it, cure breast cancer, will come to an end. Fair and just treatment?

Dr. Bretz,

I reviewed the letter you sent to ████████████

You are not in non-compliance, you are in non-practice, pended status. Any non-practice time will extend your probation.

You are currently on probation with the Medical Board of California for a period of three years.

I believe everyone has been hit hard, in one way or another due to the coronavirus pandemic. You are on probation and must abide by the terms and conditions of your probation.

You are required to work at least 40 hours in direct patient care per month. If you had seen 40 to 60 patients in a month, your practice monitor would have reviewed 6 to 9 charts per month. So that would be 18 to 27 charts per quarter. If you saw less than 100 patients per month, your practice monitor needs to review 15%, not 10% of your patients seen.

In Quarter 1 – 2020, your practice monitor reviewed four charts. Since his report states that represents 10% of your patients for the quarter, I am assuming you saw 40 patients in three months, or in the 1st Quarter. This would be non-practice.

In Quarter 2 – 2020, your practice monitor reviewed two charts. Since his report states that represents 10% of your patients for the quarter, I am assuming you saw 20 patients in three months, or in the 2nd Quarter. This would be non-practice.

In Quarter 3 – 2020, your practice monitor reviewed one chart. Since his report states that represents 10% of your patients for the quarter, I am assuming you saw 10 patients in three months, or in the 3rd Quarter. This would be non-practice.

In Quarter 4 – 2020, your practice monitor reviewed three charts. Since his report states that represents 10% of your patients for the quarter, I am assuming you saw 30 patients in three months, or in the 4th Quarter. This would be non-practice.

Please continue to send in your patient list, either monthly or quarterly.

Thank you.

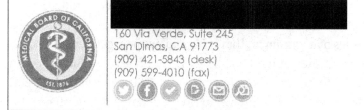

160 Via Verde, Suite 245
San Dimas, CA 91773
(909) 421-5843 (desk)
(909) 599-4010 (fax)

In the middle of writing this memoir, I got to see Diana, one of my poster Lavender girls. As of April 14, 2021, she is now seven years out from Lavender and cancer-free, but there is a story behind this. She is probably the only woman on the face of the earth with THREE cancers in one breast yet still has that breast. She is of Puerto Rican descent, and back in the day, she could have given Miss Puerto Rico a run for her money. In any case, her story started in 1994. At age forty she developed an invasive left breast cancer at about two o'clock in the upper outer quadrant. This was operated on by another surgeon in town. She went until about 2003 when she developed a local recurrence at the original site. Under my care then, I had advanced to using APBR. You can see a picture of how this looked in my paper on page 1.

Basically, it's like a foley catheter with a balloon attached that is blown up with saline, and the catheter provides a route for the radiation source to go down it and provide the area with target radiation. The rationale was that about 90% of local recurrences are within 1 centimeter of the lumpectomy site. It provided twice daily radiation for five days instead of five days a week for six weeks of external beam.

It also cut way back on breast shrinkage from radiation and the skin changes that accompany it, specifically peau d'orange. For me, it was a breath of fresh air after decades of dogma about how you had to radiate the entire breast because there was cancer all over that you couldn't see, etc.

I came up with that new surgical procedure called "The Autologous Free Fat Transfer" published in ASTRO. Now standard of care and the "book" say you can't radiate a breast again once radiated, and the breast must, therefore, come off. Well, both Diana and her husband wanted her breast saved if possible. I knew there was no "evidenced-based medicine" to say that using APBR after external beam radiation was acceptable. But again, just like Lavender and Tamoxifen, I reasoned (from decades of experience) that if I could, with targeted radiation, kill that recurrence, then at least locally with the breast, she should be fine. She had to be then one of the only women in the world to be treated outside standard of care in this manner. I have always maintained that once being informed of all the options available and given time to reconsider, that whatever the patient decides to do, that is what should be done. I thought in our country every patient is free to choose (even against medical advice or all the data in the world) what that particular patient receives in the way of treatment or not. But some people apparently don't believe that.

We went ahead with re-lumpectomy and APBR and she went until 2014, then developed a THIRD cancer in the same breast. Only this time, it was on the opposite side around nine o'clock. It was about 5 millimeters in diameter. Being able to pick up a recurrent cancer at about 5 millimeters is a reflection of one of the many positive side effects of seeing patient's decades after treatment. Now I'm about to really break the rules and say she is probably the only girl on earth who developed THREE cancers in the same breast and still has that breast. For those who haven't guessed, yes, I was doing Lavender Procedure then, and that's what both Diana and her husband opted for (after discussing ALL options, including standard of care, requiring for sure this time to do a mastectomy). Folks, that was seven years ago, and she still feels great, like a whole woman intact and cancer-free. In my estimation, the proof's in the pudding. Is it worth anything to anybody to know that this is possible instead of just lopping off the breast and moving on to the next hernia operation and never seeing that patient again?

Wow, at least my wife is really impressed, having personally seen the horrendous results of other surgeons' attempts at breast surgery. I can't tell you how gratifying it is that I had the vision and knowledge to care for Diana as I did. Seeing these girls seven years out from Lavender and cancer-free means more to me than any certificate, including from the American Board of Surgery or Fellow of the American College of Surgeons (FACS), another organization I'm not allowed to broach because of my iniquities. I hope you're asking yourself if this guy can do it, how come everyone isn't at least trying to replicate his findings? How come he's not on the cover of *Time* magazine?

So, I will leave it up to the people across this great land to decide what to do about anything. My main reasons for writing this book were to give my grandchildren something to read about how I was if I'm not here when they come of age. The other reason with the publishing of my paper, to get the word out to the women of this land in the hope that something will take hold to demand change because every woman's life matters.

NEWS FLASH (it seems they just keep coming, folks):

On JUNE 27, 2021, I wrote a letter to the Food and Drug Administration (FDA) and asked them to provide definitive statements on cryoablation. Either I would have been wrong all the while and I would issue an apology, and take my medicine without further debate, or someone else was wrong, then what should happen? Below is my letter so there is no misunderstanding of what I asked of the FDA. Following that is their response. I might add here that the FDA, for its part on ANY dealings with me from my initiating the breast cancer prevention trial to this letter, has always treated me with respect, dignity and responded to me.

Having read the two letters, hopefully you will come to the same conclusion I did. Namely, that this letter from the highest authority in the land (the US Food and Drug Administration) concerning medical devices and their use puts the final nail in the coffin of the false accusations, negative inuendo, lies and preordained predictions that didn't come to pass; like I was at fault for not doing a lymph node dissection or my NCI Principal Investigator's number was outdated and defunct or the cryo procedure I performed on the lady from Romania was not indicated.

Please pay particular attention to the strong wording in the FDA's letter in the fourth paragraph under Section 1006. They don't mince words about the AUTHORITY a health care practitioner has to help a patient assuming both are in control of their faculties.

First, my letter.

From the Desk of Phillip Bretz, M.D.

6-27-21

Dear FDA:

I am hoping you can clear up a question that people skirt around but should be crystal clear for everyone including doctors who use cryoablation and Medical Boards that determine whether a particular technology is 'EXPERIMENTAL' or not. The question is, is destruction of breast cancers using either the IceSense or Sanarus systems deemed by the FDA to be experimental or not? Also, can it be used outside of ANY clinical trial or protocol for killing breast cancers. This is particularly relevant as many doctors are using whichever system 'OUTSIDE' of any clinical trial or protocol just treating patients in the office. The next question is, are all these doctors using cryoablation in their offices in conflict of any law or somehow using cryoablation in violation of any edict by the FDA?

I have included information concerning 510Ks and advertising by these companies. It seems pretty clear with their ads and 510Ks that it is cleared (that means any doctor can use it to kill malignant tumors in various organs including the breast), right or wrong? Just because not many doctors are using cryoablation doesn't make it 'experimental' it's just that not many want to venture into this technology even though it is cleared to do so, that is killing breast cancer in the office setting.

I would very much appreciate a succinct answer to my questions. If you need to speak to me, feel free to call my cell.

Regards,
Phillip Bretz, M.D.

Next is their response.

Support at FDA/DICE Re:FW: ORP Mail Received [ref:_00Dd0fegA._500t0p05NP:ref]
2 messages

Tue, Aug 10, 2021 at 2:34 PM

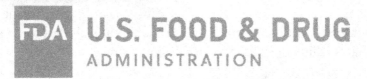

Dear Dr. Bretz:

Your letter of June 27, 2021 was forwarded to the Division of Industry and
Consumer Education (DICE) at FDA's Center for Devices and Radiological
Health (CDRH) DICE@fda.hhs.gov e-mail account.

The FDA does not have an "experimental" designation for medical
devices. Medical devices are cleared [510(k) or approved (PMA) for
specific intended uses (what the device does) and indications for use
(intended patient population, use environment, etc.).

However, the FDA is not involved in interactions between patients and
health care providers under the Practice of Medicine: Regarding
prescription of medical devices, Section 1006 of the Federal Food, Drug
and Cosmetic Act (FD&C Act) states:

*Nothing in this Act shall be construed to limit or interfere with the authority of a
health care practitioner to prescribe or administer any legally marketed device to
a patient for any condition or disease within a legitimate health care practitioner-
patient relationship. This section shall not limit any existing authority of the
Secretary to establish and enforce restrictions on the sale or distribution, or in the
labeling, of a device that are part of a determination of substantial equivalence,
established as a condition of approval, or promulgated through regulations.
Further, this section shall not change any existing prohibition on the promotion of
unapproved uses of legally marketed devices*

The Practice of Medicine permits a healthcare provider to use a medical device for an intended use or indication for use that was not in the cleared or approved intended uses and/or indications for use. This is known as "off-label use."

The FDA cannot address the effectiveness of off-label use because the data received in the premarket application only addressed the use/s for which the cryoablation devices were cleared or approved.

Insurance companies might consider off-label use to be "experimental." That designation is determined by individual insurers.

Please note that although healthcare practitioner may use medical devices off-label, the manufacturers of those devices may NOT label or advertise off-label use/es of the device. Device companies may only promote their devices for their cleared or approved uses.

Here is a link to guidance about off-label use:

Guidance for Industry Responding to Unsolicited Requests for Off-Label Information About Prescription Drugs and Medical Devices: Draft Guidance

https://www.fda.gov/files/drugs/published/Responding-to-Unsolicited-Requests-for-Off-Label-Information-About-Prescription-Drugs-and-Medical-Devices.pdf

"Off-Label" and Investigational Use Of Marketed Drugs, Biologics, and Medical Devices: Guidance for Institutional Review Boards and Clinical Investigators

https://www.fda.gov/regulatory-information/search-fda-guidance-documents/label-and-investigational-use-marketed-drugs-biologics-and-medical-devices

The above guidances are only in draft form. Draft guidance is issued for comment purposes only. However, draft guidance can give people an idea of the Agency's thinking on a topic. Medical devices can be used off label in clinical trials if the appropriate Investigational Device Exemption (IDE) regulations in 21 CFR 812 are followed.

The content of that FDA letter is very important for my defense. If the FDA of our great country says (reading between the lines) what transpires between a health care provider and the patient in order to help said patient is totally and only between said patient and their doctor, not any other authority. Like I said before, if the patient, after all options have been discussed and given time to decide, wants to eat two pounds of blueberries to cure her cancer (although no doctor would advocate that) because she read it on the internet, *then that's what should happen.*

All this, as I said, assumes the health care provider is competent, knowledgeable enough and is acting in good faith. And that the patient has been given time to understand all options and has chosen whatever they want to do irrespective of any other authority anywhere or any standard of care. Now, if the Medical Board had on their website in 2014 a section on the dos and don'ts of cryoablation (and we need to know when it was put up, because it will be now) and I was negligent in not accessing their website about cryoablation, then case closed against me. But if they don't, please re-read the letter from the FDA under "oncology." It says, "The system may be used for ablation of cancerous or malignant tissue." It doesn't get much clearer than that. That is the FDA's wording on the 510(k) of IceCure and it says as plain as day that their device (almost the same wording for Sanarus) is cleared for use to treat cancer. And the FDA didn't restrict its use to any specific organ either.

Further, in the third paragraph on the second page the FDA states, "Insurance companies might consider off-label use to be 'experimental.' That designation is determined by individual insurers." To me, the use of "experimental" is totally inappropriate in the case of cryo and I wish people would stop dancing around it and start trying to cure cancer with this technology all the while preserving mind, body, and spirit. That's my hope anyway, is it yours? Then you have to do something about it to shake the very foundations of the medical industrial complex so all women are treated right. To my thinking/experience the only way to do this is through the Lavender Way/Procedure, out of the hands of functionaries.

So that competitor surgeon was wrong to say it wasn't cleared to treat cancer or what I was doing was not in the best interest of any of the patients. I did act in the best interest of my patients and the cancer-free survivors are the proof. The FDA says it's no one else's business. Or have we come to the place where individual desires are supplanted by some committee? Why have doctors anymore? Meanwhile, this competitor surgeon destroyed me and my good name. That surgeon didn't have the courtesy to research any of the statements in the letter to the Medical Board which were half-truths and lies. If that competitor surgeon had not written that letter or threatened and harrassed Mrs. Smith, by now I would have California the world's leader in cryoablation of breast cancer, obviating surgery, chemotherapy, and radiation. But that isn't happening unless the governor has enough guts to re-open my case. It won't do any good to write the Medical Board, in my case it would be akin to the governor (and the governor only) staying my execution, reinstating me and expunging all negative references to my name and requesting I return to help however I could. That could include working with the Medical Board to detail a statement on cryoablation and under what circumstances it should be carried out. Then I could still do it.

Another thing to consider here is I started doing cryoablation as self-taught and these cases were my first experiences, but look at the results. If I was enabled to do hundreds of cases and hone my skill even more (and every other doctor that could be taught), and yes, I would include the competitor surgeon, then we might see the true potential of the Lavender Procedure.

On October 14, 2021, I executed the form from the Medical Board of California to "Surrender of License While on Probation." I did this because my probation would apparently last forever because of being in "non-practice." As a last-ditch effort to preserve my station in life I have fought so hard for, I have attempted to answer the question they posed which is, "Reason for License Surrender." I sent a hard copy to the President of the Board who holds a degree in Doctor of Jurisprudence (JD). I wonder just how much the Attorney General (present at my interview with the Board which consisted of two people) actually knew about any of these important details, like the original competitor surgeon's letter or the fact that Mrs. Smith (name changed), the patient who filed the "complaint," in her letter of retraction said, "not in a million years," would she file a complaint against me if she wasn't extremely intimidated into signing a document that she really didn't understand. I never got the chance to see this document Mrs. Smith originally signed. Because if a lawyer would have read that letter of retraction, right away they would have discovered what had occurred as to why Mrs. Smith felt she was compelled to sign some official looking letter. I won't tell you; you'll have to read my response below and see if you can guess what that surgeon might be guilty of. Now we come to the final pronouncements of my fate. The following is a form for "Surrender of License While on Probation." In it there is a small space for the doctor (in this case me) to say why he is surrendering his license. In that space I say, "See attached," then my letter follows.

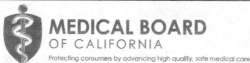

MEDICAL BOARD
OF CALIFORNIA
Protecting consumers by advancing high quality, safe medical care.

Enforcement Program
2005 Evergreen Street, Suite 1200
Sacramento, CA 95815-5401
Phone: (916) 263-2125
Fax: (916) 263-1692
www.mbc.ca.gov

Gavin Newsom, Governor, State of California | Business, Consumer Services and Housing Agency | Department of Consumer Affairs

REQUEST FOR SURRENDER OF LICENSE
WHILE ON PROBATION

Pursuant to the Decision and Order, if you cease practicing due to retirement, health reasons or are otherwise unable to satisfy the terms and conditions of probation, you may request the surrender of your license.

Once your application has been filed, the Medical Board (Board) will review and evaluate your request for surrender. The Board reserves the right to evaluate the request and to exercise its discretion whether or not to grant the request or take any other action deemed appropriate and reasonable under the circumstances. If accepted, the Board will prepare a formal Agreement for Surrender of License for your signature. Until this document is signed by you and the Executive Director of the Board, the license surrender will not become effective and the Board's case will not be closed.

Full Name: PHILLIP DeEVANS BRETZ

Medical License No.: ▮▮▮▮▮

Address: ▮▮▮▮▮▮ NA STEB LeQUINTA, CA 92253

Telephone Number: ▮▮▮▮▮

Last Date You Practiced Medicine: 10·31-21

Reason for License Surrender: SEE ATTACHED

Signature: _____   Date: 10.14-21

Printed Name: PHILLIP BRETZ

Received by: _____   Date: _____

From the Desk of Mr. Phillip Bretz
    Reason for license surrender?
    Is this a rhetorical question?
    Since the Board has renewed my license for 40 years without
question, with me doing thousands of sometimes very complicated
surgical cases (including the First Lady and Secret Service personnel),
and for the last 33 years as a dedicated breast cancer surgeon/
researcher (the most litigious outside obstetrics with 0 lawsuits) with
over 13,000 patients from all over the world, and carrying a Principal
Investigator number with the NCI renewed yearly last time January
2021 with the active number of 17790, (incidentally the Boards
"expert" was wrong when he declared my five digit number was no
longer valid), and considering I was the author of a truly ground
breaking clinical trial, our country's first large-scale breast cancer
prevention clinical trial using the drug Tamoxifen FDA IND 34,223,
the results of which showed Tamoxifen reduced the risk of breast
cancer by 50% and now untold numbers of women worldwide are
preventing breast cancer because of that trial (did something good
there). I had the vision to found the first comprehensive breast center
in the Coachella Valley (1988 when there was no such thing), and
one of the first in the country and have pioneered multiple ground
breaking techniques like Accelerated Partial Breast Radiation (APBR)
including inventing a new surgical procedure using an autologous free
fat patch for APBR (published), and pioneering The Lavender Way
and Lavender Procedure (cryoablation), which portends a totally
new paradigm in diagnosing and treating breast cancer (now having
cancer-free patients over seven and a half years out from a 20 minute
office procedure) saving breasts, lives and hundreds of thousands of
dollars for the system, and since I served as Chairman of the Cancer
Committee Eisenhower Memorial Hospital and since the governing
board at Eisenhower renewed my privileges for all those thirty years,
without restriction, specifically looking into my outcomes, conduct,
professionalism and ethics as stated in their letters and since I served
as the field liaison officer for the American College of Surgeons at
EMH and since I was awarded the Carnegie Medal for an outstanding

act of heroism when I answered the most ethical question ever asked, "Would you sacrifice your life for someone you don't even know," and since I have letters of commendation from the White House, the erstwhile Soviet Union, a former US President, a former Governor of California, the Commanding General of the Marine Air Ground Combat Center at 29 Palms, General R.H. Sutton and C.S. Chitwood, Commander of the Navy at 29 (where I was a civilian physician covering the emergency room for three years), and I'm at the height of my career, why the hell would I want to surrender my license to practice medicine, the most coveted license mankind has to offer? The simple answer is I don't want to.

However, because I have been in so-called "non-practice" for 18 months (which by the way covers all the COVID down time when all physicians were all in non-practice) and since because I have previously detailed the reasons why I'm not seeing 20 or so patients daily where I had before including but not limited to not being on a hospital staff since 2009 thus no referrals there, not advertising, my Medicare patients come from all over and many are still afraid to fly or are actually restricted, and summer in the desert brings weeks of temperatures in excess of 110 degrees where local authorities tell people to stay indoors (especially older senior population) and half the population leaves.

Page 2

I see virtually no "new" patients now as if one is referred, they Google me and find out I'm on probation and negligent thus not making an appointment, and since most of my patients are senior Medicare age the most susceptible to COVID and with current restrictions many are still afraid to venture out except for food, etc.

The only reason I am forced to surrender my license is the Board has said that because of my "non-practice" issue my probation would be extended "indefinitely" also at a cost of over $6,000.00 per year including quarterly meetings with my "probation officer," quarterly reports handed in on time and my "practice monitor" reviewing my cases, it becomes untenable for me. Some might see this as cruel and unusual punishment given my reasons why I don't see a lot of patients now.

This is all disappointingly enigmatic and difficult to understand since the Board's action against me was initiated by a competitor surgeon in the valley, not a patient. The Board knows who that is. That letter was full of negative innuendo (like I was trained in Mexico, not true, I went to medical school in Mexico, I did my surgical training at Loyola University Medical Center in Chicago). It was full of totally false statements (like I would destroy the patient's breast and nipple and leave her with a hard lump in her breast) none of which happened. Further, the Board should know I never got the chance to refute any of these false statements or meet the competitor surgeon face to face with the Board because I was never informed of its existence. I only found it perusing thru discovery material my attorney had sent me after the verdict was in. (I understand that's the attorney's fault). Further, the Board should be aware that the competitor surgeon in question made multiple harassing and threatening phone calls to my patient who was successfully treated with the Lavender Procedure. That surgeon told my patient that she would die if she came to me and that if the patient didn't sign a complaint against me that the surgeon would file a lawsuit against her and take her to court. This is conduct unbefitting a licensed physician and highly unprofessional and highly unethical and the Board should look into this including questioning the patient. Alternatively, the Board can read the extensive letter of retraction the patient wrote on my behalf when she found out what I was going through as she wrote, an "unnecessary investigation." Because if that harassed patient never signed that complaint form provided for her, the Board would never have had any issues with me, I reckon. And since I had at the time probably the most experience in the State of California using cryoablation (an FDA approved device for treating cancer, approved in 2010 four years ahead of when I started to use this technology), I was extremely disappointed and numbed that I didn't get the opportunity to explain to the Board's "expert" the multiple decisions I made regarding the treatments I performed on my patients. The verdict just came down. Cryoablation and the Lavender

Way and Lavender Procedure offer a totally new way to diagnose and treat breast cancer which should not have been subjected to the old paradigm since Lavender renders the old paradigm obsolete. I say this now since as already discussed, many of my patients are over seven and a half years out treated with the Lavender Procedure and cancer-free. Now either I guessed right on all those patients or just perhaps I had brought something to the table after 40 years of trying to find an answer to breast cancer no one else envisioned. How could that be? It's the same thing that happened when I was the first to author the Tamoxifen prevention trial. No other researcher in the land from Harvard, to Sloan Kettering to MD Anderson to Stanford had the slightest inkling that Tamoxifen could be used for active breast cancer prevention, it was just me.

Page 3

I readily admit my thinking throughout my entire surgical career has been out of the box yet in all those years, yet CNN found my researched intriguing enough to do a three-part series on me, Vogue magazine also among others, but the Board never contacted me about anything I was doing that certainly back then wasn't standard of care like the Tamoxifen trial.

Where do breakthroughs in cancer care and thus saving lives come from? I can assure you it's not from doing the same thing for decades on end. That's why the deaths from breast cancer have been the same for over 40 years and over 40,000 yearly.

I wonder since it's breast cancer awareness month if anyone would be interested in my outcomes of the cancer-free patients treated in an office setting in 20 minutes? They all resumed normal activity immediately treated with no need for surgery, chemotherapy or radiation. How did I do that? No one asked. Would anyone anywhere would want to know how I achieved those outcomes of very grateful patients and let cryoablation (aka The Lavender Procedure) see the light of day and start saving all our women, let them see it. You know you can talk to my patients. We are all concerned with and hope for a defeat of cancer.

Just this weekend I noted while watching NFL football games all the hats and some of the t-shirts the coaches were wearing said:

CRITICAL CATCH
INTERCEPT CANCER

The NFL is calling for us (meaning researchers) to intercept cancer? Well, that's exactly what I did and can prove it. I thought we were all in this together? For all these reasons and under the current circumstances, I find it impossible to continue as a licensed physician in the State of California. If, however, after considering all this and how it fraudulently started, and reviewing the letter of retraction (which————MD received, not sure if any other Board members, i.e., Investigator ████ or the Attorney General received that letter which———- MD should have forwarded, I never heard a thing), but if the Board wishes to re-open my case, I could help the Board with guidelines for cryoablation and let California lead the way in breast cancer diagnosis and treatment of breast cancer. If not, then the Board has done what it set out to do from the outset I fear (because you believed that letter sent by the competitor surgeon whose motives include, unprofessional and unethical conduct I want you to investigate).

The letter of retraction is interesting for a couple of reasons. First, the patient never intended to file a complaint against me (as stated in her letter, "not in a million years") and only did so under extreme intimidation and threat of a lawsuit (with untold consequences for my patient) by that competitor surgeon that would take her to court if she didn't sign a complaint against me. I have the letter if you are unable to find it and would be happy to forward it to the Board. The word escapes me but Ms. ████ being a Doctor of Jurisprudence (JD) would surely be able to provide it, where intentional intimidation of a person is used to obtain something of value. Then too, the recent letter I received from the FDA is also interesting, a copy of which is provided.

Page 4

You have destroyed me and a sterling reputation in my community I spent forty years achieving, hurt my family, my patients and everything I have stood for in my entire surgical career. Many many people are proud to say I am their doctor and they are proud of my meager accomplishments because they know the truth. You can put another "notch" on your gun. There is a TV commercial everyone knows about "Californian's dream big." That's exactly what I did to show the NCI that people from my state just aren't from the land of "fruits and nuts," as they called us back in the day. Denzel Washington has said, "If you fail, fail big." I wonder if Denzel would question these entire proceedings?

Regards,
Mr. Bretz

CC – to———————, JD, - President of the Medical Board of California

Subject	NCI RCR Registration Approved for Dr. Phillip D. Bretz (IVR-17790) Request R000148410	
From	<RCRNS@nih.gov>	*roundcube*
To	<drbretz@visionarybreastcenter.com>	
Bcc	<RCRNS@nih.gov>	
Date	2021-02-05 16:35	

Dear Dr. Phillip D. Bretz (IVR-17790),

The Cancer Therapy Evaluation Program, NCI has approved your registration packet for request **R000148410.**

You are currently registered as an **INVESTIGATOR** with an **ACTIVE** registration status. Your registration expiration date is **21-Feb-2022.**

Comments:

Next are the last couple communications with the Medical Board of California. I sent my final letter to the Medical Board "return receipt requested" so as to document they actually received it. Following that is the letter from which you can draw your own conclusions. Mine is only that twenty days have gone by without a word. Today is the 6th of November 2021. As you see, I let my license expire on, of all days, Halloween. I did this since the Board had informed me because I was, according to them, in "non-practice," (even though the office is open 9 a.m. to 5 p.m. weekdays and on weekends as needed) and my probation would be extended indefinitely. You can review my letter to the Board outlining the reasons why I am not seeing the requisite number of patients.

I said, some people might consider my never-ending probation to be cruel and unusual punishment. The Board told me to "volunteer" to get the number of patient visits at an acceptable level. Of course, the Board knows that with the public disclosure of my "probation" for being negligent, there was no way in hell that anyone would even let me volunteer and even if they did, for how long would I have to do that? I hope you can understand my frustration at this and the reason why now if you see me, just call me Mr. Bretz. Actually, Phil is fine. I never made an issue out of someone having to call me "doctor."

From the Desk of Mr. Phillip Bretz

10-27-21

Dear—-

I am writing today since my previous correspondence of days ago has not been acknowledged. As you may know, I have not renewed my medical license which is due to expire on the 31st (Halloween, how appropriate!). If you received my previous letter along with the form to "surrender of license while on probation," you know I sent a copy to Ms. ====== (with return receipt requested), as I wanted her to weigh in on my proceedings. All along I felt like my life was being trifled with or otherwise being treated in a frivolous and condescending manner. You guys have been trained well to accomplish your set goals. That all my 40 plus years of serving people (as their go to surgeon) in the Coachella Valley and around the world (literally) didn't amount to a hill of beans to steal a quote from the movie Casablanca. And while I recognize the need to "policing" of my profession for "bad apples," it seemed like there were no checks and balances anyone paid attention to like one of the founding principles of our country to govern people fairly like the Legislative, Judicial and Executive branches of our government keeping tabs on each other. In my particular case, I found it very disconcerting that one person as the term (I) was used instead of the Medical Board (implying more than one person) was to make the decision that my probation would extend into the future indefinitely. In essence, saying that all through COVID which is where my 18 months of apparently being in "non-practice" would have taken me where every physician in this land was in "non-practice," that fact made no difference and that I had to abide by the rules of my probation, really? This on top of the fact that I paid $4,800.00 for the yearly privilege of being on probation and that next year the fee goes up to over $6,000.00 at a time when the Federal Government is doling out billions of dollars to sustain people because of COVID is very difficult to justify, seems to me. But who am I but just a proverbial "disposable cog in the wheel?"

So, while my time as a licensed physician is apparently being allowed to just run its course so I disappear, I would like the following facts to be noted. Am I worried that I can't be re-instated even though my license was not renewed? I should say not. The Medical Board can do anything they want to do to anyone at any time, isn't that true?

Page 2
I would like the following facts to be noted:

1. That the original complaint against me was filed not by a patient (and never would have been), but by a competitor surgeon in town who might have done this capricious activity before (please check).

2. That the original letter from that surgeon was full of half-truths and falsehoods.

3. Probably most important is that I was never apprised of that letter. And the only reason I know about the letter is after the verdict came in that my treatment was an "extreme departure from standard-of-care" and my license was revoked stayed etc, that my attorney forwarded material and I found it there.

Further, because of that I was never given the opportunity to face my accuser in front of the Board to refute the entire letter as to the lies it contained sentence by sentence. And that this abomination has resulted in my good name being dragged through the mud before my entire community to now ridicule me after 40 years of saving lives.

4. That I never was given the opportunity to account for my actions concerning the treatment of my patients with the Lavender Procedure. That is, once the Board's "Expert" had made his pronouncements, I was never called in to sit across from him to explain anything concerning what Lavender means and why I did or didn't do certain things. For example, he denounced the fact that I didn't perform axillary lymph node dissections. The reason I didn't was the fact that I knew the genetics of these tumors, how small they were, the patient's personal history and biology of the tumor and clinical status of the patient's lymph nodes under ultrasound guidance. Further that I used 40 years of experience in diagnosing and treating breast cancer to make my decisions. Not just that but as you are aware, I follow all my patients for decades, many well over 30 years unlike the vast majority of surgeons doing breast surgery that never see the patient again. Also, cryoablation portends a totally different set of guidelines as opposed to the old standard. If one hasn't done a cryoablation case or bothered to follow the patients, how can one make a judgement about cryoablation? I was never told the Board's "Expert" either had done many cryo cases or none and was therefore judging me on the old standards. He portended that since I didn't perform axillary lymph node dissection, my patients would be riddled with axillary cancer and by extension eventually die because of my negligence. The fact is, almost eight years later in the patients I performed Lavender on that I followed diligently, not one of them in groups 1 and 2 has any axillary involvement with cancer. So, either I guessed right on all of them or perhaps like I said I had opened the

door to a new kind of treatment for all women with breast cancer where we didn't have to destroy their bodies and none of the bad things portended by breast cancer happened to them.

Page 3

5. A real problem for me is the fact that the patient who filed the supposed complaint (and the Board knows who that is) never wrote those words that appeared on the original correspondence by the Board concerning the complaint. I believe if you check under oath, it was the competitor surgeon who typed the complaint letter out and threatened the patient with a lawsuit and being taken to court if she didn't sign that document. In the patient's letter of retraction (which I have and can supply anyone at the Board with if they don't have it) it is clear that the patient didn't know what she was signing and signed it under extreme duress and fear of the lawsuit. I think there is a name for that but I'm not a lawyer. As I said before, I am fairly sure that at least the Board's surgeon who was present when I went to be before the Board received the retraction letter. I'm not certain if the other two (the investigator and the attorney from the Attorney General's office received it) and if they didn't, that's a problem with communication between them since someone's reputation and ability to earn money are at stake. And at least to me it's a real problem that the Board took it that the patient wrote those words instead of the competitor surgeon. I never heard from the Board they did receive the letter or retraction or not.

6. I must reiterate that the further marginalization of me and my character by the Board's "Expert" that my Principal Investigator's number 17790 issued by the National Cancer Institute was not current and invalid was wrong. I included in my prior letter, the receipt from the NCI where I had to renew the number yearly including January 2021 and my number

is good until January 2022. Do or did I get a correction or apology from the Board or the "Expert," no, further marginalizing my character which I can assure is substantial being asked and permitted to operate on First Lady Betty Ford and a contingent of President Reagan's Secret Service, not to mention that I was the Principal Investigator at Eisenhower Medical Center for the National Surgical Adjuvant Breast Project, the largest breast cancer research group in the world. There's more I could add, like being sought out by an Olympic Gold Medal figure skater to provide care, but I guess none of that makes any difference, even though I was awarded the Carnegie Medal for an outstanding act of heroism.

7. Lastly, this part disturbs me a lot. The Board's "Expert" decreed that my treatment in one of the patients was "not indicated." I have treated thousands of patients in 40 plus years of caring and always explained all options to my patients, but I always knew who made the final decision and that was the patient whether or not it was standard-of-care.

Page 4

It was the patients right and choice. With the "Expert" saying my treatment was not indicated have we entered a time when some entity decrees what a patient should or should not have in the way of treatment? That patient happened to try and escape from state imposed Olympic training during the Nicolae Ceausesu (Romanian Dictator) regime, was caught, put in a gulag and raped over and over.

After Ceausesu was shot, she was released and immigrated to the US and was married. The husband died and she suffered from PTSD to the extreme. She was treated by the same competitor surgeon and had retained cancer at the lumpectomy site necessitating another surgery which she wouldn't consent to but she would cryoablation. She wrote that surgeon a blistering letter following her partial treatment. I treated her via the Lavender Procedure because that was the only thing she would consent to. And that's what I took an oath to do to the best of my ability, help people. Or would the Board rather I just sent here on her way to eventually die from no treatment? I can't wrap my head around the "Expert" saying my treatment wasn't indicated. George Orwell here we come.

I guess none of what I say makes any difference so I'll let the chips fall where they may.

Mr. Phillip Bretz

CC:——————, JD - President of the Medical Board of California

The following is the final blow from the Medical Board. Having read the two letters I wrote specifically to the President of the Board making it plain just what transpired from day one, I guess I expected a little more than the final dismantling of my character in such a perfunctory way, like I was worthless at best, not worthy to even stand in their presence. As you'll read, I can't even call myself a doctor anymore (after over forty years of healing people), even though that's an earned degree and not from the Medical Board. Some lawyer somewhere will have to tell me they actually have the authority to impose an edict like that, stripping away, as it were, the authority of the medical school who granted me my MD, to just strip it away? What about the rights of the medical school? Can somebody somewhere strip your Bachelor of Arts degree from you after your four years of attending a university and passing the tests? Talk about a dangerous precedent! I would think medical schools knowing this now would take some action and regain their turf. Over the years, I have treated at least two lawyers that never passed the "bar exam" but they graduated with a law degree from law school and are still called lawyers. They just can't practice law.

Is there anything more they could do to me to strip me of my dignity, humanity and healing abilities? You'd think at least they would have a fellow doctor to bring down the last sentence instead of someone who probably never did more medical treatment than applying a Band-Aid. I can guarantee you the Executive Director of the Medical Board never has been able to walk out of the OR (and know that feeling) after a six-hour trauma surgery in which you saved a life or a twenty-minute breast cancer procedure (Lavender) and talked to the family. Oh, I'm sorry, in the case of the Lavender Procedure you don't have to walk out to talk to the family because they were there all along seeing the cancer killed. If anyone close to you ever develops breast cancer and is treated within the "system," ask the surgeon if you as a family member can come in and watch and ask questions. I'd bet my medical license on the fact you would be rebuffed. Wait a minute, I no longer have a medical license. No wonder they are afraid, just like in the movie *The Accountant,* that said, "You're different and sooner or later different scares people." I'm so glad I did it. And I'm glad I'm out from under the "sword of Damocles" posture of the Medical Board. This should give all licensed physicians in the State of California and you as a patient pause, that your doctor has to get up every morning knowing that a disaster like what happened to me could befall them at any moment (by an anonymous letter), and that there is no way to stop it, or is there? That should give you pause about the extent of authority and how it is used.

I'm sure they'll try to retaliate after reading my book. In fact, I told a few of my patients when saying goodbye that if they put me in jail, they'll have to visit me and bring donuts. They just asked if I wanted chocolate donuts?

I suppose I could conclude with pages of rant but I promised myself I would refrain from that journalism. In fact, I thought I'd close this chapter with the following quote from the Medical Board on their letterhead.

"Protecting consumers by advancing high quality, safe medical care."

Really? I hope you'll agree now having read my story that both the Lavender Way and Lavender Procedure are indeed extreme departures from standard of care.

Don't ask me, ask my Lavender girls. Lavender in my opinion is of the highest quality and the safest manner and finally a way to treat all women as they should be treated with dignity, caring and the will (by their doctor) to preserve their bodies, not like the numerous correspondences you have read where they are afraid, worried and feel abandoned. I did my best to reverse all of it and you will have to ask my Lavender girls if I succeeded. Heck, at this point ask yourself.

As I said elsewhere, there are only three things in play here. First, that after renewing my medical license for over forty years (without incident) they finally caught up with me, and thank G-D they did so you can sleep now. Two, at the end of what some would say is a sterling career practicing the healing arts (as Jeff Levine said), I suddenly turned into Mr. Hyde and it's a good thing they stopped me from doing further damage upon the women of this state and the world. Or three, there was something else afoot all along. The following are the final letters from the Medical Board. On one of the pages it says, "TO ALL PARTIES," I guess that includes the reader. Be my guest to this public self-defacement of me and everything I ever stood for. I stood for and still stand for you.

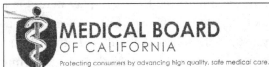

MEDICAL BOARD
OF CALIFORNIA
Protecting consumers by advancing high quality, safe medical care.

Enforcement Program
2005 Evergreen Street, Suite 1200
Sacramento, CA 95815-5401
Phone: (916) 263-2525
Fax: (916) 263-2473
www.mbc.ca.gov

Gavin Newsom, Governor, State of California | Business, Consumer Services and Housing Agency | Department of Consumer Affair

November 5, 2021

Phillip De Evans Bretz, M.D.

Dear Dr. Bretz:

This is in reference to the "Request for Surrender of License While on Probation" that you completed on October 14, 2021. You have elected to surrender License No. A 32596, to practice medicine in the State of California, along with your D.E.A Certificate. The consequence of this action is that you can no longer practice medicine in this state, nor can you refer to yourself as an M.D. or licensed physician. You may wish to consult with your attorney in this matter.

Enclosed are two copies of an "Agreement for Surrender of License" document. Please sign them at the bottom and have them witnessed. One original of this Agreement should be returned within thirty (30) days, to the address shown below, along with your wall license and wallet certificate. The second copy may be retained for your records. As with any license surrender, this Agreement constitutes a public record and will be disclosed to the public and reported to the National Practitioner Data Bank.

Once the Medical Board (Board) receives the signed document and has obtained your physician's and surgeon's wall license and wallet certificate for cancellation, the Board will close the case. Please send your D.E.A. Certificate to the Drug Enforcement Agency for cancellation.

Sincerely,

Executive Director

enclosures

cc:

Case No. 800-2015-017972

BEFORE THE
MEDICAL BOARD OF CALIFORNIA
DEPARTMENT OF CONSUMER AFFAIRS
STATE OF CALIFORNIA

In the Matter of the Accusation
Against:

         Case No. 800-2015-017972

Phillip De Evans Bretz, M.D.

█████████████████████

         AGREEMENT FOR
Physician's and Surgeon's **SURRENDER OF LICENSE**
Certificate No. A 32596

       Respondent.

TO ALL PARTIES:

IT IS HEREBY STIPULATED AND AGREED by and between the parties to the

above-entitled proceedings, that the following matters are true:

  1. Complainant, ██████████ s the Executive Director of the Medical

Board of California, Department of Consumer Affairs ("Board").

  2. Phillip De Evans Bretz, M.D. ("Respondent") has carefully read and fully

understands the effect of this Agreement.

  3. Respondent understands that by signing this Agreement he is enabling

the Board to issue this order accepting the surrender of license without further

process. Respondent understands and agrees that Board staff and counsel for

complainant may communicate directly with the Board regarding this Agreement,

without notice to or participation by Respondent. The Board will not be disqualified

from further action in this matter by virtue of its consideration of this Agreement.

  4. Respondent acknowledges there is current disciplinary action against

his license, that on October 31, 2018, an Accusation was filed against him and on

October 25, 2019, a Decision was rendered wherein his license was revoked, with

the revocation stayed, and placed on 3 years' probation with various standard

terms and conditions.

5.   The current disciplinary action provides in pertinent part, "Following the effective date of this Decision, if Respondent ceases practicing due to retirement, health reasons, or is otherwise unable to satisfy the terms and conditions of probation, Respondent may request voluntary surrender of Respondent's license." (Condition #14).

6.   Upon acceptance of the Agreement by the Board, Respondent understands he will no longer be permitted to practice as a physician and surgeon in California, and also agrees to surrender his wallet certificate, wall license and any D.E.A. Certificate(s) for an address in California.

7.   Respondent fully understands and agrees that if Respondent ever files an application for relicensure or reinstatement in the State of California, the Board shall treat it as a Petition for Reinstatement of a revoked license in effect at the time the Petition is filed. In addition, any Medical Board Investigation Report(s), including all referenced documents and other exhibits, upon which the Board is predicated, and any such Investigation Report(s), attachments, and other exhibits, that may be generated subsequent to the filing of this Agreement for Surrender of License, shall be admissible as direct evidence, and any time-based defenses, such as laches or any applicable statute of limitations, shall be waived when the Board determines whether to grant or deny the Petition.

///

Having received the above, I authored my last letter to the Executive Director of the Board. I have waited for a couple of weeks now and no response. Actually, it's now January 14, 2022 and no response. Seeing my life's work destroyed and seeing how my patients uniformly feel about me, I couldn't help but write this last letter. From the Desk of Phillip Bretz, no MD after. I wrote this in part because my experience with the Medical Board of California is much like the old saying now of "What happens in Vegas stays in Vegas." It seems what happens in one department stays in that department and just verdicts come out. Remember, I didn't think for one minute that the person representing the Attorney General ever was privy to the first letter written by the competitor surgeon or the letter of retraction or that that person bothered to check that the complaint sent to me wasn't written by the patient at all but by that competitor surgeon intimidating my patient into signing the "official" looking document. As I say in the letter below, I didn't expect the Executive Director to meddle in the everyday workings of the people below him, so like the person from the Attorney General's office, I don't suspect the Executive Director knew the nuances of my case. But with this letter, he does now.

Just one final question to the Board. Is it true that during my period of probation, that there were three different supervisors? That the two earlier ones knew about my not seeing a horde of patients and never said a word about my being in "non-practice"? That it was only the last supervisor that decided apparently unilaterally that I was in "non-practice"? If that's true, then it seems to me that's a lot of power to place in one person's hands to destroy someone. It seems to me that a decision to essentially stop a doctor from a lifelong practice of caring, that that should be a decision made by a number of people, not just one. Did the Executive Director know about the decision to keep me on probation forever because of my supposed "non-practice"? And having successfully removed me from my principal source of income, that last supervisor knew it would be the final straw, that is, keeping me on probation where I was forced under duress to surrender my license. I guess it's good to be the king.

From the Desk of Phillip Bretz
11-16-21

Dear Mr. ████████
Executive Director,
Medical Board of California

Enclosed you will find the executed forms for surrender of my license to practice medicine in California. However, before you process these documents, I wish you to know just what transpired in my case from the get go, and for you to judge if this is exculpatory evidence enough to reverse the current edict. It is not expected as part of your job that you monitor or nitpick the daily work of the people below you but you need to know in my case the falsehoods and inaccurate pronouncements that occurred. In the attached you will find exhibits A-F, each with its own special reference to these falsehoods and preordained pronouncements which didn't come to pass.

Exhibit A - (The letter written to the Board by Dr. ███████) - Is the original letter to the Board lodged by a competitor surgeon in town having seen the TV segment on the Lavender Procedure. This letter that I was never apprised of by the Board (I only found it by happenstance) is full of half-truths and outright falsehoods. I was never given the opportunity by the Board to sit across from Dr. ███ to refute the entire letter sentence by sentence. One example is that I was doing the procedure 'for cash of course.' Well, I was charging cash (initially $2,500.00) because at the time I started, there were no codes for billing with any insurance company or Medicare. The $2,500.00 barely offset the cost of doing the procedure. The probes cost $1,300.00 apiece and my ultrasound tech charged $300.00 per case and the liquid nitrogen was $130.00 per case and the local anesthesia, drapes etc, were about $50.00. That left me with a profit of $820.00 for potentially curing a breast cancer in 20 minutes in an in-office procedure vs around $250,000.00 for traditional care including possible multiple surgeries, chemotherapy and radiation. Now there are doctors charging $8,000.00 for the procedure. I generally don't use the word cure but I do have multiple patients in groups one and two who are approaching 8 years out cancer free. Their breasts look like they were never touched.

Another thing Dr. ███ said in ███ letter is that I would 'undubtely have to destroy the nipple.' ███ spelled undoubtedly wrong. How dare ███ have the audacity to preordain my surgical ability. Of course, Mrs. ██████ is now over five years out and as far as I know cancer free with her breasts intact. I can refute and prove the falsehoods in each sentence of Dr. ███ letter including the following, "I think you should also be aware that Dr. Bretz has lost hospital privileges, trained in Guadalajara" – First, this intimates that I somehow (after 30 sterling years on the active surgical staff at Eisenhower) did some horrendous act that caused my dismissal.

Page 2

The fact is, after nine years as first assistant on the open-heart team at EMC, (we had the lowest mortality rate in the country 0.6% and they don't let stumblebums or negligent surgeons operate on the First Lady), I had given up general surgery to concentrate on breast cancer research and participate in many clinical trials. In fact, I brought NCI clinical trials to the Coachella Valley. I didn't need the hospital and didn't want to pay the exorbitant fees of malpractice so I just let my privileges lapse. It had nothing to do with any malpractice issues or disciplinary issues as intimated. And I didn't train in Guadalajara, I went to medical school in Mexico but trained at Loyola University Medical Center in Chicago successfully and faithfully completing a five year straight surgical residency as my certificate says. ██ makes it sound like I'm a second-class citizen because I went to medical school in Mexico. ██ owes all Hispanic doctors and Hispanic people an apology. I doubt ██ had ever attempted a cryoablation case and then acts like an 'expert.' This letter is unacceptable with all its falsehoods and for the Board to essentially swallow it hook line and sinker is unacceptable. But what was really unacceptable was the Board never notified me of that letter and had ██ sit across the table so I could face my accuser and refute everything. After over forty years of the Board renewing my license without incident, you'd think I'd be owed that much instead of hiding that letter from me and letting things just snowball leading to my demise. I could continue to refute each sentence and ██ ineptness but I know your time is valuable.

Exhibit B – (The letter of notification of a complaint) - Let's look at the actual letter I received from the Board with Mrs. ██████ supposed complaint. It says, "Dr. Bretz is performing experimental cancer treatments called the Lavendar Procedure (Dr. ██ misspelled Lavender). Wait a minute you say, this was a complaint written and filed by Mrs. ███████. What if I could prove it wasn't from Mrs. ███████ and that Mrs. ███████ never had any intention of filing a complaint against me? To continue (still quoting) "which is not the standard of care nor an approved treatment for cancer. The treatments are being performed in the office of Dr. Bretz as he has lost his hospital privileges. The procedure involves placing a cryoprobe into a tumor." We have previously discussed the issue of losing hospital privileges so you know I didn't. And the reason I was performing the procedure in the office was not because I had lost privileges at the hospital. Cryoablation is specifically approved by the FDA for the doctor to perform the procedure in the office setting. The only thing true in this supposed complaint is that (A), I was performing the procedure in my office (as it is specifically cleared by the FDA for just such a purpose) and (B) The procedure involves placing a cryoprobe into a tumor.

If you check, Dr. ████ misspelled Lavender (Lavendar) in both ██ original letter to the Board and when ██ wrote the complaint that Mrs. ██████ never wrote and never intended to write. While it is true that cryoablation of breast cancer is not standard of care, it is FDA approved as we will see in Exhibit D.

Page 3

I can't help it if surgeons are not using whatever FDA approved devices that are out there. Now let's get to the heart of the matter. I believe Mrs. ██████ never wrote that complaint and never intended to. She was coerced, harassed (Mrs. ██████ own words, see her letter of retraction Exhibit C), and threatened and was told she would die if she didn't have surgery. Is Dr. ██████ conduct behavior unbecoming? How do I know she was coerced, harassed, threatened and intimidated? All we have to do is read Mrs. ██████ letter of retraction.

Now I believe her letter of retraction was sent to all three members of the Board where I was questioned. But I'm not sure since I never received any notification about that letter from the Board. But I believe ████████ MD, FACS did get it. And as a member of the Board interviewing me, and knowing what an impact that letter might have, he should have made sure that Investigator ██ and the lady from the Attorney General also received that letter of retraction. My contention is that Mrs. ██ never wrote that complaint, Dr. ██ did. Mrs. ██ never intended to write a complaint (since she did so well) but that Dr. ██ wrote it, sent it to Mrs. ██ and threatened her with a lawsuit and being taken to court (as you'll see Mrs. ██ words) if she didn't sign what looked like an official letter. In fact, In Mrs. ██ own words and I quote, "I never in a million years would have thought that it was a letter to accuse dr. Bretz of being a bad surgeon." As you'll read, Mrs. ██ was scared and already had been through so much and when the letter (written by Dr. ██) arrived looking official, she was so intimidated that she just signed it not wanting to be involved in a lawsuit and court proceedings. This is all on top of Dr. ██ saying she would die if she didn't have surgery. How can Dr. ██ make a statement like that seemingly without ethics and certainly without professionalism?

Exhibit C (Mrs. ██ letter of retraction grammar uncorrected) – While I expect you to read the entire letter, I'll just mention a few lines I deem most important. "He was a god send . . . we had an excellent meeting where he went above and beyond to explain everything that his treatment entailed." "The surgeon who was also a friend of my niece sent her a very angry text message telling her that her aunt was going to die if she didn't get surgery and what was she thinking?" "I started getting continuous phone calls from ██ office and from god knows who but I got so nervous and already dealing with so much.. I panicked when a week later I receive a letter in the mail that looked pretty official telling me if I didn't sign it I would be going to court for backing out of surgery" "I never thought that it was a letter to accuse dr. Bretz of being a bad surgeon. I have only recently become aware that he has been accused supposedly by me. I'm devastated to think that for two years this dr. Who saved my life.. was kind.. and extremely professional has been going through an uncalled for investigation."

There is so much to say about all this but you get the idea, I hope.

Page 4

Exhibit D (The 510K from the FDA approving IceCure's cryoablation device on November 29, 2010 four years before I starting using cryoablation). I didn't include the entire letter for as much brevity as possible. If you read under 'Oncology,' you'll see the following, "The system may be used for ablation of cancerous or malignant tissue." Now unless I can't read English the FDA says that cryoablation in essence is not experimental and can be used to treat cancer and it doesn't limit the tissue it can be used on.

Exhibit E (A letter from the FDA) - The bottom paragraph is what is important here relating to my using cryoablation. Unless in 2014 the Medical Board of California had on their website specific guidelines relating to the use of cryoablation not to include for instance breast cancer, I was following the highest authority in the land concerning the use of any medical device. The FDA uses words like not to 'limit' or 'interfere with' the authority of a health care practitioner to prescribe or administer any legally marketed device to a patient for any condition or disease with the legitimate health care practitioner-patient relationship. Pretty straight forward. Of course, that's just my opinion.

Exhibit F (renewal authorization from the National Cancer Institute of Principal Investigators number) – I included this since it was a way to prove that the statement made by the Board's 'expert' who reviewed my cases said in effect that I claimed to carry a Principal Investigators number with the NCI but he was certain my five-digit number was not valid any longer. He knew the NCI had given up the five-digit number some years ago. Really? That may be but it is probably because I've held a Principal Investigator number with the National Cancer Institute for so long, I'm probably grandfathered. I include below the notification from them saying my Principal Investigator number 17790 is current and active until February 2022.

Page 5

It seems to me; the Board's expert was wrong about that and didn't bother (nor anybody else from the Board) to check with the National Cancer Institute. In addition, the Board's expert said that my treatment was an extreme departure from standard of care as I didn't perform lymph node dissections on these patients. That is true but I never got the chance to sit across from the Board's expert and tell him why I didn't perform lymph node dissections, the verdict just came down. And more than seven years out from their Lavender Procedures, none of the patients in groups 1 or 2 have had any occurrence of cancer in their lymph nodes meaning they are cancer free. How can that be when the Board's expert preordained as it were lymph node metastasis in these patients?

Simple, I was finding these cancers before they had the ability to metastasis and I knew the genetics of the tumor, the patient's personal history and the lymph nodes under physical exam and ultrasound were negative. So, either I guessed right on all these patients or I perhaps have indeed opened the door to better care for all women with breast cancer.

I was able to treat breast cancer patients successfully without surgery, chemotherapy or radiation. The Board never asked me how the patients were doing. I'd like to know just how many cryoablation cases the Board's 'expert' had done with how much follow up to make judgements like he did. You see, comparing cryoablation to the dogma of traditional surgery is like comparing apples and oranges. It's a whole different set of criteria and if you're not versed in it thus holding cryoablation to the old standards, then how can a decision be made that is just? I invited Investigator ■■■■ out to my office on multiple occasions to see videos and review the entire process to achieve some understanding but he never acknowledged that or came out.

Another thing the Board's expert said was one of the patients I performed the Lavender Procedure on, that the procedure was not indicated. In all my years of caring for patients many critically ill, I always knew who I was working for. Let's talk about a patient with breast cancer. To put it another way, if the patient has been given ALL the options and possible complications of whatever procedures (assuming the doctor is not corrupt, and is acting in accordance with ethical standards of the profession), then if the patient says, "Thanks doc but I read in the internet that if I eat two pounds of blueberries every day, my cancer will go away. That's what I want to do," then so be it. It is always the patient's choice to proceed or not with any procedure. See below.

Page 6

The first 10 amendments of the U.S. Constitution, known as the Bill of Rights, were outlined to protect citizens from infringement on their basic freedoms, e.g., freedom of speech, the press, religion. A corollary to the basic foundation established by the Bill of Rights is the common-law principle of self-determination that guarantees the individual's right to privacy and protection against the actions of others that may threaten bodily integrity.[1] An extension of self-determination includes the right to exercise control over one's body, for example, the right to accept or refuse medical treatment. It is expected that when one freely accepts or refuses treatment, he or she is competent to do so, and is, therefore, accountable for the choices made. Prim Care Companion J Clin Psychiatry. 1999 Oct; 1(5): 131–141.

I can go into more detail about this but like I said I know your time is valuable. If taking what has been presented here has not given you pause then so be it. I guess the Medical Board of California and I can agree to disagree on how doctors should behave and treat patients. You can easily dispose of me now but if there is any justice to be had with the Board, then Dr. ███ should be brought to task for writing a letter that was inaccurate, claimed to be written by the patient (knowing it was a lie to the Board) and in so doing took a good doctor out of the loop of saving lives and may have committed a criminal act. I think there is a term used for what she perpetrated on Mrs. ███ to in essence force Mrs. ███ to sign that falsified document. Dr. ███ took advantage of my vulnerable frightened patient.

Of course, I'm not a lawyer but one can't intimidate a person into doing something to gain something of value. In my case that something of value was Dr. ███ acknowledgement to ███ that ███ singlehandedly sunk that bastard Bretz, I showed him who was boss and who is 'THE' breast cancer surgeon in town. Yeah, ███ may have accomplished ███ goal, but all ███ had to do was call me and I would have invited ███ to sit in on a couple of cases and would have been happy to teach ███ how to do a Lavender Procedure. Of course, there is a word used in psychology that describes people who act capriciously, shooting from the hip as it were causing great harm and who show no remorse.

Below is what I dared to do and I'm proud of it.

Imagine being able to know enough about breast cancer to find ultra-small tumors and treat them in about 20 minutes in the office under local anesthesia with relatives able to be present holding and comforting the patient while both see the cancer being killed before their eyes? I found I made it possible to take away all the dread, fear, anxiety and loss of hope that the diagnosis of breast cancer portends. You've taken that achievement from me and hundreds of women from all over the world who I could have helped. At the end, the breast is left intact virtually without a scar (a minute 3mm stab wound for the probe entrance) and they resume normal activity immediately (without a single stitch). They have remained cancer free for over seven years. There are a few with local recurrences that under the 'system' should have had a mastectomy but didn't are alive, happy and cancer free to tell the tale. It's called the Lavender Procedure because usually right after the case if the patient was hungry, we would walk over the Lavender Bistro for lunch or dinner, because they felt great and wanted to celebrate (as Mrs. ▮▮▮▮ did with her family). And yes, we toasted with a glass of Chardonnay (incidentally Dr. ▮▮▮▮ also misspelled Chardonnay in ▮▮ letter to the Board). We toasted because none of the terrible things that usually happen with breast cancer treatment that have plagued women for eons ever happened to my patients.

Page 7

It is a miracle and one day it will be known as such and people will ask why it took so long to see the light of day and who delayed it? The Lavender procedure was almost a euphoric experience that lasts years instead of dread, depression, physical disfigurement, nerve damage, lymphedema, husbands leaving, bankruptcies and families destroyed and for what? It's because of arrogance of those who are in essence held hostage by the system or else thus afraid to step outside of the box to provide better care.

I sincerely hope none of your loved ones ever develops breast cancer and have to endure possibly unnecessary surgery, chemotherapy and radiation which is the order of the day of what Dr. Azra Raza in her book The First Cell calls the slash – poison – burn approach the system demands. All this takes place because of the assumed rightness of the way things are done, unwilling to learn and change.

You should know I am the author of our country's first large-scale breast cancer prevention clinical trial using the drug Tamoxifen FDA IND 34,223, 1990. It was I who thought to do that, not any other researcher in the country from Sloan Kettering to MD Anderson to Stanford. That was an extreme departure from standard of care (giving a pill to prevent cancer) ending up in the LA Times, CNN and the White House. Yet I didn't hear a peep from the Medical Board of California. I was even asked by the State of California to testify in the hearing on Tamoxifen which I did happily as I was a team player. I have the letter thanking me from the state.

I will end now and will say again, if you're happy with the conduct of all your people then so be it. On the other hand, if you want to right a wrong (in my opinion anyway) with both me and the Board ending in a win/win situation, including my helping the Board with cryoablation guidelines, and have California lead the way, give me a call. You'll find I'm not really a bad person. 760-███████ or e-mail me.

VOIR DIRE

Phil

I'll close this with four of the many letters I continue to receive apparently on my character, conduct, professionalism and ethics, otherwise all these women would not have written a single word. Again, you be the judge.

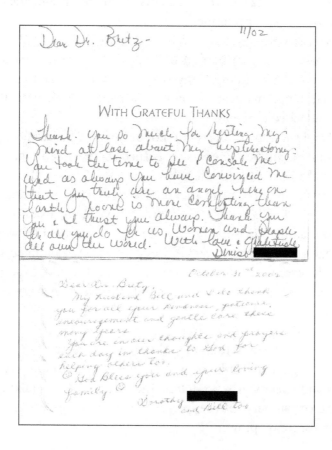

November 4, 2021

███████████████ President
California Medical Board
2005 Evergreen Street
Suite 1200
Sacramento, California 95814

Re: Dr. Phillip Bretz, Case #

Dear President Dr. ████████ and Members of the California Board of Medicine:

I have been a patient of Dr. Bretz since 1995. His dedicated care to *all* his patients has been unbelievable and I have told hundreds of people, that Dr. Bretz has "dedicated his life to finding a medical way to alleviate breast cancer treatment."

I am 79 years old, and have always had dense breasts. At 28 years old, (1970) I had to sign papers that the surgeon could do a mastectomy, if the lump was malignant in my right breast. It was benign, but that began mammograms every 6 months for years, even with the «old balloon» attached to the x-ray machine.

In 1995, I went to Dr. Bretz and not only would he carefully go over my mammograms, but if he was concerned about something, he would immediately do an ultrasound in his office

Do you know how much that alleviated my fear of breast cancer, *again that was in 1995*. Since that year, I traveled long distances to have Dr. Bretz read my mammograms (even if the mammogram were done in Arizona or Washington state), to be physically examined by him. Usually the exam included an ultrasound, and I would be so relieved and grateful to him for my piece of mind. This went on every year with my last visit in February 2021.

Through the years he shared with me some exciting procedures to recognize very small tumors and state of the art breakthroughs in treatment. Again, I would copy and share his achievements to my relatives and friends. Always, telling them, if a doctor is talking about breast cancer surgery, please, please make an appointment with Dr. Bretz for a second opinion.

I was excited when he went to China to deliver his findings in breast cancer treatment, and thought it fantastic, that finally, he was recognized for his dedication to helping women with breast cancer. I read the articles written in Rancho Mirage Health news, and celebrated that finally women had a choice in treatment of small tumors that would not destroy their breasts and/or their physical and mental health.

To my dismay, I read that "crappy article" of a surgeon challenging his findings, and then your board putting Dr. Bretz on probation and then . . . unbelievable, sanctioning him and shutting down valuable research for breast cancer.

In my opinion, your board DID NOT research this alleged claim, and should have interviewed the outrageous claimants!

* I would love to be contacted regarding the outstanding care provided by Dr. Bretz since 1995.

(760) ███████

Your negative decision made me:

- Sick to my stomach

- angry

- Seriously search media to have someone recognize your terrible decision

- Wondering how much research was done by your board. Who was the Expert to what?

- Wish I could testify under oath to Governor and Attorney General

- Hope I can contact Cancer Research Organizations and inform them of your lack of knowledge on up-to-date breast cancer research.

- Very, very questionable on WHO instigated this claim.

- Were any doctors and/or scientists contacted for information regarding "Cryoablation" or RAS publishers, "Oncology and Therapy Journal."

I urge you to reopen this decision, as I am positive, that this case needs to be re-examined. Especially, if a competitor surgeon opened the claim. (What research was done on this surgeon "crying wolf?). As a retired school counselor, I have found that "people do crazy things when greed and profession are threatened!"

I am so upset over your decision, that I'm going to spend my time searching for people that will look into your terrible, uninformed decision regarding a doctor that has spent his life (not only professional, but includes his family) searching for ways to treat breast cancer without surgical destruction of the breast, radiation, chemotherapy and destruction of quality of life.

Again, I, please, urge you to reconsider this case. I consider such action to be very important to research and treatment of Breast Cancer.

Sincerely,

Linda ███████████

███████████████

███████████████

cc:
Honorable Governor Gavin Newsom of California
Honorable Rob Bonta, Attorney General of California
Honorable Kamala Harris, Vice President, United States of America
Karen E Knudson, PhD, Chief Executor Officer, American Cancer Society

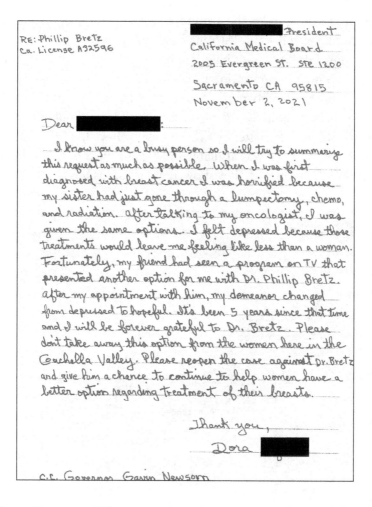

RE: Phillip Bretz
Ca. License A32596

███████████ President
California Medical Board
2005 Evergreen ST. Ste 1200
Sacramento CA 95815
November 2, 2021

Dear ███████████:

I know you are a busy person so I will try to summarize this request as much as possible. When I was first diagnosed with breast cancer I was horrified because my sister had just gone through a lumpectomy, chemo, and radiation. After talking to my oncologist, I was given the same options. I felt depressed because those treatments would leave me feeling like less than a woman. Fortunately, my friend had seen a program on TV that presented another option for me with Dr. Phillip Bretz. After my appointment with him, my demeanor changed from depressed to hopeful. It's been 5 years since that time and I will be forever grateful to Dr. Bretz. Please don't take away this option from the women here in the Coachella Valley. Please reopen the case against Dr. Bretz and give him a chance to continue to help women have a better option regarding treatment of their breasts.

Thank you,

Dora ███████████

C.C. Governor Gavin Newsom

I hope I've proved I'm not an incompetent or negligent milquetoast but perhaps the doctor you wish you had. Or should I just go fishing? This is only half the story of my efforts to help all women. If you halfway enjoyed reading this book, then you will want to read *Sacrificing America's Women II* to see how your tax dollars are spent to defeat cancer.

Sacrificing America's Women II is the story of how I came up with the idea to do our country's first large-scale breast cancer prevention clinical trial using the drug Tamoxifen. It was quite a ride. It made me feel like Huck Finn and James Bond all at once. It was thrilling to get up in the morning to lay the groundwork and see it take on a life of its own. I think you will enjoy learning how I intended to change the world, and see how I did it. It ends based on my original idea with our country doing a $68 million prevention trial with Tamoxifen, the first time ever we had a way to possibly prevent cancer with a pill. I wasn't going to let any information about *Sacrificing America's Women II* out but you need to see Dr. John Link's letter below. Can you believe the gall of the cabal to cut me out of what was arguably the biggest most important clinical trial ever (I thought up)? They showed me who was boss.

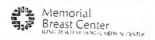

Memorial
Breast Center
LONG BEACH MEMORIAL MEDICAL CENTER

2880 Atlantic Avenue, Suite 100
Long Beach, California 90806
(213) 595-3838

January 29, 1992

Phillip Bretz, M.D.
Desert Breast Institute
39-800 Bob Hope Drive, Suite C
Rancho Mirage, CA 92270

Dear Phil:

I hope things are going well with you and your Breast Center. As you are surely aware, the NSABP is forging ahead with their breast prevention trial based on your original idea and protocol. The Memorial Breast Center was accepted as an institution and recently we attended an orientation meeting in Pittsburgh. I had planned to see you at the meeting but was extremely surprised to learn that the NSABP had decided not to use the originator of the idea for the trial.

In any event, I wanted to congratulate you that "your baby" really has been born and the trial actually looks quite exciting. Clearly it is where the NCI and the government should be putting their clinical research dollars rather than trying to discover a new poison.

Wendy Schain and I met recently and discussed our own conduct of the trial and we were wondering if somehow we could collaborate with you or make some type of outreach to the Desert area to include potential patients on the trial. We would be happy to brainstorm regarding this and wanted you to give it some thought. The actual beginning of the trial will not occur until probably April 1 or slightly later. Please give this some thought and I will try to contact you within the next several weeks to discuss the matter further.

Warmest regards,

John S. Link, M.D.
Medical Director

JSL/sec

It turned out I was absolutely right in my prediction that Tamoxifen would prevent breast cancer in high-risk women. I would call that changing the world. It turns out it lowers the risk by about 50% in high-risk women. How did we find out who is high-risk when about 90% of women who develop breast cancer have no demonstrable risk factors like family history? Functionaries at insurance companies have made the edict not to pay for any genetic tests if there is no family history. When about 90% of women who develop breast cancer have no family history, how stupid is that? All women should be tested period and I'm not talking about BRCA 1&2 which is only good for about 10% of breast cancer patients. I'm talking about risk tests like OncoVue or BrevGen Plus. This is especially important now with at least two medications (Tamoxifen and Evista) that lower the risk by about 50%. Right, the only way to determine high risk is via a network of Lavender Centers that do genetic risk testing on every woman (who wants it) as the starting point. Then everything evolves individually from that finding.

It might interest you to know that after I received my Investigational New Drug Application (IND) from the FDA 34,223 and did all the groundwork (or, as Dr. Bernard Fisher said "groundbreaking"), I was then invited to the erstwhile Soviet Union (to also make the world safer) and then the FDA hearing, not only was I not afforded the privilege to conduct the trial, since I thought it up (when every other researcher in the country was not thinking out of the box), but I wasn't allowed to even participate. How's that? It's a cool tale. Lastly, the only person who can change things is the President of the United States. By now you know, expecting change to the system, it will never happen.

Alternatively, if a multi-millionaire reads this and wants to write a check, that would be alright too.

Take time now and review possible answers to the questions posed at the outset. That is, that only three things are in play here, do you remember them?

Lastly, I highly recommend Dr. Azra Raza's (world class hematologist at Columbia University) book *The First Cell*. You'll find I'm not the only one who wants change in the system. In fact, let me quote from her book. Her message is vitally important and maybe somebody in a position to change things will listen to her message while not paying attention to mine. It's utterly imperative and so important the reader understands exactly what Dr. Raza is declaring after forty-plus years of being on the front lines of our war to cure cancer and why we are not going anywhere soon. It is also important to demand meaningful change so that cancer doesn't become our number one killer which it is on pace to do. Take these passages to heart. As well, see if I have tried on my own to do exactly what she calls for, going after the first cell, not the last (with the innovative Tamoxifen prevention clinical trial) and now with Lavender. These quotes are taken from her book with my comments interposed as needed. These quotes are not in consecutive order but understandable. I did ask permission to do this.

Why quote her and tout her book? Because she is the only one of rank that has had the guts to tell it straight and true. And because as I've said before and all along, it's not about me. It's about the message of hope for all women. But yes, I guess my message is important too because not only have I come up with a plan, I executed it and have the seven-and-a-half-year cancer-free survivors to prove the Lavender Way/Procedure deserves to displace the current model's period. Here's her quotes.

"With minor variations, a protocol of surgery, chemotherapy, and radiation- the slash-poison-burn approach to treating cancer-remains unchanged. It is an embarrassment. Equally embarrassing is the arrogant denial of that embarrassment. Technologic advances and the cure of cancer in animal models are loudly proclaimed as if those successes have had anything to do with treating disease in humans. No one is winning the war on cancer. It is mostly hype, the same rhetoric from the same self-important voices for the past half-century. The gaping disconnect between knowledge about cancer biology and the capacity to use this knowledge to benefit patients is staggering. The disease is fantastically complex. More fantastic is the reductionist conceit that targeting a single genetic abnormality with a single drug will be curative. This "magic bullet" concept becomes especially entrenched because of a couple of early successes.

"Chronic myeloid leukemia and Acute promyelocytic leukemia come to mind. These two success stories seemed to confirm a paradigm: cancer results from a genetic mutation that can be cured with a drug. Unfortunately, most common cancers have proved to be more complex, with many more biologic aberrations driving the malignant phenotype. The failure rate for drugs brought into clinical trials using such preclinical drug-testing platforms is 95 percent. The 5 percent of drugs that reach approval might as well have failed, since they prolong survival of patients by no more than a few months at best. Since 2005, 70 percent of approved drugs have shown zero improvement in survival rates while up to 70 percent have been actually harmful to patients."

That's why all the TV commercials you see about drugs spend half their time telling the listener about all the side effects and usually in the mix is death.

"The consensus today is that prevention is preferable to treatment. Yet actions to make this happen are obscenely lagging behind." Not by me if I may point out that the prevention trial was thought up in 1989, a long time ago. "How good are the solutions we offer if we constantly have to ask ourselves whether the cancer or the treatment, we prescribe will kill the patient? After fifty years of developing cancer drugs this way, is it time to reassess the preclinical model? No. it is time to abandon the strategy altogether. The new strategy is to stop chasing after the last cell and focus on eliminating the first. Better still, prevent the appearance of the first cancer cell by finding its earliest footprints. The new strategy must go beyond early detection as practiced currently through mammograms and other routine screening tests."

"Too many lives are being lost because of our own unshakable hubris, convinced as we are that we possess the power to untangle the intricacies of as complex a disease as cancer. It is like saying we will cure aging." I could go on and on here but the reader should by now grasp the focus of Dr. Raza's arguments against the status-quo. To support myself, I think I've done what she has asked and started a couple of decades ago with Tamoxifen prevention and now with Lavender however severely my conduct, diagnostic and treatment modalities are criticized and I am beaten back. Does it sound like we need sweeping change at the top of the leadership in its war on cancer? Here is an idea. Leave the self-appointed hierarchy in place and start a new paradigm with a new mission statement and give those people five years to see how far we can come in achieving our goal. Again, any billionaire out there instead of funneling enormous funds into a black hole with no results, try something completely different.

News Flash – I just saw Rosie. She was the third case I did on my first day of doing Lavender Procedure. She had implants and it was character building to say the least. She is the one referred to in the complaint to the Board from the competitor surgeon. She just had her mammogram now seven and a half-years out having had no surgery, no chemotherapy, and no radiation. As well, she looks to be cancer-free and no involved lymph nodes. So, was someone wrong in jumping the gun not asking how the patients were doing? I hope you know the answer to that one. Just for the record, I saw Rosie's mammo report come over the fax and I cringed when I saw her name (because that weight never leaves my shoulders).

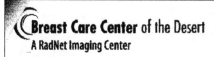

Breast Care Center of the Desert
A RadNet Imaging Center

Breast Care nter of the Desert
35800 Bob Hope Drive Suites 150A & 150B
Rancho Mirage, CA 92270
Phone: (760) 770-1920
Fax: (760) 324-0848

, ROSWITHA
MRN: 1293947BR1
DOB: 05-02-1962   Sex: F
Phone:

Ordered By
PHILLIP D BRETZ, MD
78034 CALLE BARCELONA, STE B
LA QUINTA CA, 92253

Date of Service: 04-23-2021

FAX: (760) 771-4749

EXAM: TOMOSYNTHESIS DIGITAL DIAGNOSTIC BILATERAL MAMMOGRAPHY WITH IMPLANTS

HISTORY: Asymptomatic 58-year-old female status post 3 left malignant lumpectomy sent cryoablation in 2014

TECHNIQUE: Mediolateral oblique and craniocaudal views were obtained using a digital tomosynthesis system (3D imaging). Implant-displaced views were also obtained. Computer-Aided Detection (CAD) was utilized.

COMPARISON: 2019, 2017

FINDINGS:

Tissue Density: There are scattered areas of fibroglandular density.

No suspicious mass, architectural distortion, asymmetry or calcification is identified in either breast. Stable asymmetry with punctate scattered calcifications seen within left breast subareolar region outer quadrant since 2017. Bilateral breast implants are present.

IMPRESSION: Bilateral stable mammogram

RECOMMENDATION: Annual mammography.

ASSESSMENT: BI-RADS Category 2: Benign.

A letter regarding the results of this study has been sent to the patient.

Your patient has been entered into our reminder system. We will notify the patient when their next breast imaging exam is due.
End of diagnostic report for accession: 27082066
Dictated: 04-23-2021 9:31:13 AM
Electronically Signed By: Patel, Hiten, MD 04-23-2021 9:31:13 AM

Confidential

Patient: ROSWITHA   DOB: 05-02-1962   Page 1 of 1

After I reviewed the report, yes, we went over to Lavender Bistro and I had a glass of Meiomi. Hope everyone is satisfied. You already saw her mammogram and ultrasound by a third party so I can't be accused of missing a cancer when I say there is none. Below is her card to me on my last day of being a doctor.

9-30-21

Dear Joan and Dr. Bretz

I am wishing you all the best
for your next endeavor.

Thank you for being so caring
and passionate.

I will be always grateful, for
what you have done for me.

Love Rosi

As you have read, for decades I have extended myself in the sole pursuit of a quest to defeat breast cancer and I have an answer. Notice, I didn't say "the" answer. I know Lavender works, the cancer-free living patients are a testament to it. All those letters you read from my patients point to an undeniable trust women around the world have had in me to safeguard their lives. I have never acted in an unethical or unprofessional manner and each step closer from mastectomy to the Lavender Procedure has been through using my G-D given talent that people from North Park to UAG to Loyola and EMC taught me. I must confess though; with the Medical Board's action, I am utterly exhausted and weary of the fight. The only way to resurrect me is for the system to recognize Lavender and change everything for the benefit of women without regard to the personal welfare the doctors supporting the system. I leave it to the American public to debate this fate.

You know, my friend and attorney Steve DeLateur said, "It's what they didn't ask you," meaning how the patients were doing. Further, he said that if that surgeon never acted, the Medical Board would have never known who you were." I would have helped that surgeon, now I can't.

I will close with one of my favorite Bible verses. It is apropos to my quest. It is from Proverbs Chapter 5 verse 19 and it says, "A loving doe a graceful dear, may her breasts satisfy you always, may you ever be captivated by her love."

The following page is again an article that I accidently ran across only a few months ago.

Topic: This is incredible! It just goes to show you that the public is acutely on to real breakthroughs and longs for the nail to be put into breast cancer's coffin like we can do with Lavender Way and Lavender Procedure. You will note the date on its appearance is 2015. I didn't run across it until six years later and the author states, "Time will tell if this procedure will truly be successful." In the next chapter you are about to read the results seven-and-a-half years out from Lavender. Then you will know the truth and hopefully raise your collective voices to give Lavender a chance at seeing the light of day. It also says that, "If it is, this guy will go down in history." I'm going down in history alright, just don't know how yet and that's up to you.

Topic: This is incredible!

Forum: Clinical Trials, Research News, Podcasts, and Study Results
—

Share your research articles, interpretations and experiences here. Let us know how these studies affect you and your decisions.

Posted on: Nov 1, 2015 09:59AM - edited Nov 1, 2015 09:59AM by ███████████

███████████ wrote:

http://www.kesq.com/news/local-doctor-kills-breast-cancer-with-unique-procedure/35985362

Sueris found this and I just had to create a thread on it hoping that many see this. This is a story on a breast cancer procedure that does not include chemotherapy, radiation nor surgery of course there can not be any spreading of the cancer for this to work. Time will tell if this procedure will truly be successful. If it is this guy will go down in history. The tumor stays with the person, it will be dead but it stays there, I wonder if over time a person's body will make it dissolve? The medical system will loose thousands of dollars on treatment but I think women will want to get tested more often so this procedure would be available to them, not to say that getting screened more often insures that the cancer will be found before it spreads. I also wonder if this procedure is applicable to other solid tumor cancers?

Make sure that you view what is on the second page which includes a small statement that the cancer must be found early. There are also additional videos, two which include statements about deaths from breast cancer.

LAVENDER IS THE NEW PINK

Next is my informed consent for the Lavender Procedure. To my way of thinking, an informed consent should be fairly exhaustive in its attempt to educate the patient on the benefits and potential complications of any procedure. Again, the reader can be the judge if I succeeded in that effort.

CHAPTER 9

Informed Consent for the Lavender Procedure

FOR

CRYOABLATION OF BREAST CANCER AKA THE LAVENDER PROCEDURE

Date:_____

This document is what is known as an informed consent. We will discuss options to care for your breast cancer so you can make an informed decision as to treatment. You do not have to do Cryoablation. Please read this document carefully. While we like to move along once a diagnosis of breast cancer is made, there is no rush to make a decision. Before reading this document you have been afforded the opportunity to discuss options with the oncologist and radiation therapist. This has been one of the cornerstones of Dr. Bretz's vision of breast care. That is, before the surgeon acts independently (as they had for decades), the patient is afforded the opportunity to visit other members of the team. This is the cornerstone of a comprehensive breast center.

Dr. Bretz or an associate has discussed in person with you options available for treatment of your breast cancer. These include; 1) doing nothing or just take an anti-estrogen pill, 2) Radical Mastectomy, a procedure where the entire breast, the chest wall muscles are removed along with a full axillary lymph node dissection, sometimes requiring a skin graft, 3) Modified Radical Mastectomy, this procedure only removes the breast and axillary lymph nodes leaving the chest wall muscles intact, 4) Lumpectomy with or without axillary lymph node dissection, this procedure involves only removal of the tumor through a small incision with a margin of healthy tissue around it. The lymph nodes are removed generally through a separate incision. 5) Sentinel Lymph Node Biopsy, this procedure allows for removal of only one lymph node called the sentinel node that is most likely to be the first to be involved with tumor spreading, it was a great advance and no arm swelling or painful shoulder 6) No follow up radiation, just a lumpectomy for instance, 7)External Beam Radiation, this procedure can cover the entire chest, axilla, above the collar bone etc, (6 weeks), 8) Accelerated Partial Breast Radiation (APBR) five days twice a day using a special catheter inserted in the office, 9) Intraoperative Radiation (IORT) radiation during surgery completes it, 10) Radio Frequency Ablation 11) Cryoablation using a liquid nitrogen probe through a tiny stab wound no real incision and doesn't remove any tissue, the body absorbs the dead cancer cells over time (a few months), 12) other treatments pre and post procedure such as neoadjuvant or primary chemotherapy used to shrink or downstage the tumor, anti-estrogen pre or post operation, 13) bilateral prophylactic mastectomies, ala Angelina Jolie, 14) participate in a clinical trial.

Understanding some history enables one to understand a statement that perhaps now we have arrived at a place in time where we can successfully treat breast cancer without traditional surgery, chemotherapy or radiation using the cryogenic probe without that statement seeming implausible. When Dr. Bretz opened the first comprehensive breast center in the valley in 1988, his mantra from the beginning was to preserve mind, body and spirit. Having an opportunity to view photos of his results vs. other surgeons, you can judge for yourself. As well this documents some of the personal achievements of Dr. Bretz during his decade's long fight against this disease. The one thing all these treatments have in common is the results (if done properly) are virtually the same with less and less aggressive treatments.

Over the years as a principal investigator with the National Cancer Institute (17790), Dr. Bretz has had an opportunity to see and participate in many clinical trials. With this in mind, in 1989 he had the vision to author our country's first large-scale breast cancer prevention clinical trial using the drug Tamoxifen (FDA IND 34,223) engaging the erstwhile Soviet Union as well. At the time this concept was met with much skepticism by high ranking cancer centers and for that matter the NCI. That idea was certainly outside the box as no one ever put forth this idea of preventing cancer with a pill before it gets a foothold. His idea worked and Tamoxifen was the first drug to be approved by the FDA for breast cancer prevention. Now we have three drugs but the entire advance was based on his groundbreaking idea.

What we learned from the prevention trial was we could stop cancer 50% of the time without any intervention except the pill. This was important in paving the way for other less aggressive treatments.

This document is more concerned with present day and what you decide to do with your breasts to get rid of the cancer. One misconception many have is that removing the entire breast or both will prevent me from dying if I have breast cancer. This stems from the original mantra of early surgeons to 'get it all.' We know that basically each tumor is unique and has the ability to change its genetic make-up rapidly making it resistant to any therapy. That's why 40,000 or more women in the U.S. continue to die yearly decade after decade. That is due to the tumor spreading or metastizing. If there are viable cells out there in the body then removing the breast makes no difference. It's like closing the barn door after the horse is out. The key to less aggressive procedures on the actual breast is dependent on the finding the cancers very early at about 5mm (like an eraser head on a pencil). At that size virtually none of the cancers will have reached the capacity to spread (even though in the future they might be very aggressive killers) and thus can be killed off with lessor procedures.

Over the decades starting in 1979 (Italy), a few surgeons wanted to see if lumpectomy was just as good a mastectomy with its attendant multiple side effects. To find out, clinical trials were established. Over thirty years later we know that lumpectomy results followed by some form of radiation yield the same results of local control and survival as mastectomy. The same can be said of almost all the other options. Actually Dr. Bretz was the first surgeon to perform a lumpectomy at Eisenhower Medical Center in Rancho Mirage. This was radical thinking at the time and again met with skepticism by the older surgeons. Their skepticism was unfounded. Less invasive options from sentinel lymph node biopsy (removing one node) to APBR (five days of radiation instead of six weeks) and now IORT (intraoperative Radiation) as a onetime event are again yielding the same results. Do you see a pattern emerging? Dr. Bretz has personally performed about 35 APBR procedures with no local recurrences at the original lumpectomy site over more than 15 years follow up. In fact, he is one of the only surgeons (if not the only one) to use APBR (to save the breast again), in the treatment of a local recurrence following lumpectomy and external beam radiation, when standard of care would have dictated a mastectomy. This points to a problem with advancing these techniques. Most surgeons are trained with one or two techniques and just stick to it and are not concerned with trying to change anything. The mind set to change things has to reside in the surgeon who is willing (safely) to explore new technology. During his involvement with clinical trials, Dr. Bretz and his team have successfully treated invasive breast cancer with just chemotherapy and radiation and no surgery at all. That data is published in ASCOs(American Society of Clinical Oncology) a peer reviewed journal.

Think about this. For over a hundred years surgeons were taught the dogma that only six weeks of external beam (treating the entire breast and sometimes more) radiation would be required to cure the patient. Then about fifteen years ago, APBR came into existence. APBR uses a special catheter to deliver targeted radiation to the lumpectomy site only. APBR lasts only five days instead of six weeks, another radical departure that is still not embraced by most surgeons.

Why? Because as I said, most surgeons just do their surgery and leave the rest to others. That's what separates a comprehensive center because we all strive to turn over every rock to see if there is another answer. If there is destined to be a local recurrence, 90% of the time it will recur within 1cm of the original lumpectomy site. APBR kills that 1cm so if done correctly, the results are the same compared to external beam radiation and arguable much better because of better preservation of the breast. Now surgeons in Italy have developed IORT (intraoperative radiation). The theory is that the patient has her lumpectomy and radiation during the same procedure right there in the OR. So when the patient awakens the recovery room she is done with her radiation and surgery. Now they are telling surgeons that twenty minutes of radiation is equal to the traditional six weeks. How radical is that to believe?

So if you are a radiation therapist that works at a company or hospital that recently invested more than a million dollars in advanced external beam therapy, how anxious will you be to not use that equipment and have to invest in an IORT machine? See how this works? And of course this delays bringing true advances to the majority of women. IORT is currently only done at a few hospitals in the Southern California area and Dr. Bretz has worked with Hoag Hospital in Newport Beach, sending them about five patients. The results are very good if not great.

This brings us to cryoablation. The only difference now between killing a targeted area with IORT or cryoablation is the method of killing. One uses radiation, is very costly and requires an operation in the hospital OR. Cryoablation is being done in the office under local anesthesia and the patient resumes normal activity immediately at a dramatic reduction in cost. Cryoablation is not new, in fact, it's been around for over twenty years but principally used on cancers of the liver. The key to using cryoablation in the breast is finding ultra-small tumors. This is where Dr. Bretz has concentrated his research for the last five years using modified digital military infrared, advanced ultrasound with Elastography, Halo and genetics (another new frontier doctors don't want to hear about). Dr. Fukuma in Japan has the most experience in the world using cryoablation having done about 40 cases over the last six years. To date he has no local recurrences or distant metastasis.

While Dr. Bretz (and others) are just starting this type of treatment, someone has to start here in American and make a real attempt to obtain validating data of cryoablation's possible future role in treating breast cancer. Even with excellent results, it may take another twenty years for cryoablation to become widespread just like lumpectomy did. Neither Dr. Bretz or you have that time. Thus far Dr.Bretz has done ____ cryoablation procedures starting in January of 2014.

The procedure is as follows: Instead of a hospital operating room, cryoablation can be carried out in our office setting in about a 20 minute procedure depending on the tumor size among other things. The area in question is cleaned and anesthetized using local anesthesia. A small 2mm nick in the skin is done and the probe inserted into the tissue. We use real time ultrasound to locate the tumor and make sure the probe is properly placed in ideal position. This may take several passes. In some cases if the tumor is close to the skin, Dr. Bretz will inject sterile saline immediately under the skin (using ultrasound guidance) to separate the tumor from the skin. This is necessary as the cryogenic probe produces a freeze ball (of various sizes) that approaches about -300 degrees Fahrenheit.

If the freeze ball touches the skin it may well damage it thus the reason for the saline injections. The toughest part of the procedure is excellent placement of the probe through the tumor. Once the probe is placed the machine is activated and the freezing begun for about 8 minutes. This is followed by about 6 minutes of thawing. The thawing changes the environment around the cancer cells so that they rupture. This is followed by another freezing period of 8 or so minutes. This completes the procedure and the probe is heated and removed. It's important to understand that the cryogenic procedure does not remove any tissue. It freezes the cancer and the body absorbs the dead cells over time in about six to a year depending on the size of the freezeball. Upon completion, not even a stitch or butterfly has been required and normal activity follows, even having dinner out at Lavender Bistro across the street, (thus the name The Lavender Procedure) immediately after.

Think about that. In the past patients undergoing mastectomy and axillary lymph node dissection were required to stay in the hospital several days. A 'Reach to Recovery' person came in to help teach you how to use your arm again, let alone recover psychologically from having the breast removed. This was of course preceded by interviews at the hospital, general anesthesia, the procedure itself (if a mastectomy and node dissection about 2 hours) and the risks incurred by that and hospital stay. All that is gone with the Sanarus Visica 2 System.

Complications from cryoablation are potentially the same as with any surgery. Infection, allergic reaction, skin damage, poor position of the probe and of course, failure to kill all the cancer which is akin to failure to remove all the tumor via the first lumpectomy. On average a second lumpectomy is required 40% of the time following the initial lumpectomy for retained cancer at the margins. The average complication rate across the country in younger women is about 30% and for older patients approaches 70%. You will be able to see (during the procedure) the kill zone on the ultrasound pictures. Another thing to consider is if an emergency develops, we will need to call 911 whereas the hospital is set to handle this type of emergency. Our oldest patient thus far is 86 and she tolerated the procedure very well.

The up side is:

no traditional surgery	no general anesthesia	no hospital
low cost	about a twenty minute procedure	no big incisions
no drains	normal activity after	no mastectomy

The down side: Not yet covered by insurance, the patient will be able to feel the freezeball for about a year. This procedure, 'The Lavender Procedure', is rightfully called experimental in terms of not having 20 years of known results now as with lumpectomy yet it is FDA approved for just what we do, in office cryoablation of the breast cancer. There aren't thousands of patients that have been done by anybody. We have no long term results but a small study showed 100% kill for cancer 1cm or less (what we are shooting for). For tumors larger 1.5cm to over 2cm, the first time kill is about 75%. It may well be that for larger tumors it may require two procedures. We don't know yet.

Even so, it would be arguably worth it vs. a mastectomy or the like. You will be one of the first in the United States to undergo this procedure. Future generations (your own daughter perhaps) depend on others before them stepping forward to advance technology like lumpectomy vs. mastectomy.

Dr. Bretz is as certain about this procedure will be the answer as he was when he thought up the Tamoxifen study when no one else did. Quite frankly, it has taken a long time to know what Dr. Bretz does about treating breast cancer and he is very happy with this procedure. It is what he has researched and worked on for over two decades. As indicated in the beginning, you do not have to choose Cryoablation but if you do, you should feel very comfortable that this is the right procedure for you, your questions have been answered and you are ready to proceed.

The freezeball created with the Lavender Procedure takes a long time to dissipate (go away). For larger tumors the freeze ball has still been palpable for over a year. This has not caused undo stress of any other problem to the patients. It gets smaller as the body absorbs the dead cancer cells.

There is preliminary evidence that as the dead cancer cells are absorbed by the body, the patient's own immune system may recognize the dead cancer cells (like the dead Polio Virus) and it may produce specific antibodies against the patient's own tumor. It will take years to see the value of this if any in terms of local recurrence or survival. We will be doing this in our own patients. About two months after the procedure a core biopsy will be done to document that all the cancer has been killed. The pathology reports should come back 'fat necrosis/infarction (dead tissue)'. Then mammography will be done at certain intervals and you will be able to see the 'cryohalo' that develops where the tumor was.

Lastly, there is the issue (as in all breast cancer cases) of the possibility that the disease has already spread and what to do about it. Traditionally, surgeons and oncologists have relied on a complete axillary (armpit) removal of most of the patient's lymph nodes to decide on systemic therapy (chemotherapy). Now with Sentinel Node Biopsy this has changed where one 'gatekeeper' lymph node is sampled to decide on a course of action. Also now we have tumor markers which help us decide how aggressive a given tumor might be. Even if the lymph nodes are negative the tumor can spread through the blood stream to other parts of the body and that is why we also rely on tumor analysis to decide the treatment plan. So even if the lymph nodes are negative the patient may still be a candidate for chemotherapy. The Lavender Procedure doesn't preclude axillary node surgery or chemotherapy either before or after, but generally we do it after. Chemotherapy has a profound effect on the cancer site in the breast. When chemotherapy is given before surgery (called neo-adjuvant or primary chemotherapy) there is an 80% reduction in tumor size and 30% of the time there is a complete response. Lavender is local treatment of the breast cancer only just like lumpectomy or mastectomy. Ideally with an ultra-small breast cancer at 3-5mm and with tumor analysis showing a non-aggressive tumor the goal is to avoid surgery, chemotherapy and radiation. Your significant other is invited to be present (usually hand holding) during the procedure.

Dr. Bretz has every faith in Lavender however, as this document pointed out in the beginning, you need to feel comfortable and that your concerns have been addressed and you are ready to proceed. You won't be treated differently if you decide to do conventional therapy. It's your choice. Lastly, the reason it's called The Lavender Procedure is that our fledgling tradition now is that if the patient wants we can all go over to Lavender Bistro and toast killing her cancer with a glass of chardonnay.

Your Lavender Procedure

Date:_____

Site:_____

Surgeon:_____

Equipment:_____

_____   _____   _____
       Patient   Dr. Bretz   Witness

VISIONARY BREAST CENTERS

PERMISSION TO FILM

Date:_____

I am about to undergo cryoablation (aka The Lavender Procedure) as part of my definitive care for my breast cancer. Dr. Bretz has asked my permission to film the procedure in its entirety. By signing below I am giving consent to film my procedure. I understand that on my wish my face will be blurred out such that no one can recognize me. I may also wish to be filmed without my face being blurred as future support for women around the world. Taking a stand on this issue is very important but not necessary for the filming. I will also grant or not permission to use my name in whole or part.

I also understand that filming this procedure has multiple purposes which by signing below indicates my support and consent. One purpose is to provide future surgeons/radiologists with a step by step instruction film on how to perform this procedure and another may be the use of the film for prospective investors in this technology. In the future it will be used as an educational film for women wanting to learn more about this procedure. Lastly, at the appropriate time and place it may be used in whole or part for a television type documentary.

Signed:_____

I wish my face to be blurred out: Yes   No

It's ok not to blur my face: ok not to blur   no, blur it please

You may use my name: No   First name only   First and last name are ok

Witness: _____

CHAPTER 10
MY PAPER

THE AUTHORS STATE they have no competing interests financial or otherwise and have received no funding. Because my original typed version will probably be easier to read, the published version is not presented except this first page. You can reach it at RASpublishers.com and click on oncology and therapy journal or go to scr@sciencerepository.org and click Surgical Case reports, Volume 4 Issue 9. As we go to press it's still up front but may be in the archives. Legends for the figures are at the end of the paper.

RAS ONCOLOGY & THERAPY

ISSN : 2766-2055

Research Article : The Lavender Way – Lavender Procedure - A Way to Defeat Breast Cancer Without Surgery, Chemotherapy or Radiation A Clarion Call for Radical Change

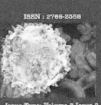

Issue Type: Volume 2 Issue 2

Author Name:
Phillip Bretz, M.D., BG Richard Lynch, D.O., (U.S. Army retired), David Mantik, M.D., Ph.D.

Corresponding Author:
Phillip Bretz, M.D., Richard Lynch, D.O., David Mantik, M.D., Ph.D

Citation: Phillip Bretz, M.D. The Lavender Way – Lavender Procedure A Way to Defeat Breast Cancer Without Surgery, Chemotherapy or Radiation A Clarion Call for Radical Change

Received Date: 18th July 2021

Published Date: 28th July 2021

Abstract:
Background
Despite advances in metabolic pathways, exosomes, ct-DNA, biomarkers, and imaging technology, breast cancer is still with us. It is a global curse with incidence set to double in the U.S. by 2030. Increasingly, researchers blame this debacle on our persistent use of unreliable preclinical testing with mouse models. Further, while basic science understanding has exploded, we know each daughter cell is genetically different, with likely increased resistance to therapy - and increased aggressiveness. Nonetheless, our current approach requires killing every one of these daughters to the last. The authors have devised a new game plan; the new goal is to kill the very first cells, not the last ones. This can be implemented globally - with dramatic cost reduction, and more lives saved while leaving the breast intact.

Methods
The authors have created The Lavender Way, which employs multiple non-radiation diagnostic modalities. This allows us to predict within ten years in a person's lifetime when breast cancer will likely manifest. Then, imaging is accelerated with modified military Infrared, ultrasound, and others to locate ultra-small breast cancers (5-8mm). Tumor analysis can determine each tumor's aggressiveness. Via a 20-minute office procedure under local anesthesia (i.e., Cryoablation, aka The Lavender Procedure), the tumor can be killed with the patients resuming normal activity immediately. It is both a dramatic change in treatment and, just as significant, a dramatic change in lifting the psychological burden of this dreaded disease.

Results
Group I - Ideal Patients Group II - Less than Ideal Group III - Strictly Palliative. All in Group I are alive after seven years except one. That one died of a fall, cancer-free, and one is alive with a local recurrence successfully treated with repeat cryoablation. Group II had one local recurrence, and one had a second primary tumor in a different location in the breast. Group III refused any other treatment and had metastatic disease. They were treated to prevent tumors from eroding through the skin. Most have died. The Lavender Way paves the way for The Lavender Procedure Conclusion

Ultra-small breast cancers with optimal bio-markers are ideal candidates for The Lavender Procedure (i.e., Cryoablation). All patients resumed normal activity immediately - without sutures. All patients in Group I and II patients have avoided surgery, chemotherapy, and radiation.

Keywords: Breast cancer, Infrared, genetic risk test, Cryoablation

INTRODUCTION

Ever since man became interested in aiding his fellow man with any medical treatment, the breast, which has always been a source of perceived beauty, sexual desire, and the epitome of femininity, has been subjected to horrendous surgical assaults throughout millennia. Fig A. Legends are on page 10.

The Lavender Way - Lavender Procedure

The Lavender Way - Lavender Procedure
A Way to Defeat Breast Cancer Without Surgery,
Chemotherapy or Radiation
A Clarion Call for Radical Change
Phillip Bretz, M.D. BG Richard Lynch, D.O. (U.S. Army Retired),
David Mantik, M.D., Ph.D
ABSTRACT

Background

Despite advances in metabolic pathways, exosomes, ct-DNA, biomarkers, and imaging technology, breast cancer is still with us. It is a global curse with incidence set to double in the U.S. by 2030. Increasingly, researchers blame this debacle on our persistent use of unreliable preclinical testing with mouse models. Further, while basic science understanding has exploded, we know each daughter cell is genetically different, with likely increased resistance to therapy - and increased aggressiveness. Nonetheless, our current approach requires killing every one of these daughters to the last. The authors have devised a new game plan; the new goal is to kill the very first cells, not the last ones. This can be implemented globally - with dramatic cost reduction, and more lives saved while leaving the breast intact.

Methods

The authors have created The Lavender Way, which employs multiple non-radiation diagnostic modalities. This allows us to predict within ten years in a person's lifetime when breast cancer will likely manifest. Then imaging is accelerated with modified military Infrared, ultrasound, and others to locate ultra-small breast cancers (5-8mm). Tumor analysis can determine each tumor's aggressiveness. Via a 20-minute office procedure under local anesthesia (i.e., Cryoablation, aka The Lavender Procedure), the tumor can be killed with the patients resuming normal activity immediately. It is both a dramatic change in treatment and, just as significant, a dramatic change in lifting the psychological burden of this dreaded disease.

Results

Group I - Ideal Patients Group II – Less than Ideal Group III – Strictly Palliative

All in Group I are alive after seven years except one. That one died of a fall, cancer-free, and one is alive with a local recurrence successfully treated with repeat cryoablation. Group II had one local recurrence, and one had a second primary tumor in a different location in the breast. Group III refused any other treatment and had metastatic disease. They were treated to prevent tumors from eroding through the skin. Most have died. The Lavender Way paves the way for The Lavender Procedure

Conclusion

Ultra-small breast cancers with optimal bio-markers are ideal candidates for The Lavender Procedure (i.e., Cryoablation). All patients resumed normal activity immediately – without sutures. All patients in Group I and II patients have avoided surgery, chemotherapy, and radiation.

The Lavender Way – Lavender Procedure

The Lavender Way – Lavender Procedure
A Way to Defeat Breast Cancer Without Surgery,
Chemotherapy or Radiation
A Clarion Call for Radical Change
Phillip Bretz, ~~M.D.~~ BG Richard Lynch, D.O. (US ARMY Retired),
David Mantik, M.D., Ph.D.

Introduction

Ever since man became interested in aiding his fellow man with any medical treatment, the breast, which has always been a source of esteemed beauty, sexual desire, and the epitome of femininity, has been subjected to horrendous surgical assaults throughout millennia. Fig A. Legends to follow paper.

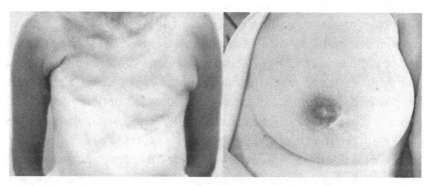

(Fig A.)

From the Edwin Smith Papyrus to Galen to Virchow to Halstead and Bernard Fisher (initiating clinical trials), we have seen an evolution of minimizing the once heralded radical surgery (1). This move from radical surgery to lumpectomy and sentinel lymph node biopsy (over the past 30 years) is being supplanted now with so-called 'Oncoplastic Surgery,' which is nothing more than an attempt by general surgeons to invade the realm of the plastic surgeon; all the while heralding the cause as cosmetic.

The United States alone has spent hundreds of millions on clinical trials that verified lumpectomy (in most cases) was the treatment of choice, less disfiguring. It took over twenty years for lumpectomy to become 'standard of care', and now it is being systematically attacked. The notion that a surgeon can go to a 'weekend' course on 'Oncoplastic' technique and become competent that effectively replaces years of plastic surgery residency is preposterous.

A naïve public and frightened women who have grown up with the notion to 'Just get it out of me,' have permitted this nonsense to be perpetuated thus reverting back to 'getting it all,' accompanied with the equally preposterous assurance that the breast will attain a cosmetic result second to none. Almost every advance in less disfiguring treatment has been met with opposition from a hierarchy of self-proclaimed key opinion leaders. Evidence-based medicine, which has come into vogue ushered in by an increasing number of functionaries, has eviscerated the 'art of medicine.'

Doctors under the constant threat of litigation or an aggressive non-understanding medical board or a restrictive H.M.O. are afraid to step out of the safe harbor of 'standard of care.' While it can be argued that evidence-based medicine has its place in documenting progress for posterity, it cannot be relied on to provide optimal care to an individual patient. Years of experience interacting with patients hones one's ability to treat cancer, adding to one's expertise as decades go by. Dogma and tradition make it almost impossible for radical change to free us from "the confident complacency of assumed righteousness in the way things are done." (2)

Having been trained by aggressive surgeons (whose motto was, 'For them it is unresectable'), we participated in the holocaust on women that dictated radical disfiguring surgery was the key in the late 1970s. Embracing lumpectomy following Umberto Veronese's seminal paper in 1979 led to further reductions in the aggressive approach including embracing Accelerated Partial Breast Radiation (twice daily for five days), Fig B, which partially supplanted the five days a week for six weeks with a booster at the end, namely external beam radiation.

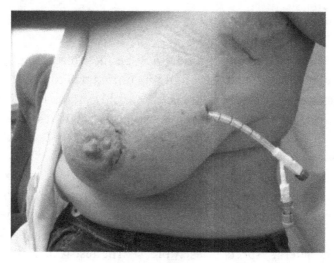

(Fig B.)

Further refinements in radiation, i.e., IORT (Intraoperative radiation), led to a breakthrough to minimize treatment (Cryoablation) and refinements in the basic understanding of the genome and infrared technology as well as other non-radiation imaging devices. Technology has caught up to breast cancer if one bothers to look. This is a core problem as hardly few doctors appear interested.

Instead of chasing the last cancer cell to kill it, we embraced the journey of finding the first cell as close as possible, thus ushering the age of The Lavender Way/Procedure. Cancer in its final display of authority over the body, "crushes hope, leaving a wasteland of grief, depression, despair and a sense of unending futility." (2)

What if it were possible to obviate everything breast cancer has wrought on us for millennia? What if breast cancer treatment could be taken not only out of the operating theatre but out of the system altogether at the cost of a few hundred dollars (depending on how much one wanted to save), save lives, and make it available to virtually every woman globally?

Methods

INFRARED

Multiple non-radiation modalities besides mammography are used to optimize our chances of finding ultra-small tumors (5-8mm). Those include modified military Infrared, ultrasound, Halo, and Sure Touch devices. The I.R. technology used is not that of the 1970s, where in the past, Infrared obtained a bad reputation. It was classified military until about 2002 when then-President Bush declassified it. The patient is seated disrobed on top, 4ft from the cooling device, which houses an 8000 BTU air conditioner. No hand ice cooling is necessary. The ambient temperature in the room is maintained at 73 degrees. First-degree mirrors are attached to the chair and placed to image the lateral aspects of each breast. The test runs four minutes (including 3000 images), and results are available immediately, including neural network (running the patient's heat signature by known cancer cases). As time passes and more cancer heat signatures are added, the result becomes that much more accurate. In the first 500 patients, the false-negative rate was 0.4%. The smallest cancer found was 4mm.

The Infrared employed is not the technology of the 1970s but rather modified military digital infrared coupled with immediate computer readout of results and analysis via a neural network (artificial intelligence). The unit is called Sentinel BreastScan developed by First Sense Medical. What is infrared? Infrared is part of the electromagnetic spectrum lying between visible and microwave segments of the spectrum. An infrared imaging camera observes and measures thermal energy emitted from an object. The higher the object's temperature, the greater the I.R. energy emitted. The infrared camera is a non-contact device that detects infrared energy and converts it into an electronic signal that is then processed to produce a thermal image on a video monitor. It also performs temperature calculations. Recent innovations in detector technology have made its use in breast imaging much more accurate. A microbolometer is used as a detector in infrared cameras. Emitted infrared energy from an object with a wavelength from 8 to 13 um strikes the detector, heating it, and changing its electric resistance. This resistance change is measured and proceeds into temperature, which can be used to create an image on the video monitor.

The microbolometer used in the FLIR A 40 is an uncooled thermal sensor. Simply put, the military uses advanced infrared technology because it works. The military uses infrared from sniper scopes to cameras onboard the Predator, to visible light video tracking systems such as THEL (Tactical High Energy Laser). By using Infrared as an adjunct, the tracked target's imaging is improved under no-light conditions or heavy cloud cover. Thus, the target's bearing, range, and elevations can be continuously updated. It is called Range Phenomenology. Modern uncooled detectors all use sensors that work by the change of resistance, voltage, or current when heated by infrared radiation.

A possible sensor assembly uses an integrated circuit with barium strontium titanate, bump-bonded polymide in a thermally insulated connection.

The FLIR A40 detector is a focal plane array, an uncooled microbolometer with 320,240 pixels. The neural network should be continuously updated. It currently uses a collection of infrared reports integrated with pathology reports and programmed into the computer. The military has a name for objects on the ground sensed by Infrared from the air: "heat signature." So too, do cancers leave a "heat signature." The neural network is designed to learn and then becomes more accurate as experience develops. The current camera has the capability of detecting heat coming from developing cancer of 1.5 mm. It also works independently of angiogenesis and has detected small (2 mm) clusters of evolving benign calcifications. See Figs C, D, E, F, G, H, I, J. All legends for figures are on pages 20-21. Halo is a liquid biopsy device that potentially alerts the doctor to nascent cancers about 2mm or less. Sure-Touch is a pressure sensing device able to identify single and multiple targets, hard and soft at 5mm. See Fig. K.

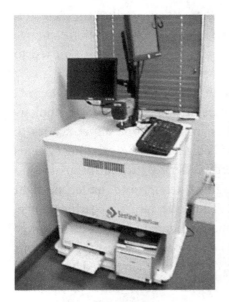

(Fig C.)

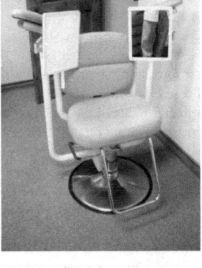

(Fig D.)

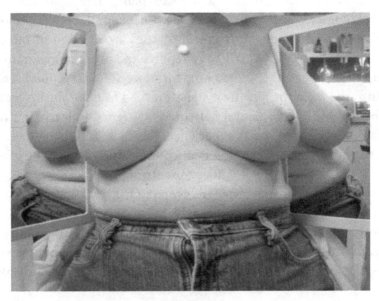

(Fig E.)

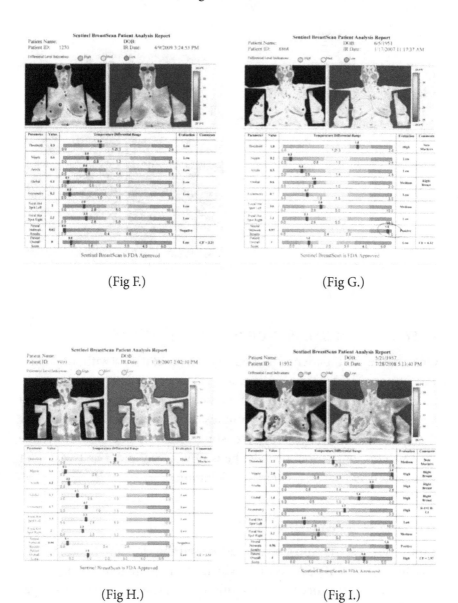

(Fig F.)   (Fig G.)

(Fig H.)   (Fig I.)

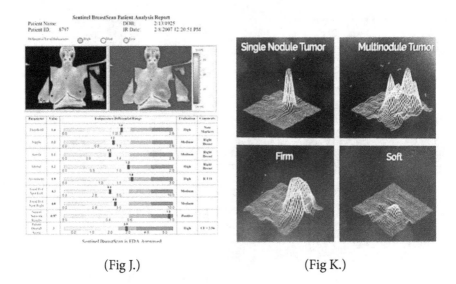

(Fig J.)   (Fig K.)

WHY IS IT NAMED LAVENDER?

One of the first patients to undergo Cryoablation (with implants) was hungry right after, and she suggested we walk across the street to Lavender Bistro (a high-end French/American restaurant in La Quinta, CA). Within twenty minutes after the procedure, she was dining on lobster salad and, yes, toasting with a sip of chardonnay, like the procedure never happened. She is now seven and a half-years out cancer-free. No surgery, chemo or radiation.

WHAT IS THE LAVENDER WAY?

Simply put, it starts with a healthy 20 something who undergoes genetic risk testing, not BRCA testing, which is only suitable for about 10 percent of breast cancer patients. It is a saliva test that singles out age-specific SNPs (single nucleotide polymorphisms), so we can predict not only lifetime risk but when that risk is likely to manifest within ten years. In most cases, this gives us decades to alter lifestyle changes and active prevention with Nolvadex or Raloxifene when a patient hits menopause. This genetic information is used to decide what imaging should be done and how often, independent of any guidelines, genuinely personalized care. Then as the time to the theorized appearance of the cancer approaches, imaging is accelerated since none of these diagnostic modalities harbors radiation. Mammography and M.R.I. are included on an as-needed basis. This approach may have saved Miss Venezuela, who died of metastatic breast cancer at age 26. She brings home the point. Yes, by herself, it is just an anecdotal case, but be assured it was not anecdotal to her family. Cancer cuts deep and is a very sobering personal experience for each person. Our task is to unload that burden.

It is not just that. Lavender is a sanctuary dedicated to educating young and older women on the journey of life's health problems and how to avoid their impact. It is giving them street smarts. The same doctor sees patients for decades (sans E.M.R.), so a real understanding of each patient's needs and real communication takes place in a trusting atmosphere.

Each patient knows what steps are being taken to diagnose and prevent breast cancer. She knows as well, if those steps are followed if cancer does ever arise, she should be a candidate for The Lavender Procedure, meaning Cryoablation, hopefully being able to avoid any surgery, chemotherapy or radiation.

This situation calls for an entirely different approach than instituting a nationwide breast screening program and hoping women flock in. Family physicians acting as gatekeepers and some self-appointed key opinion makers dictate thru some 'national guidelines' when and how often a woman undergoes what type of imaging. This approach must stop. We must abandon the one size fits all and replace it with a truly personalized caring environment. There are increasing numbers of women deciding to avoid mammography altogether for various reasons, including the fear of radiation. The Lavender Way would be effective here with genetic testing and the use of multiple non-radiation modalities. Otherwise, this burgeoning population of women would just come in with advanced tumors. The treating breast doctor must be beyond fluent in reading mammograms (actually viewing each one along with the patient), trained to be multi-talented and able to act (if necessary) the same day, i.e., ultrasound-guided core biopsy. The sine qua non of Lavender is that the patient leaves the center armed with the knowledge that generally would sometimes take weeks to learn and what will be done about it. That is, the very same doctor she has seen for sometimes decades can carry out treatment after all options and second opinions are explored.

The current system in the U.S. is not geared to finding ultra-small cancers, and major cancer centers must deal with whatever palpable cancer walks through the door. It is their fatal flaw.

This perpetuates the "slash-poison-burn" approach as Dr. Raza so eloquently puts it. Another sine qua non is no waiting. If the patient needs to be seen that day, she is. No gatekeeper stands in the way of alleviating the oppressing distress that finding a 'lump' brings. The Lavender Way paves the way for The Lavender Procedure.

WHAT IS THE LAVENDER PROCEDURE?

Simply put, it kills a DCIS or invasive breast cancer in the office in about 20 minutes under local anesthesia using a liquid nitrogen emitting probe to engulf the tumor under real-time ultrasound. Fig L, M, N, O, P, Q. In a play on words like the sign that read, "All Ye who enter here abandon all hope," to understand the Lavender method, the sign needs to read, "All Ye who enter here abandon all previous dogma on breast cancer treatment." Starting with a blank sheet of paper was/ is the order of the day. A sterling example is that for decades, surgeons, pathologists, oncologists, and radiation therapists have fretted about obtaining 'clear margins' and exactly what that constitutes. In Lavender, the tumor is never removed, so margins never come into play in the traditional sense. The operating surgeon knows the genetic potential, family history, markers, and size of the tumor to ensure an adequate P.K.Z. (peripheral kill zone) which can be altered at will to engulf the tumor and surrounding tissue. This process is easily seen on ultrasound.

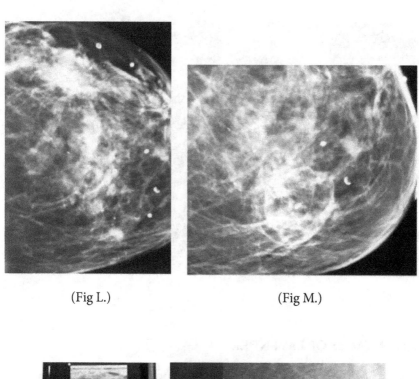

(Fig L.) (Fig M.)

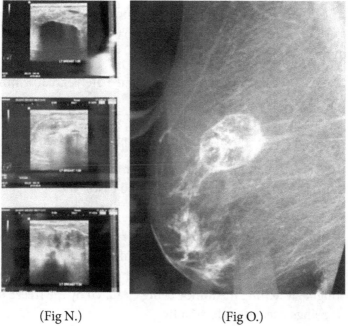

(Fig N.) (Fig O.)

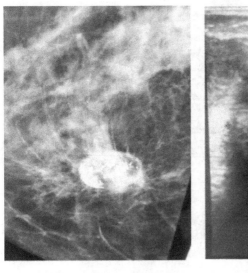

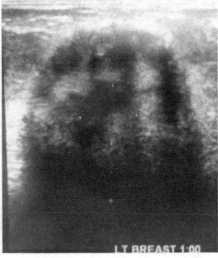

(Fig P.)   (Fig Q.)

ADVANTAGES OF LAVENDER

- It is a 20-minute in-office procedure outside the OR and system, hopefully avoiding surgery, chemotherapy, and radiation.

- Patients resume normal activity immediately, no downtime.

- No suturing is necessary.

- Lavender saves on environmental concerns and time.

- Lavender does not preclude either chemotherapy (pre or post-therapy) or radiation in selected cases.

- Patients are awake throughout the entire process. Once the probe is placed, a significant other may enter the room to hold the patient's hand or just observe. It dramatically changes the frightening experience (waiting in the hospital) to an almost "high," watching the tumor being engulfed by the freeze ball. It brings needed understanding.

- There is no general anesthesia.

- The aim is no axillary dissection (depending on ultrasound, genetics, and markers).

- There is a low chance of infection.

- There is a dramatic reduction in cost, the entire process from diagnosis to treatment costing a few hundred dollars to a few thousand (depending on how much is to be saved) vs. about $125,00 for an average breast cancer case from diagnosis to treatment in the U.S. There is the potential to save over 10 billion dollars annually.

- It would be available to the entire population, thereby leveling the playing field for the underserved.

- Any doctor in a country where surgeons or radiologists are not plentiful can be trained.

- In countries with remote populations, i.e., Africa, the entire process could be achieved on an 18 wheeler offering (if need be) diagnosis and treatment in one day.

- Because The Lavender Way is efficient at finding ultra-small tumors, most will be hormone positive and susceptible to an anti-estrogen of choice to complement the procedure. While tumors will generally become more aggressive as they grow, finding an ultra-small tumor usually means less aggression and positive hormone receptors.

- There is increasing evidence that upon resorption of the dead tumor cells, the patient's immune system responds in producing specific antibodies against the tumor. Long-term analysis of this phenomenon needs follow-up for any recurrence prevention, e.g., The Abscopal Effect.

- The Lavender Procedure can be repeated without sacrificing the breast.

- Cost in 3rd world countries could be drastically reduced, allowing treatment of all women.

- Multiple tumors in one breast can be treated the same day. We call it the "snowman" since one freeze ball will be on top of another. This option is limited, and perhaps one additional tumor close by is acceptable, not scattered multiple tumors.

- Mammography/ultrasound and core biopsy are performed two months post Lavender to ensure total kill of the tumor. Should any residual tumor be present, the patient has the option of a repeat Lavender or moving on to more standard care. This option is not open if mastectomy has been performed. Essentially, no time is lost as the patient is usually on anti-estrogen therapy.

- Lavender can be performed on patients with breast implants.

- Lavender can be performed on elderly patients so as not to impede their quality of life.

- Instead of the patient's relentless depressing mood with traditional therapy, the extremely positive outlook expressed by the patient and their families is second to none.

- Last but not least, it is virtually impossible to tell the breast was ever touched. We have seen the long term positive emotional and psychological implications for the patient, partner, and family.

DISAVANTAGES OF LAVENDER

- The doctor must be trained/skilled in real-time ultrasound probe insertion.

- In most cases, there would be no "in hospital" code team should the patient arrest.

- This is not for every patient, especially larger tumors, 2cm, and above.

- Potential skin damage because of contact with the nitrogen freeze ball is avoided with an infusion of saline acting as a buffer and utilizing warm saline compresses to help protect the skin.

- As in lumpectomy, it may require a second procedure.

- There is possible pain on insertion of the probe, which is generally well controlled with local anesthesia.

- Potential for infection; however, none so far going into the 6th year.

- Most patients end up with a few millimeters residual freeze ball, at times palpable.

- In 2020 this procedure is currently not covered by insurance.

PATIENT SELECTION

Since this is a fledging endeavor for most doctors, limiting patients with tumors 1cm or less and easily seen on ultrasound should portend success. However, before attempting a live case (as the patient and family are present), practicing skewering an olive or the like with a probe under ultrasound guidance is recommended. A turkey breast serves the purpose.

The nodal situation could be dealt with performing a needle biopsy of an axillary node via ultrasound, if possible. If tumor analysis dictates a less aggressive tumor (which is what Lavender Way portends), e.g., low Ki-67 and clinically negative nodes, and benign appearance on ultrasound, we have avoided any node surgery including Sentinel. Thus far, there have been no positive axillary lymph nodes years later. Generally, most of these smaller tumors will still be hormone-positive, and patients started on an anti-estrogen of choice depending on age. An ultrasound technician may assist until expertise is developed.

INFORMED CONSENT

A thorough informed consent should extol the virtues of each option from mastectomy to Cryoablation. The patient should not be 'talked into' Cryoablation but embrace it after considering all options with their pros and cons.

RESULTS - *Praesessi Pro Se Loqui*

Between January 2014 and August 2016, I have performed 25 procedures on 21 patients. One patient had multiple synchronous bilateral cancers and refused any treatment but Cryoablation. Because of her and others refusing any other treatment, we performed Lavender on larger tumors, up to 3.5cm. Most of those patients ultimately died of metastatic disease. We have divided the patients into three groups. Group I are ideal patients that we felt disease in the breast could be controlled. We do not use the word cure. Group II patients had less than desirable targets, i.e., DCIS (no precise solid mass on ultrasound) and Group III are patients who refused traditional treatment with larger tumors where we knowingly had no real chance for control except for preventing skin invasion and considered these palliative procedures.

Group I (11 patients)	Group II (4 patients)	Group III (6 patients)
Ages – 43 – 86	65-75	38-81
Tumors – 5mm – 1.1cm	Tis (DCIS) – 8mm	Tis (prior lumpectomy) - 3.5cm
Breast – UOQ – 6, UIQ – 2, LIQ – 2, LOQ - 1	UOQ – 3 LIQ – 1	UOQ – 5 LOQ - 1
Markers – ER+ 8, PR+ 8, Her 2- neg (7)	ER+ 4, PR+ 3, Her2+	ER+ 3,PR+ 1, Her2+1

Ki-67 mostly very low	N/A	no data
Nodes – all clinically and U/S benign	all clinically neg/ U/S benign	all palpable nodes
Freezeball – 4-5cm	3cm	5cm
Saline – 7 yes, 4 no	2 yes, 2 no	all
Anti-estrogen – most all	most all	mostly refused
Sequence - usually 6-10-6	usually 6-10-6, one 4-10-4 (recurrence)	multiple attempts
Old Local Recurrence – 2 (FROM IDC 2003 & 2007)	2 one DCIS and another second primary	1

Anesthesia - .25% Marcaine without epi uniformly

EBL – Minimal	Minimal	Minimal
Complications – 0	0	0
Alive cancer-free – 10	3	1
Deaths – 1 from fall not breast cancer	1 – from primary lung not breast	One died we can verify as some in Group III were from foreign countries where we lost contact.

EQUIPMENT LIST

- A table to place the patient in semi-Fowler's position

- Sterile half sheet and scissors to cut an appropriate hole for the breast

- 2 pillows (one for the patient's head and another to prop up the patient's side)

- Mobile tray with a sterile cover

- Local anesthesia of choice (.25% Marcaine without epinephrine)

- Liquid nitrogen (ensure enough for scheduled cases)

- Tuberculin syringe (to create a skin wheal)

- Five loaded 20cc syringes with sterile saline with 25ga. needle (for buffer)

- 4x4 gauze, and 2-inch Transpore tape to prop up the breast as needed

- Betadine

- 11 blade knife with Ethyl Chloride to spray skin before local anesthesia is applied.

- Ultrasound machine – cryoablation unit

- Sterile water (for probe testing)

- 2 probes (one held in abeyance should the primary probe fail)

- Signed consent for procedure and filming, including whether face should be blurred.

- Smelling salts in case of a vaso-vagal reaction

- Medium hot water soaked 4x4s for warm compress (changes as needed to protect skin)

- Sterile gloves

- Antibiotic ointment and 2x2 gauze with Transpore tape to cover probe entrance site

- Camera

- Dedicated personnel to provide warm compresses and change Dewar

FOLLOW UP LIST

- A phone call to the patient the day after for status check

- The patient is notified (again) to contact the office for any problems

- Office visit one week later for a recheck and perform ultrasound

- Mammogram/ultrasound with core biopsy two months later to ensure a total kill

- Mammogram every six months for three years/ultrasound every six months for five years then yearly

- Document patient taking anti-estrogen

- Continued data collection and publication of results are critical

DISCUSSION

If breast cancer were as lethal as a bite from a Black Mamba (a highly poisonous snake), then patients in Group I should all have died from metastatic breast cancer. However, some going into the 7th year they have not. Perhaps Lavender has shown another way to diagnose and manage breast cancer that can put breast cancer in the history books. Countries must first decide just how important women are and institute an environment like Lavender to change the paradigm. Most in Group I had invasive breast cancer, and some would say treated outside of 'standard of care,' yet (all technology is F.D.A. cleared) they are all alive except one (from the fall) and cancer-free into the 5th and some beyond 7 years. As would be expected, these very early cancers are usually hormone positive and lower Ki-67, thus permitting no axillary dissection. Thus far, there is no positive nodal involvement. The procedure can be performed on patients with implants and is an ideal alternative for elderly patients with limited mobility, which might be exacerbated with axillary dissection and subsequent nerve damage. The cosmetic result is indeed second to none in preserving a woman's natural breast. Since only two months go by after Lavender (with the patient usually on an anti-estrogen) when mammography and biopsy are done, essentially no valuable time is lost if a residual tumor is found to proceed with another attempt or move to lumpectomy. Lavender has been successfully used on local recurrences where tradition dictates mastectomy. In each case, the breast was able to be preserved. One patient has had three cancers in one breast stemming from cancer in her early 30s, where lumpectomy and external radiation were employed. This was followed by a local recurrence 14 years later, and APBR (Accelerated Partial Breast Radiation) was employed and yet another cancer, 15 years later, in another part of the breast and Lavender was employed.

This was well outside of 'standard of care;' however, she is now more than seven years out and thus far cancer-free with an intact body. Patients (where possible) have been followed for a minimum of five years and some more than 7.5 years in groups 1 and 2 including those treated with a local recurrence.

Another critical issue is that implementing Lavender Centers nationally would help obviate the known discrepancy of decreased survival and developing more aggressive tumors earlier in life between African-American women and all other races.

Lavender would level the playing field overnight. The key to this entire endeavor is the foreknowledge of when the cancer is most likely to strike and to accelerate the non-radiation modalities to find these nascent tumors amenable to Lavender, thus obviating surgery, chemotherapy, and radiation. To ensure success at the outset, one should limit their foray into Lavender with very easily and sharply defined targets on ultrasound.

Group II patients are examples of less-than-ideal targets with less-than-ideal results. Experience will dictate the limits of Lavender. We were self-taught as there was no one six years ago providing instruction. We have learned both the limits and the unlimited potential of Lavender. Group III was solely palliative in nature to prevent these tumors from eroding the skin.

The other side of the coin is the horrendous psychological battles that rage relentlessly in a patient just diagnosed with breast cancer. As a patient recently wrote, "It's like staring into an abyss without means of comfort thinking the worst, leaving your children and family behind." Not so with Lavender. The psychological turnaround is dramatic. There is no downtime, and bodies are intact (unscathed from side effects of surgery, chemotherapy, and radiation). This positive turnaround is seen, especially with the patient and her family being able to watch the entire procedure. They can watch the cancer being killed right before their eyes. It is dramatically euphoric. Lifting this burden from women that have haunted them for many millennia is finally within reach. The status quo needs to be challenged.

The Abscopal Effect – While complicated, a simple explanation is that under certain conditions, a combination of immunotherapy with Cryoablation not only kills cells locally but may effectively kill cancer cells in the periphery. With the dawn of the revaluation that Cryoablation under certain conditions may obviate the decade's long disfiguring surgery, comes the revaluation that killing cancer with Cryoablation (liquid nitrogen at -180 C or -300 F) may well activate the immune system to kill cancer cells elsewhere in the body. The investigation of this phenomenon is in its infancy. That said, there are some facts known. Cancers can and do escape the immune system's response, and one of the known ways to prevent this evasion is through immune checkpoint inhibitors. "Cryoablation causes cell death by necrosis induced by cold temperatures and by apoptosis in cells found in the periphery of the tumor. Cells dying from apoptosis do not stimulate T-cells. It is theorized that intracellular contents of cells killed by necrosis stay intact. This may result in an immune response which may well kill cancer cells distant from the primary site. This is the Abscopal Effect. The trick is to enhance this effect. Preliminary investigation indicates this can be done by affecting the signals produced by the intracellular contents of the cells killed by necrosis. The intracellular contents cause mature dendritic cells which fully activate T cell receptors.

This is so-called signal 1. Signal 2 involves the interplay between programmed death receptor 1 (PD-1) on the T-cell and programmed death ligand 1 (PD-L1) on the tumor cell. T-cell activation (and thus anti-body formation) is blocked if signal 2 is suppressed. Thus, the cancer cell escapes death. However, if anti-PD1 antibody is used, that inhibiting signal is blocked allowing activation of the T cell.

Another immune checkpoint inhibitor, anti-cytotoxic T lymphocyte-associated protein 4 (CTLA-4), also has been shown to enhance the immune response" (3)(4). Further investigation into the enhancement of immunostimulatory and immunosuppressive responses is needed to elucidate the potential of the abscopal effect fully.

The Tulip Procedure – We have used the Lavender Procedure on multiple old local recurrences, and those patients are now over five years out without evidence of re-recurrence. All the while, her body, and mind remain intact. It has been dubbed "The Tulip Procedure" because just like a tulip comes through the ground every spring, cancer does what it does, and that is, at times, recur. While treating doctors can differ on the ideal treatment for each patient, what they can't differ on is that there is a time interval (different for each patient) when a tumor is born and when it attains the capacity to metastasize. This is when the cancer is most amenable to conservative treatment, including Lavender. Likewise, with a nascent recurrence, that same time frame (different but real for each patient) comes to be. Since these patients are watched so closely, it has been our experience to re-Lavender these patients (after due consideration for alternative more standard of care procedures), and they have done well. More experience will dictate how many Tulip Procedures are feasible.

One final aspect is the psychological impact on the operating doctor. In traditional therapy, the blame for a patient not doing well could be passed around, so to speak. The surgeon did not get clear margins, the oncologist did not use the right drug, and the radiation therapist did not use the right portals. With Lavender, there is only one person to blame, and one must be able to withstand the pressure each time one of these patients undergoes mammography.

Conclusion

In the beginning, a clarion call was issued for radical change in the standard of care in the diagnosis and treatment of breast cancer. A different standard of care will be called for if The Lavender Way and Lavender Procedure have a mainstream presence. The gist of all this is that embracing Lavender, bodies, lives, and families can be saved without enormous cost, and any trained doctor could do it. A large cancer center is not needed to execute this endeavor. While there are more emerging articles about Cryoablation, we are not aware of any entity that has figured out a way to ensure the successful outcome that finding ultra-small breast cancer portends like The Lavender Way. That is the key. We all have to decide just how important women are and act on it. "Since 2005, 70 percent of approved drugs have shown zero improvement in survival rate while up to 70 percent have been actually harmful to patients.

The issue is not so much that there has been little progress in cancer research, the question is why there is so little improvement in treatment. With minor variations, a protocol of surgery, chemotherapy and radiation - the slash-poison-burn approach to treating cancer – remains unchanged. It is an embarrassment. Equally embarrassing is the arrogant denial of that embarrassment." (2) A search of the literature reveals almost 4 million papers published on cancer. The question is who reads all these papers?? Who is in charge of implementing any change on a nationwide or global basis?

It is clear that confronted with this regimen, how will change, and a cure for cancer ever come to pass? In the United States of America, at least, only one person has the legal and moral authority to break this stranglehold on cancer research, and that is the President of the United States.

Recently, the Space Force was authorized as a separate entity among the various armed forces of the U.S. The President could enact a new and separate research agency with a new vision, separate and apart from existing health agencies such as the N.I.H. and NCI.

Alternatively, a forward-thinking country could initiate The Lavender Way and Lavender Procedure and publish their results. The first country to do this will bring a new paradigm to the detection and treatment of breast cancer. Ultimately, women and their caregivers must demand this change in the standard of care.

As final thoughts, it is apropos to revisit some writings of Dr. Vincent T. DeVita Jr as his experience should open our eyes to just how innovation takes place and what hinders it, especially in a disease like cancer. Taken from an article published in the New Yorker on December 7th, 2015, "The breakthroughs made at the N.C.I. in the nineteen-sixties and seventies were the product of a freewheeling intellectual climate. The social conditions that birthed a new idea in one place, impeded the spread of that same idea in another. When the cancer researcher Bernard Fisher (R.I.P.) did a study showing that there was no difference in outcome between radical mastectomies and the far less invasive lumpectomies, he called DeVita in distress. He couldn't get the study published." This is a sterling example of people's uptight nature reluctant to change even when positive results are staring them in the face.

This example of Fisher's problem getting his study published points to another problem of American cancer researchers. What isn't mentioned in DeVita's article or in the publication of Fisher is that Fisher's trial's initiation was based totally on Umberto Veronesi's landmark article. Simply by our American researchers embracing a well-done study by the Italians and getting this new, less disfiguring treatment out there immediately, we had to do yet another six-year-long re-do. Even when results verified Umberto's, it took about twenty years for lumpectomy to be accepted. Now with functionaries leading the way with ever-mounting regulations and insistence on 'evidence-based medicine' as the only way, no wonder women are continually sacrificed.

DeVita further states, "Clinical progress against a disease as wily and dimly understood as cancer, DeVita argues, happens when doctors have the freedom to try unorthodox things – and he worries we have lost sight on that fact." Another sterling example is his association with Dr. Freireich at the N.C.I. This is how intrathecal injections of an antibiotic came to save lives of people with leukemia and Pseudomonas Meningitis. "The first time Freireich told me to do it, I held up the vial and showed him the label, thinking that he'd possibly missed something. It said right there, Do Not Use Intrathecally. I said. Freireich glowed at me and pointed a long bony finger in my face "DO IT." "He barked. I did it, though I was terrified. But it worked every time." No evidence-based medicine here.

Concerning breast cancer, specifically, DeVita writes, "Years ago, women with all stages of breast cancer had radical mastectomies, leaving just tissue over bone and a painful swollen arm. Then they died. Look how far we've come."

The question now is, have we come far enough to see the light, or are we reverting to 'getting it all' with oncoplastic surgery, with the simultaneous incrimination of Cryoablation and advanced non-radiation diagnostic modalities?

Considering the entrenched opinions of a key self-appointed hierarchy, our assertion that the only person to break this tumult is the President of the United States - by authorizing a new research agency and deployment of a pilot study of Lavender Breast Centers.

Compliance with Ethical Standards

All three authors report no conflict of interest
No animals were used
Informed consent was obtained from all patients
These proceedings were carried out with ethical standards set down in the 1964 Helsinki declaration and its later amendments.

REFERENCES

1. Larhthkia Ritu, A Brief History of Breast Cancer, Sultan Qaboos University Medical Journal, 2014 May; 14 (2): @ 166-169

2. Raza Azra, The First Cell, Hachette Book Group, October 2019, page 35

3. Abdo J, Immunotherapy Plus Cryoablation: Potential to Augmented Abscopal Effect for Advanced Cancers, Front Oncol, 2018 Mar 28; 8:85

4. Aarts B.M., Cryoablation and immunotherapy: an overview of evidence on its synergy, Insights Imaging, 2019 Dec; 10:53 Department of Radiology. The Netherlands Cancer Institute

FIGURE LEGENDS

A - This photo depicts the aggressive surgery of the 1970's compared to Lavender on the right just about two minutes after the procedure with a dab of antibiotic ointment, no suturing ever.

B - This photo depicts APBR with a lumpectomy and Sentinel node incision.

C - This photo depicts the infrared machine set up

D - This photo depicts the chair with first degree mirrors

E - This photo depicts a patient in the chair with mirrors reflecting the lateral aspect of each breast

F - This is the report generated immediately. It has multiple readings including threshold both depicted above left and below on the colored bars showing temperature differential. The threshold above left shows the most reluctant tissue to cool down; it is either the small or big circle and either green, yellow or pink.

The photo above right displays lines drawn by the operator to direct the computer where to analyze. The locations and which breast are seen on the left, followed by the temperature differential; then evaluation and lastly the comment section will identify right or left breast U.O.Q. etc. It is better to be in the green. The evaluation section is either low or high and the neural network is either positive or negative (indicating it has seen this heat pattern before and likely a cancer). The comment section is critical. If there is an indication of what breast and where in the comment section, it usually means the sensors have identified an area which demands attention. Lastly, while this report is a negative (83.8% were), it does show a cancer (not in the breast). Can you find it? It's a basal cell carcinoma in the neck. We call it the 'Ruby Sign.'

G - This report depicts a patient with a probable cancer in the right breast in the U.O.Q., can you tell why? Look at the neural network and threshold image.

H - This report shows a target in the left breast at six o'clock. However, unlike the mammogram which called it suspicious for cancer, it is telling us the lesion is benign and so it was on biopsy. The false negative rate for mammography in our series was 24%. The lesion was actually just about a 3mm focus of evolving calcifications. This report also demonstrates that I.R. can pick up targets without neo-vascularization. Reports such as this also demonstrate that combined with other modalities, especially genetics risk, we can potentially limit breast biopsies (of which there are over 700,000 in the U.S. annually and about 80% are benign).

I - This report demonstrates a large right breast cancer with multiple findings.

J - This report demonstrates a cancer in the right breast or does it? Look at the images and read the graph, evaluation and comment sections. A work up of the breast including M.R.I.

failed to demonstrate a cancer in the right breast. Where could the cancer be? It was in the right upper lobe of the lung.

FIGURE LEGENDS CONTINUED

K - This is a Sure-Touch representation of typical targets identified using this pressure sensing device. It can identify targets as small as 5mm. The patient (once instructed) could do this at home to complement self-breast exam and the report sent into the cloud.

L - This mammogram shows a CC view of the left breast and a cancer medial (see arrow). This patient is significant in that she first developed breast cancer in her early thirties and lumpectomy and external beam were preformed (architectural distortion laterally). After about 14 years she had a local recurrence at the original site. It was treated with re-lumpectomy and APBR, not mastectomy, as standard of care would dictate. She went another 15 years and then had a second primary in the same breast (three cancers in all), well medial from the original site. The patient was adamant in trying to preserve her breast. Five years ago, she underwent The Lavender Procedure, i.e., Cryoablation and has been cancer free, breast intact and on Nolvadex for over five years.

M - This is her mammogram five years out with the typical residual 'cryo halo' with no evidence of cancer. See arrow. It remains clinically palpable but only about 5mm. The original lateral position has been submitted to two core biopsies over the years also without a recurrence.

N - This series of ultrasounds depicts the tumor below; the middle image is the cryoprobe skewering the tumor and the top is the growing freezeball encompassing the tumor and P.K.Z. (peripheral kill zone) well beyond the tumor margin. The operator controls the size and location of the freezeball so excision of the tumor with verification of negative margins is not necessary. The total kill is confirmed on core biopsy two months post procedure.

O - This mammogram depicts a typical freezeball years after the procedure. Most patients end up with a small (few millimeter) nodule as a remnant of the original freezeball.

P - This mammogram depicts a more calcified freezeball which often happens but is usually small.

Q - This ultrasound image depicts the typical liquefaction following Cryoablation and it usually stays like this for about 3 years on ultrasound.

Before we move on to Chapter 11, I thought I would include some images of surgeries I've done, and surgeries done by competitor surgeons in town. These images are not so horrendous but some still disturbing like the surgeon who told the patient he didn't have time to do a circumareolar incision. You will see that outcome.

Here is an image of the reverse fistula I helped pioneer at Loyola and later at Eisenhower. A fistula is needed so the patient's vein can withstand multiple venous punctures for dialysis when the kidneys fail. Below this image you can see the vein under the skin which over time becomes like an artery.

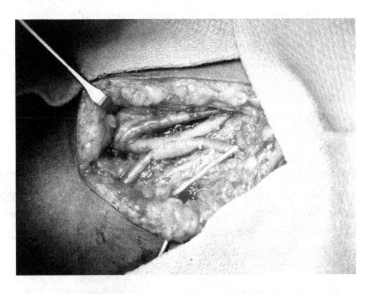

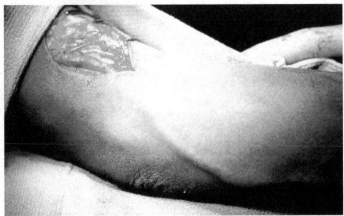

Below are a couple of bad lumpectomies, no need for this disfigurement if the surgeon knows how to avoid it and leave the breast basically untouched. I guess that's asking too much.

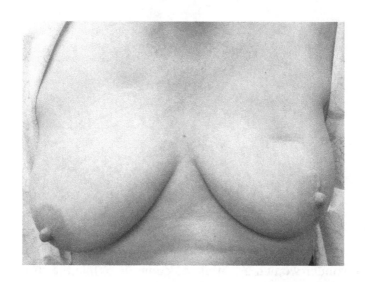

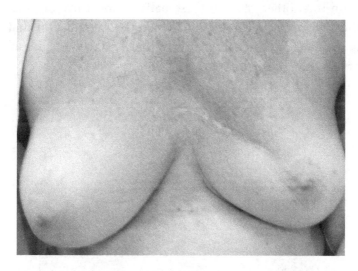

Where do these guys/girls come from? Unacceptable! The next patient is an otherwise beautiful 30-year-old. Did she deserve the slash technique?

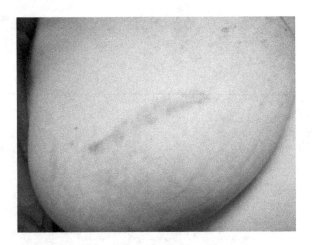

No wonder women are afraid to come in. While the surgeon just moves on to another case, all these patients must live out their lives with the disfigurement caused by a system that is rigid. One that is not willing to change and apparently, with images like these, doesn't care. It's not like changing a tire, is it.

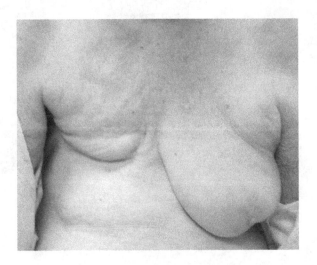

The next one is one of my "cosmetic lumpectomies" with the circumareolar incision. As I said, I was after her to get the incision tattooed but she won't because it reminds her of me. Can you believe that? I'd rather have that accolade than any certificate. This image reminds me of a similar patient that had her post lumpectomy photo taken and sent to Playboy for a centerfold. I thought she could do more for women's rights with that one photo than all the pink ribbons have ever done. I could just see every woman going to visit her surgeon and holding up the centerfold lumpectomy photo and saying, "This is how I want to look." I guess I'm guilty of that outrageous thought.

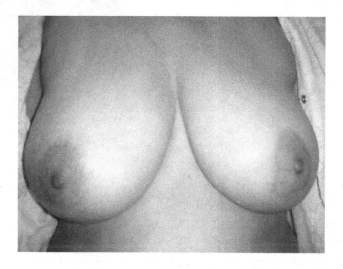

I just had to put the next patient in again as it is so egregious and unnecessary. Monkey see monkey do.

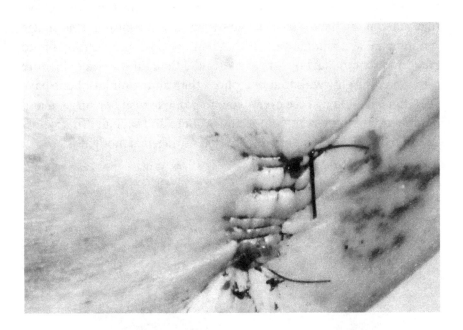

Next this is a patient who had ductal carcinoma in situ (DCIS). Decades ago we used to treat DCIS with a mastectomy because by definition, the cancer hadn't spread and it was a 100% cure. Now there are doctors just monitoring DCIS as we now know that not all DCIS becomes invasive and spreads. However, this patient was talked into bilateral subcutaneous mastectomies with reconstruction. She is on her third surgery to correct the problem. It was performed at a major hospital on the west coast. You can judge for yourself if they are making progress or not.

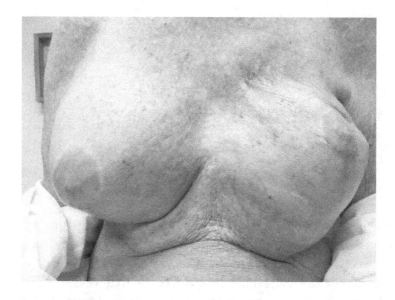

The next image is a little more tolerable. It's me suturing in the 'fat patch,' so the patient can undergo APBR.

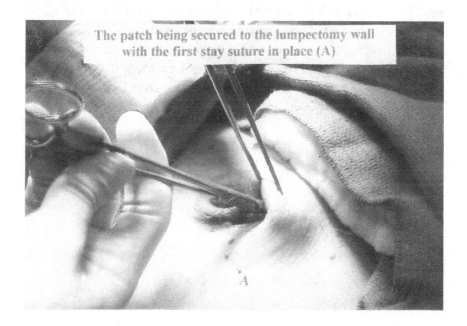

The patch being secured to the lumpectomy wall with the first stay suture in place (A)

The next page is intentionally left blank. The reason is the page after that has a very disturbing photo of a woman with breast cancer. If you don't have a strong stomach, I suggest you skip the next two pages. If you do choose to see it, I hope it convinces you that we need a complete overhaul of our current breast cancer diagnosis and treatment system. There are a lot of very smart people, it just needs someone who gives a damn. A woman such as this in America today should be impossible to find. It's a disgrace. But we have found several women that are so afraid of the system and what it will do to them, they end up like this woman, a tragedy that could be avoided with a proper system in place that would not only save and preserve women's lives but save billions of dollars yearly. If you've had enough, you know what needs to be done. You and millions of women in America need to make their voices heard.

This page intentionally left blank.

This page intentionally left blank.

This page intentionally left blank.

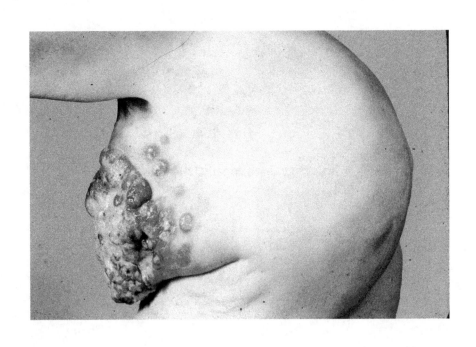

This page intentionally left blank.

This page intentionally left blank.

This page intentionally left blank.

Here is another patient who obviously let her cancer grow for years and years. She refused treatment and was putting horse urine on the tumor to make it go away but, of course, it didn't. We have women like this in America because they are afraid of the system. I have presented another approach. She also has osteoporosis with the common Dowager's hump.

The image below is a ductogram or glactogram where I injected dye through the nipple into a duct that was leaking fluid and it imaged an entire lobe. There are about ten to twelve lobules in each breast and the white lines are the ducts that carry milk and where about 90% of the cancers arise, which is why it is called an invasive intraductal cancer. The white puff balls are the actual terminal lobules that make the milk. The image on the right depicts an intraductal tumor (inside the duct) surrounded by contrast material. You can see how big these ducts can get with a tumor growing inside. I just injected the duct and sent the patient for a mammogram. This is what we actually see on a mammogram (white tissue) but we don't see the actual ducts unless a ductogram is performed. It's a very delicate procedure as the probe can pass directly through the ducts and you get a puddleogram instead of a cool image as below.

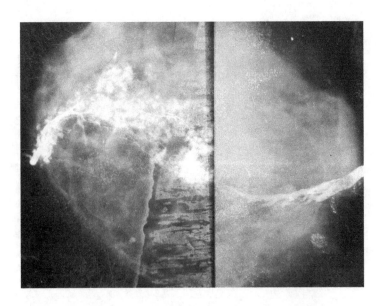

CHAPTER 11
PATIENT LETTERS AND SUPORTING DOCUMENTS

N OW WE COME to Chapter 11, wherein I present just a spattering of the many letters I have received about my care to patients over the decades. Some of these documents are from leaders in industry who meet daily with distinguished people yet took the time to acknowledge my conduct. As you read each of these letters, you'll come to realize that these just aren't Hallmark cards with a signature at the end, but many are handwritten (indeed personalized design), so the person had to put thought to it, they were that motivated. Ask yourself, how many times are you motivated to sit and write a letter of appreciation because someone went out of their way to assist you? Also, over the years I have never received one derogatory letter about my skill as a surgeon, any outcomes or nefarious conduct period.

As well included in this chapter are just a few of the many inquires I received from all over the world by women and their families that were so dissatisfied with the proposed care in whatever country they wanted to fly to me. I averaged before Board action about four a week and now it is almost zero as if you Google me, you'll find first thing the Board's implication and decision that I was negligent. My ability to help and direct care of patients in other countries is obviously lost.

I recognize there are a lot of letters, however, they are really my only defense where I can't really defend myself any other way. And either I was so slick for decades on end deceiving all these women and their husbands and I somehow stumbled through all those thousands of surgeries in a mediocre fashion or I'm exactly what they portray in each and every one of those letters. When you read these to the end, I want you to ask yourself, "Hey wait a minute, what the hell went on here?" What have these authoritative bodies become, or was their action indeed justified?

The last section of this chapter illustrates my various publications in peer-reviewed journals. My first one was published in the American Society of Clinical Oncology, the largest oncology group in the country. This was the abstract on the Compass Treatment. What was curious was with successfully treating breast cancer without surgery, just chemotherapy and radiation, no one ever contacted me about how I accomplished my results.

I've had the opportunity to present my results all over the world in places like the erstwhile USSR, China, Brazil, Canada, Austria, and Mexico. And all over the world I've been treated with respect and an outpouring of wanting to hear what I have to say.

We'll start with my certificate from Rutgers Medical School in New Jersey.

COLLEGE OF MEDICINE AND DENTISTRY OF NEW JERSEY

Know all men by these Presents, that

Phillip DeEvans Bretz

after completing medical studies at
Universidad Autonoma de Guadalajara, Mexico
has served one academic year of clinical training and responsibili
Muhlenberg Hospital, Plainfield
10 September 1973 - 29 June 1974

in medicine, surgery, obstetrics, gynecology, pediatrics
and psychiatry, and is therefore awarded this

In testimony thereof we have hereunto subscribed our names
and have affixed the Common Seal of the College at Newark,
30 June 1974

PROGRAM DIRECTOR

PRESIDENT OF THE COLLEGE

HOSPITAL DIRECTOR OF PROGRAM

REGISTRAR

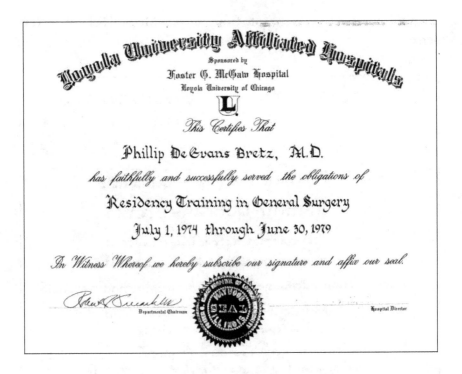

This was as close as I ever got to become a fellow in the American College of Surgeons.

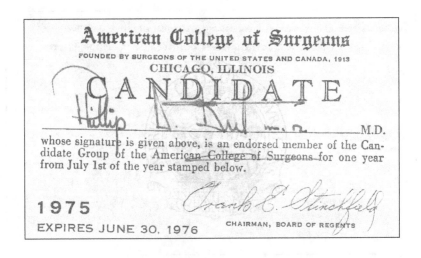

I guess they changed their minds about me but, yes, I was the Field Liaison officer for the American College of Surgeons at Eisenhower.

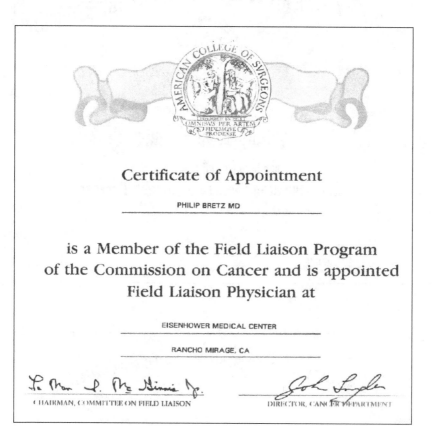

Certificate of Appointment

PHILIP BRETZ MD

is a Member of the Field Liaison Program
of the Commission on Cancer and is appointed
Field Liaison Physician at

EISENHOWER MEDICAL CENTER

RANCHO MIRAGE, CA

CHAIRMAN, COMMITTEE ON FIELD LIAISON   DIRECTOR, CANCER DEPARTMENT

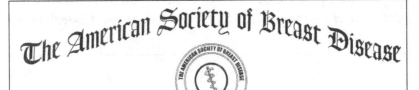

The American Society of Breast Disease

This is to certify that

Phillip D. Bretz, M.D.

has been elected a member of

The American Society of Breast Disease

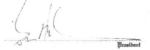

President

Admitted   2006

Department of Registration and Education

State of Illinois

CERTIFICATE NO.

This is to certify that   PHILLIP D. BRETZ, M.D.   36-55297

IS A LICENSED

PHYSICIAN AND SURGEON

REGISTERED UNDER THE PROVISIONS OF THE LAWS OF THE STATE OF ILLINOIS
AND IS ENTITLED TO PRACTICE MEDICINE IN ALL OF ITS BRANCHES

In Witness Whereof, The Director of the Department of Registration and Education has hereby affixed his hand and the seal of the said Department this   11th   day of   AUGUST   A.D. 1977

Attest

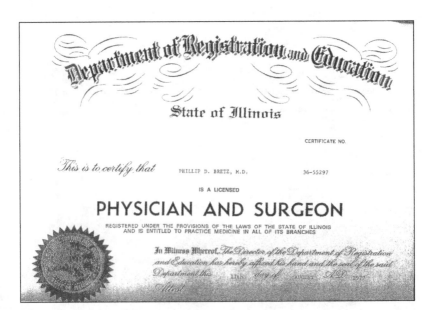

The Board of Medical Quality Assurance
of the State of California

This is to Certify, that ___Phillip De Evans Bretz___ a graduate of ___Autonomous University of Guadalajara Faculty of Medicine___

having shown to the satisfaction of this Board that __he possesses the qualifications required by law, and having successfully passed an examination by this Board as to h15 qualifications, is hereby granted a

Physician's and Surgeon's Certificate
To Practice Medicine and Surgery
in this State

In Testimony Whereof, THE BOARD OF MEDICAL QUALITY ASSURANCE *of the* STATE OF CALIFORNIA *has issued this* CERTIFICATE *and caused the same to be signed by its* PRESIDENT *and* SECRETARY-TREASURER, *and its* SEAL *to be hereto affixed this* __17th__ *day of* ___July___ A. D. 19__78__

The Board of Medical Quality Assurance
OF THE STATE OF CALIFORNIA

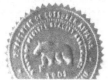

No. A 32596

_____
President

_____
Secretary-Treasurer

This document shows that the State of California came to me to give testimony concerning their investigation of Tamoxifen. I was glad to do it and be included as a team player for the State of California.

California Environmental Protection Agency   *State of California*

Pete Wilson, *Governor*

OFFICE OF ENVIRONMENTAL HEALTH HAZARD ASSESSMENT

November 22, 1995

Phillip Bretz, M.D.
Desert Breast Institute
39800 Bob Hope Drive, Suite H
Rancho Mirage, California 92270

Dear Dr. Bretz:

    I would like to thank you for taking time to review and comment on the Office of Environmental Health Hazard Assessment's Draft Hazard Identification document on Tamoxifen and related materials. Your comments will be useful to the objective scientific evaluation of the carcinogenic potential of tamoxifen, as required under Proposition 65. We will include your comments in our administrative record and also forward them to members of the Proposition 65 Carcinogen Identification Committee and staff in the Reproductive and Cancer Hazard Assessment Section for their review.

    Should you have any questions, please contact Catherine Caraway at (916) 445-6900. Thank you for your interest.

Sincerely,

Olga Martin Steele, Deputy Director
Regulatory, Outreach, and Support Programs

cc: Thomas M. Mack, M.D., M.P.H.
       Joseph R. Landolph, Ph.D.
       Richard A. Becker, Ph.D., D.A.B.T.
       Lauren Zeise, Ph.D.

EISENHOWER MEDICAL CENTER

June 25, 1979

Phillip D. Bretz, M.D.
1202 Woodbine
Oak Park, Illinois 60302

Dear Doctor Bretz,

It is a pleasure to inform you that acting upon the recommendation of the Medical Executive Committee, the Board of Trustees has appointed you to the Associate Staff, Department of Surgery, Section of General Surgery, of the EMC Medical Staff.

In the near future, you will be invited to a Medical Staff orientation program. This will give you an opportunity to meet with representatives of the medical support services and become familiar with some of the policies of EMC. In the meantime, if you desire information concerning the hospital or the medical staff organization, Doctor Richard Mahler, President of the EMC Medical Staff, or Bill Parente, Associate Administrator, will be happy to help you.

In accordance with a protocol prepared by CMA and CHA, you may elect to participate in an arbitration program by signing the enclosed arbitration agreement card. Whether or not you plan to participate, it is important we know your intentions, and I ask that you return the card to Beverly Winegar, Medical Administration.

A brief explanation of the parking facilities, mail boxes and paging system is enclosed for your review.

In a short time, your requested clinical privileges will be reviewed by the appropriate medical staff departments and you will be advised of the privileges granted to you.

I am pleased to welcome you to the Medical Staff of EMC and look forward to a long and happy association.

Sincerely,

L. M. Vandervort
Executive Director

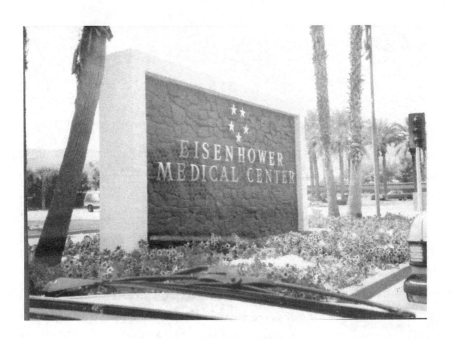

10-30-98

Dear Dr. . . .

B rilliant

R eliable

E xcellent

T rustworthy

Z any

Just a note to tell you how grateful I am that you're my doctor.

— Deborah Folsom

All these letters I hold dear and value more than any certificate (except my wedding certificate, did I get that right?). And I value one not more than another, they are all specially written by very special people who can see through any ruse. They are in no particular order. They run for decades including 2021. The proof for a surgeon is in one's conduct out in public, not some certificate on the wall.

GERALD R. FORD

May 20, 1988

Dear Dr. Bretz:

Both Mrs. Ford and I were deeply touched by your letter of April 21st. We appreciate your thoughtfulness to us personally as well as the Betty Ford Center.

By all means, please go ahead and bill Blue Shield Insurance Company of your services. Our subscriber number is 102 R00006467. Upon receipt of the payment, we will forward our check and copy of the benefits statement to your office.

After a couple of rough sessions, Mrs. Ford is now recuperating beautifully and we are looking forward to spending the summer at our home in Beaver Creek, Colorado. We thank you, Dr. Bretz, for your superb participation on her surgical team. We are so grateful to you and all of the physicians who have insured her healthy future.

Warmest, best wishes,

Phillip D. Bretz, M.D.
Suite 203, Probst Building
39000 Bob Hope Drive
Rancho Mirage, California 92270

THE WHITE HOUSE
WASHINGTON

January 13, 1985

Dear Doctors Kopp and Bretz:

I would like to thank you both very much for the care and attention afforded Special Agent Dana Brown during his surgery at your facility. We are very appreciative of your care, concern and timely reaction to this situation.

In our travels, to various cities, we are concerned with the capabilities of hospitals. Your expertise has only increased our confidence in Eisenhower Hospital Medical Center to provide care to the President of the United States and his staff.

Again, on behalf of The White House and White House Medical Unit, thank you for excellent cooperation.

Sincerely,

T. Burton Smith, M.D.
Physician to the President

PROCLAMATION OF
TECHNICAL EXCELLENCE

10 years!

THE INFRARED TRAINING CENTER RECOGNIZES

Phillip Bretz

WITH GRATITUDE AND APPRECIATION FOR YOUR OUTSTANDING CONTRIBUTION TO THE ADVANCEMENT OF APPLIED INFRARED THERMOGRAPHY THROUGH A TECHNICAL PRESENTATION AT **INFRAMATION 2009 ON OCTOBER 19-22, 2009.**

Robert P. Malding, Chairman   Gary L. Orlove, Chairman

InfraMation   ITC INFRARED TRAINING CENTER

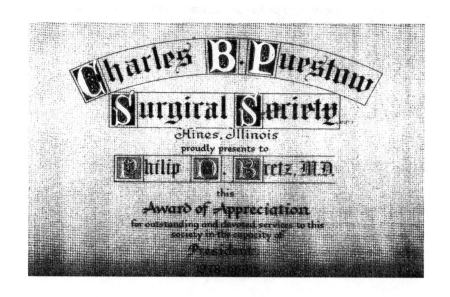

Flying Physicians Association

Having fulfilled prescribed requirements for membership, as set forth in the Constitution and By-laws of the Flying Physicians Association.

Phillip DeEvans Bretz, M.D.

is accordingly granted this certificate of membership with all of the rights and privileges appertaining thereto.

June 1, 1973

President

Secretary

Charles B. Puestow Surgical Society

Hines, Illinois

proudly presents to

Philip D. Bretz, M.D.

this

Award of Appreciation

for outstanding and devoted services to this society in the capacity of

President

To say the least, I am very confused and concerned. All my life I've embraced natural intuitive living. I am a believer in conservative or natural methods of treatment whenever possible, surgery would be the absolutely last resort, in my opinion.

Finding your TED talk and Visionary Breast Center web site was a breath of fresh air, it felt right on par with my approach to life and health. I cried when you got emotional on stage: my God, you really care! I've met so many cold and unsympathetic doctors, when my mom refused chemo and used natural FDA-approved methods to support her with stage III ductal carcinoma for 9 years, doctors who butchered her breast and created more issues than solved, doctors who finally devastated last of her body resources at the operating table during unnecessary 8-hour surgery, 24 hours later my mom passed away. To be honest, I'm terrified to get back into this system of mainstream medicine that nukes the house to get rid of the cockroaches.

I am seeking an advice and would like to know if I might be the candidate for cryoablation, or if I should do the surgical biopsy first (which I remember left my mom with a hematoma larger than the original tumor and caused more issues down the road). What would my next steps be? Could I get a consultation at your Center?

Attached are two pathology reports. I wish I'm just overreacting, and it turns out to be benign, but I would like to know for sure, and if possible avoid surgery.

Even if I'm not your patient, I want to say thank you that you exist, that you care, thank you from all of those women you saved!

With the deepest sympathy,

This letter is from one of my Lavender girls.

Dear Dr. Bretz,

"My Lavender Experience"

I shall begin when I met Dr. Bretz @ 20 years ago. He was introduced to my husband and I while treating a friend with breast cancer. Our friend was so excited and impressed with Dr. Bretz's approach and philosophy in the treatment of her breast cancer. What was so impressive was that Dr. Bretz was in the process of and determined to forge a new innovative way of approaching and curing breast cancer, thus saving his patient's life and preventing mutilation of her body. Dr. Bretz treated my friend and cured her cancer and saved her breast. I am happy to say that she has led a productive life and is still living her dream with her body intact. I knew at that point with Dr. Bretz at the helm I would never fear breast cancer.

My second experience was with a very dear friend. She called me sobbing as she was diagnosed with breast cancer and was scheduled for a mastectomy in 2 weeks. I told her not to worry because I had such confidence with Dr. Bretz. My husband and I accompanied our friend to her first appointment and thereafter . Dr. Bretz called her cancer "a garden variety" which was a slow growing cancer, her treatment was chemotherapy to shrink the tumor. Dr. Bretz performed a lumpectomy. The scar was barely visible. Dr. Bretz not only saved her breast, but her dignity, as my friend was 80 years of age. She also had a very productive life with her breast intact.

Spring forward 17 years to my wonderful "Lavender Experience" with Dr. Bretz. At this time I want to give a big thank you to his loving and very supportive wife Joan as she stood by my side and, very lovingly, held my hand and wiped my tears away.

Yes, my friends, when cancer strikes you, it is a horrifying experience!!!!! I brought all of my records to Dr. Bretz with confidence. I knew in my heart that if he could not cure me, then no one could. My husband and I put our complete trust and faith in his prognosis and treatment!!!

After several genetic blood tests, it was determined I was a candidate for cryoablation. This procedure was completed in his office. I had very little discomfort. I avoided, thanks to Dr. Bretz, chemotherapy, a lumpectomy, radiation and herception treatments.

My husband and I are so thankful to Dr. Bretz and his wife for all their endless hours of research and dedication to fight breast cancer.

I urge you, if you have been diagnosed with any type of breast cancer, please contact Dr. Bretz. I know that he will navigate the best possible treatment designed for your individual case. Ladies, we do not have to lose our breasts being treated the old way. Let's embrace the new way, the only way, the "Lavender Way"!!!!

Your friend,

3/18/2015

9-17-99

Cher Docteur Bretz

J am not sure if J have ever expressed my gratitude To you.

You are such a caring, loving Doctor. You are part of the Woman's World. You read our eyes and you feel our unspoken fear. Your dedication for humanity is well felt. Your sensitivity and your loving support is exceptional and so appreciated.

J thank God J have met you.

J drive 2 hours to see you, and maybe someday J will cross the ocean to meet you. J Know my life is in the hand of God. but J also Know my trust is *Beaucoup!* in you.

A million time " Merci beaucoup
Merci Infiniment "
avec Affection
Josette

Dear Dr. Bretz:

I am so grateful for you and your hard work and dedication, in finding an almost non-invasive treatment for my breast cancer, and, one that did not leave me with any disfiguring and ugly scars.

On July 9th I was diagnosed with breast cancer and if it had not been for you, I would have been a total mess. I've watched numerous friends and family members suffer, emotionally and physically, from the results of surgery and radiation or chemotherapy. Not only it hard on the patient it very difficult for family members as well. I did not want to go through this type therapy nor put my family through it.

Thank you for performing your Lavender Procedure (Croablation-Sanarus) on me. Just as you told me, your procedure was quick with very little pain and minimal scaring. And, because of you and your Lavender Procedure, my last mammogram showed no signs of cancer at all.

Due to the I-10 Freeway being close, the day you performed the procedure on me, we had to detour through Glamis to go home. I felt so good afterwards that my husband and I stopped at the Red Earth Casino for a celebratory drink and dinner.

I will always be grateful to you, and your wife Joan, for allowing me the opportunity to successfully experience your Lavender Procedure. I will continue to help spread the word, about your amazing treatments, to as many people, friends and family members as I can.

In my eyes, and my husband's eyes, you are a Life Saver!

Sincerely and gratefully,

Barbara Martin Nadeau

Barbara Martin Nadeau

This letter is from Frank, Corinne's husband. She had breast cancer over ten years ago and had a lumpectomy and external beam radiation by another surgeon. When she developed a local recurrence, I had just received the cryoablation machines and Corinne was my first Lavender girl. She was the first case I did. She had Alzheimer's by then and couldn't remember my name. But she knew I didn't hurt her so she let me do Lavender. She is the one who fell getting up at night and expired before the paramedics got there. But she died cancer-free and Frank wrote this letter.

To: Dr. Phil + Joan:

We wish to take this opportunity to thank you for your recent phone call and your thoughtfullness as well as your kind words in the passing of Corinne.

It's a blessing to know that her favourite Doctor had given Corinne such good attention... and personal care, which was a true comfort in all respects.

God bless you and Joan for all your good work, and it's been a privillge to have you as our Doctor and friend.

Sincerely

Frank

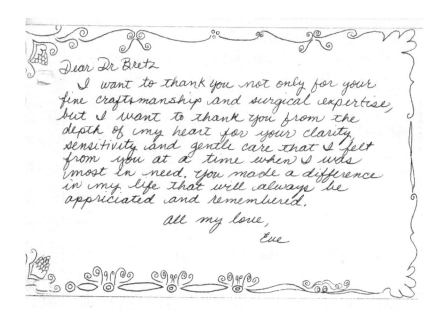

Dear Dr Bretz

I want to thank you not only for your fine craftsmanship and surgical expertise, but I want to thank you from the depth of my heart for your clarity, sensitivity and gentle care that I felt from you at a time when I was most in need. You made a difference in my life that will always be appriciated and remembered.

all my love,

Eve

10-28-87

Dear Dr. Bretz,

I take back what I said about not liking doctors... I like you.

Thank you for the excellent way you and your office staff dealt c̄ me. Listening is the most important skill practiced and you all do it beautifully.

Thank you...

Thank you...

Thank you.

Dee

a gift to you too for the "extra"
comfort you give your patients.
I think you deserved something
as great as that to happen in
your career.

　　　　　　marilyn

Indeed a very special thank you
for your dedication and care of
our Mom, callie L.

The Lord blessed us by you being
there when the need was so great.

May God bless you and keep you.

Jan 13, 1981

Dear Dr. Bretz,

I read about your patient, Velva Eddy, and you in the local newspaper last week!!

I just wanted to compliment you on your compassion and dedication. You've really been blessed in the way you touch your patient's hearts and lives.

You don't know me, but I hope you're at EMC if I ever need you! God's blessings always and warm wishes,

Sandy Walton

Dear Dr. Bretz:
Enclosed is my check for the balance of your fee. I appreciat your allowing me to make payments.

Thank you for your kindness your understanding & most important, your expert surgery

May God continue to guide you & to bless you in all your endeavors.

Sincerely,
Ruth de Cuir

YOU AND JOAN!

Dear Dr. Bretz & Joan,

Cards and words cannot express our appreciation for all the loving care you have given us. Because of your devotion as a physician and someone who is constantly pushing the envelope of the cutting edge of breast cancer and preventing mutilation of one's body and mind!

We thank you for all your 40+ years of reasearch that will benefit me and all the sisterhood of the "Bretz" survivors!

We love you both,

2014

Dear Phil Bretz MD –
Thank you for the peace of mind you gave me! You are a rare breed of physician – very direct bright and skilled – yet thoughtful and gentle.
I sincerely appreciate the time and care you gave me this past week.

Karen Maas

Patti , R. N.

Phillip D. Bretz, M.D.
78-034 Calle Barcelona
Suite B
La Quinta, CA 92253

17 Dec 09

Hi Honey Pie!

#1 – WOW! You're like E. F. Hutton . . . when you speak . . . everyone listens! After seeing you last week and your mention of the bruit . . . I cut my smoking in HALF within one week! What is your 'POWER'? Byrd, Barton, etc., etc. have mentioned my smoking, but you're the only M.D./friend whom I actually heard! I'm presuming it's our 'Mid-West language' (Chicago and St. Louis).

#2 – I saw Ryszard Skulski, M.D. per your recommendation this AM . . . he's an absolute DELIGHT with a fab+ personality. I'm presuming it's due to he being Polish and my being a 'French-Pollock'! FYI! He said, 'I asked Phil about your breasts and he said 'They're GOOD'! That was hilarious. I said, 'It's only due to Phil taking care of them for the past twenty-five+ years! I trust my 'tits' to no one but Phil!'

#3 – I know you'll receive his report and I'll see him every Dec. He'll be OK with my smoking five (5) or less cigarettes per day. He's realizes I'm old and not easy to change my lifestyle.

#4 – I heard from ████████ (she & I've been friends X 20 years) that she had the 'Infrared' and is having a biopsy = hope you're performing the biopsy, as I reiterated to her, 'NO ONE CHECKS MY BOOBS, BUT P. BRETZ, M.D., as he's the ONLY M.D. I COMPLETELY TRUST with them!

Thank you for being such a caring M.D. and friend. I definitely 'lucked out' with meeting you thirty years ago. Joan is so lucky to be married to you and she's outstanding+++++++!

Very fondly,

Dr. Bretz, Margaret, Ruth and
Sylvia ~

I don't have the words to express
my gratitude and love for all of
you. You have helped me through
some pretty tough times, both
physically and emotionally.

In this day and age, it's so
difficult to find the combination
of both medical expertise and the
caring and compassion for individuals
that all of you seem to possess.
Too many times, in other situations,
I have felt like a number ~ not
a real person with real pain and real
fears.

I have never felt that way with
you.... I believe that knowing the
people that are taking care of you
really care, is imperative for a cancer
patient. Of course, knowing that they
are "the best in the business" ~ as I
believe you are, helps a great deal too.

I am looking forward to many
years of wonderful friendships with
all of you ~ thanks to all of you.
Without you, I wouldn't have so many
things to look forward to ... ♡

...and I just want
you to know
how much I appreciate
all you've done for me.

You are the best, all of you.

Love,
Lisa

Was very pleased with the immediate & efficient
care I received at Eisenhower Hospital. Also
very happy with the attention and care
Dr. Bretz gave me ~ and the excellent
recovery I've had ~. Highly recommend him
and the hospital ~.

Barbara J.

Flora ████
████████████████
Palm Springs, CA   92264

June 22, 1990

Dear Mr Bretz.

I would like to be able to
express myself better, a
simple "Thank You" is not
enough.

Your professionalism and
courtesy extended to me is
greatly appreciated! You are
very kind, a job well done!

I wish you great success
in your new project. Thank You,
Flora ████

Dear Dr. Bretz,   10/89

I thank God daily for putting me in your skilled, caring hands! I thank you for applying those skills in my behalf. How moved I am to find a professional who has managed to maintain that sensitive intent to achieve the best result possible each step of the way. Thank you again for your focus on my health.

God bless you.

Donna Campbell

1-29-98.

Dr. Bretz.

Your the greatest. I really can't say enough kind words about you. That was very thoughtful of you to call and give me the report on my X-rays. As soon as I get a different insurance I will be in to see you. Also thank Kathy your lucky to have her she is a very special lady

Love,
Sandy Karas.

May 22, 1995

Dear Dr. Bretz,

I try to always let people who have been especially good to me know that I appreciate them.

I want to thank you for being both the kind of person and physician you are. Your kindness and your warmth didn't go unnoticed and comforted me a lot.

It must be pretty difficult to tell patients that they need further tests or treatments for cancer. I want you to know how very grateful I am that I had someone like you for my doctor and someone special like Maria too. I don't know if you know how much you're needed. I know your other patients feel this way too! You're the best they say!

I don't think it was accidental that you were the doctor to share in my gift from God last Thursday when you were able to cancel my stereotacis biopsy. I feel it was

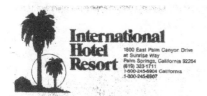

International Hotel Resort

1800 East Palm Canyon Drive
at Sunrise Way
Palm Springs, California 92264
(619) 323-1711
1-800-245-6904 California
1-800-245-6907

OCTOBER 22, 1987

PHILLIP D. BRETZ).
39000 BOB HOPE DR. .E
PROBST PROFESSIONAL BUILDING
SUITE 212
RANCHO MIRAGE, CALIFORNIA 92270

DEAR DR. BRETZ:

BEFORE CLOSING THIS NOTE, I WANT TO THANK YOU SINCERELY FOR STEPPING IN WITH SHORT
NOTICE AND PERFORMING THE SURGICAL PROCEDURE. I, NATURALLY, FELT MUCH RELIEF AND
CONFIDENCE (AS ONE NORMALLY FEELS A CERTAIN AMOUNT OF "JITTERS" PRIOR TO ANY SURGERY)
HAVING BEEN TOLD ABOUT YOUR PROFESSIONAL SERVICES — I WAS VERY GLAD THAT YOU AGREED
TO DO IT. I LIKED YOUR PROFESSIONAL ATTITUDE, AND THE FACT THAT YOU TOOK TIME
TO EXPLAIN THINGS TO ME IN DETAIL. THE SURGERY ITSELF WENT FINE, AND I FELT IMMEDIATE
RELIEF. I WAS LEFT WITH LITTLE (IF ANY) SCAR.

THANKS AGAIN FOR YOUR SERVICES. IF I KNOW OF ANYONE NEEDING THE SERVICES OF A GENERAL
SURGEON, I'LL BE HAPPY TO REFER THEM TO YOU!

MOST SINCERELY,

LEONARD

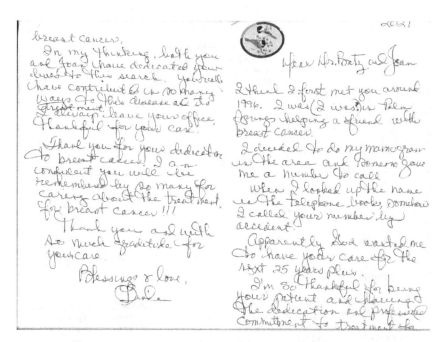

[Handwritten note, dated 2021]

Dear Mrs. Bretz and Joan

I think I first met you around 1996. I was (I was) in Palm Springs helping a friend with breast cancer.

I decided to do my mammogram in the area and someone gave me a number to call. When I looked up the name in the telephone book, somehow I called your number by accident.

Apparently God wanted me to have your care for the next 25 years plus.

I'm so thankful for being your patient and having the dedication and professional commitment to treatment of breast cancer.

In my thinking, both you and Joan have dedicated your lives to this search. You really have contributed in so many ways to this disease and its treatment. I always leave your office thankful for your care.

Thank you for your dedication to breast cancer! I am confident you will be remembered by so many for caring about the treatment for breast cancer!!!

Thank you and with so much gratitude for your care

Blessings & love,

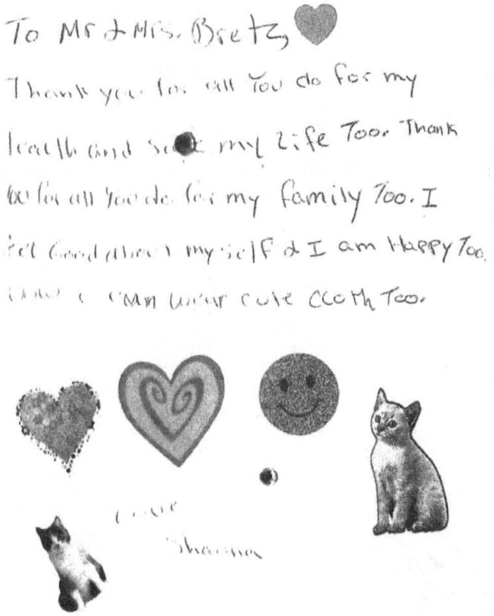

[signature]

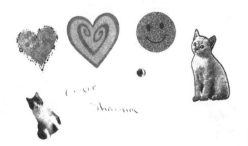

[Second handwritten note]

To Mr. & Mrs. Bretz, ♥

Thank you for all you do for my health and save my Life Too. Thank you for all you do for my family Too. I fel Good about myself & I am Happy Too. I also can wear cute cloth Too.

Love,
Shauna

LLOYD M. CAPLAN, M.D.

A Professional Corporation
1080 N. INDIAN AVENUE, SUITE 204
PALM SPRINGS, CALIFORNIA 92262
TELEPHONE (619) 320-4554

July 20, 1987

Phillip D. Bretz, M.D.
Suite 203 Probst Bldg.
39000 Bob Hope Drive
Rancho Mirage, Calif. 92270

Re: ███████ ████████

Dear Phil,

Thank you so much for your report on ████████, and thank you for your consideration and communication during the course of your involvement with her treatment. I wish that all physicians were as conscientious and thoughtful as you have been. I look forward to working with you again.

Sincerely,

Lloyd

LLOYD M. CAPLAN M.D.

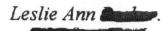

Leslie Ann ▮▮▮▮▮.

▮▮▮▮▮▮▮▮▮▮▮▮
Knightsbridge, London
SW1X OAZ
Home Phone: ▮▮▮▮▮▮▮▮

Receiving Fax #: ▮▮▮▮▮▮▮▮▮▮
Sending Fax #: ▮▮▮▮▮▮▮▮▮5

16 April 1998

Dear Dr. Bretz,

It is always a pleasure to see your face and to be in your care.....it is also a GREAT relief when the visit is over! I know you understand.

My stay in the desert was brief and I did not have the opportunity to return to your office as we discussed for you to review my recent bone density scan. I did have my report mailed to you on March 19th and I have retained a copy. To my untrained eye it looks good. Well done Fosamax! Do you suggest I continue my daily dosage, a maintenance dosage(to be determined) or stop all together? As always I remain in your hands!

The details listed above contain my fax number. Thank you once again for your care.

Kindest regards,
Leslie ▮▮▮▮

P.S. It is 36 degrees and snowing...want to trade places?

May 22, 1992

to you — Mike

Mr. Charles Mechem
Commissioner
LPGA
2507 Volusia Avenue, Suite B
Daytona Beach, FL   32114

Dear Charlie,

Congratulations on a successful Mazda LPGA Championship. I
think it's great for Betsy to win and set so many records
along the way. You probably won the Pro-Am as well!

Charlie, I am somewhat remiss in not getting the enclosed
letter to your attention sooner. I apologize. This letter
is from Lisa's lead doctor caring for her cancer problems.
I introduced you to him and I think you chatted briefly with
him about his ideas at our media party.

His idea is certainly an action plan relative to the
increasing awareness of breast cancer. Dr. Bretz has strong
credentials and is certainly one of the leaders in this
country with regard to the many aspects of breast cancer.
For Lisa and I he has been an unbelievable source of
confidence, hope and care. Without his honesty and support
I don't believe Lisa would be handling this problem as well
either physically or emotionally.

When you have some time I encourage you to think this over
and see if there is a "fit" for the LPGA. Confidentiality is
requested by Dr. Bretz at this time.

Charlie, if I can be of any help please do not hesitate to
call me. Thanks.

Best regards,

1/98

Dear Dr. Bretz
and staff,
I'm sure there are never
enough words written or spoken
in appreciation of the great
qualities of your work and the
sincere compassion you show
to all of your patents.
My family and I thank
you for going out of your way
to fit your schedules of tests with
my schedule of time. It's easier
to be miles away with my mind
at rest knowing you're in charge.
Thank you all for being
there for my mom and treating
her special. (She is special.)
Sincerely,
Sue L

October 16, 1986

Mr. George Elmore, Administrator
Eisenhower Medical Center
39000 Bob Hope Drive
Rancho Mirage, California 92270

Dear Mr. Elmore:

I would like to take this opportunity to thank you and your wonderful staff for taking such fine care of my wife. She entered the hospital on May 31st and I was able to bring her home on October 8th — and what a wonderful day that was.

I want to extend my thanks to all the fine nurses, doctors and other personnel which gave my wife such fine care. The staff in ICU were absolutely wonderful, showing care and kindnesses which she so appreciated. Even some of your girls which do the clean-up work were tremendous — especially the little girl named Debbie.

I also want to take this opportunity to extend my many thanks to Doctors Phillip Bretz, Karl Schultz and Scott Aaronson for their wonderful job as well as all the kindnesses and caring they showed my wife.

In addition, I just want to add one note here. Both Doctors Bretz and Schultz have been at our house several times to check on my dear wife Helen. This is a service above and beyond the call of duty for which we will always be eternally grateful.

Thanks again for everything.

Sincerely,

715

Hello Debbie & Dr. Bretz,
I feel wonderful
and am already sunning
topless again! No scar!
Thank-you so much for
your helpfulness, pulling
strings, ect. You're both
wonderful and I can
truthfully say I enjoyed
myself.
This is all I can
afford right now, I'm very
sorry I can't pay the whole
thing off. Thank-you again

Sincerely,
Carrie

Dear Dr. Bretz

This thank you goes way back

I appreciate what you have
done for me —
Taking time from your very
busy schedule -

your giving Heart seems limitless "

much Love
Anita

Wishing you well & the following... //

3/2005

Dear Dr. Bretz & Joan...

Thank You

Dear Dr. Bretz...
Four years ago I picked your name
out of a phone book — I loved the
d. From there you've shown me nothing
it kindness & warm feelings — You are
+ true angel of healing. You helped me
hm I was down, charged me $100" for
3 Cyst — that is unheard of "Now a days"
ion there you inspired me to get health
verage — which brought me back to see
me again 😊 Words cannot express
Just how Wonderful you are —
　　　　　a true Dr...

Just... a note of thanks
right from the heart!

ONE Love & Respect
　　　Cynthia
　　　　　U

P.S. I read youre poem
and I say M.O. stands
for My Doctor.... ♡

Dear Dr. Bretz!

Please accept my sincere
Thank's for your help, kindness
understanding and compassion
you gave my daughter Michele
during her difficult time.
You are truly a beautiful
caring person and a great
surgeon. Michele can now
start her life whole again. —
May God bless you always.

Your staff made us feel
comfortable and is most
efficient, Rita, Cathy, Kathrine
and Maria you are all
wonderful.

December 9, 1993

Dear Dr. Bretz:

A note to let you know how grateful I am for
your dedication to preserving mind, body and
spirit of those who pass through your life as
a doctor/surgeon. This, along with your superb
abilities and your association with Dr. Dreisbach
and his expertise, are so appreciated and fill me
with thankfulness that I was "lucky" enough to
walk through the doors of the Breast Institute
this last August.

May your pursuit of excellence be ever more
and more rewarding to you.

Gratefully,

P.S. And, how nice to awaken from surgery to
the cheerful presence of your office staff --
very special and thoughtful! All of you make
a good team, and all of you are great support!

But there's everything nice about you!

Dear Dr Bretz —

I greatly appreciate your treatment and care for me during my surgery.

I think you are one of the best and most wonderful Doctors in the State of Calif.

Thank you for your attention and

2261

Desert Breast Institute,
39-800 Bob Hope Dr.,
Suite C
Rancho Mirage, Ca. 92270

ATTENTION: DR. BRETZ

Dear Dr. Bretz:

     I wish to thank you for your kindness and consideration
in examining my Daughter, Jan   :. The 7:00 A.M.
appointment on a Saturday morning and the thorough examination
and explanation was very much appreciated. HOW WONDERFUL TO
FIND A DOCTOR WHO CARES!

     I also wish to thank Pat for her pleasantness and efficiency
in handling the appointments. A BIG THANK YOU to Starr
for coming in on a Saturday and taking Mamograms and X-Rays.
How wonderful for all of us to now have "Piece of Mind."

     Jan said she was fortunate that she decided to come to
your Institute for your examination and opinion, and found so
many wonderful caring people.

Dear Dr Bretz + Staff)
    Just a little note to say thank you.
I know my surgery was only minor, but
your caring and kindness was most
appreciated. We have dealth with a
great many doctors and their office staffs
but you and yours are the best.
    I also want to thank you for taking
care of my wife so quickly and efficiently
and putting her mind at ease.
    We have had a very bad year, but
knowing you is a good start for a better
one as we feel so confident in your
care.
    We also sent a letter to E.MC.
to thank all the staff involved in my
care; they were terrific.
        thank you again.

Dear Dr. Bretz,

Thank you very much for keeping me breast cancer-free.

Please keep up the good work.

☺

Dear Mr. Bretz, 2/18/93

Thank you so much for all your help. I feel very fortunate that I was referred to you. I was also touched by your compassion during surgery by holding my hand. I always assume Dr.s tend to be "business as usual" so I didn't expect any compassion or kindness. I also was very impressed at how you want women to be informed + take charge of some of their health care vs being ignorant & at the mercy of the medical profession. I think many drs. should take lessons. (HaHa)

Lastly, I was wondering if I could have a copy of the blood results. I'd like to know certain figures re: potassium, magnesium & cholesterol levels if that info. is on there. Please send ASAP. I want to follow-up on my "fatigue" level. ☺ Thanks again. What could of been traumatic was an "adventure"! God Bless, ♡ Phillip

Dear Dr. Bretz!

Please accept my sincere Thank's for your help, kindness understanding and compassion you gave my daughter Michele during her difficult time.

You are truly a beautiful caring person and a great surgeon. Michele can now start her life whole again. -

May God bless you always.

Your staff made us feel comfortable and is most efficient, Rita, Cathy, Kathrine and Maria you are all wonderful.

EISENHOWER MEMORIAL HOSPITAL

February 25, 1992

Phillip D. Bretz, M.D.
39800 Bob Hope Drive, #C
Rancho Mirage, CA. 92270.

Dear Dr. Bretz:

On behalf of the Center for Healthy Living, thank you for your excellent presentation and for participating in the Physician's Lecture Series.

The audience was most enthusiastic in their praise of your talk, and expressed their appreciation to you for giving them the benefit of your knowledge.

It is because of your generosity and willingness to participate that we are able to offer community education at its very finest. I hope that we have an opportunity to work together again. And, please do not hesitate to contact me with suggestions and ideas you may have for future programs.

Thank you again, Dr. Bretz, for your contribution to the success of our program.

Sincerely,

Susan Heggie
Coordinator
Center for Healthy Living

facsimile
TRANSMITTAL

to:	DrPhillip Bretz
fax #:	001441712351105
re:	
date:	January 16, 1996
pages:	_2_ page(s) total, including this cover sheet.

Dear Dr. Bretz,

Just hearing from you has given me a sense of confidence regarding my recent mammogram at the Lister Hospital and thank you for sharing your knowledge of Lister. I had no idea it had such an illustrious history.

Your suggestion to have a follow up test is well taken although at times I think I would rather walk in front of a moving car rather than have to go through more agonizing tests. Still we should all be grateful for today's advances and doctors like you.

I have been thinking of a return trip to the Desert and should any further treatment be needed I will be camped on your office step. In the meantime if you want me to look up any past acquaintances etc for you while we are here I would be glad to do so. Bill and I plan to make London our home, but some things are just too hard to give up... a doctor you have confidence in!

Wishing you a most happy 1996.

Sincerely,

Leslie

May 3, 2003

Dear Dr. Bretz,

Just a quick note of thanks to you for doing such a wonderful job on my surgery back in March. The doctors here in Alaska are very impressed with your work and the way it looks! I'm half way through with my radiation treatments and they seem to be going well.

Fishing season is getting underway here in Alaska so I thought you might enjoy looking at our magazines.

Have a great summer and I'll be in touch.

Sincerely,
Kathy

Every organization has intermittent issues and while I forget the exact nature of this one, apparently, we handled it well.

VALLEY ANIMAL CLIN

May 20, 1992

Desert Breast Institute, Inc
Phillip D. Bretz, M.D.
39-800 Bob Hope Dr., Suite A
Rancho Mirage, CA 92270

Dear Dr. Bretz:

LeeAnn and I would like to extend our thanks for the courtesies that were extended to her following the incident at your office.

LeeAnn was very upset about it when she returned home. Your staff did an excellent job handling the situation. Your personal phone calls were an extension of your professional courtesies.

Owning our own business, we have situations that are upsetting to us. Your attention to this matter has expressed your individual attention to your clients. LeeAnn was very impressed with your facility.

We appreciate your immediate attention to the situation.

Sincerely and with thanks,

Gary L. Homec, D.V.M.

Desert Sierra Breast Cancer Partnership

A member of the Inland Agency family of programs

6235 River Crest Drive, Suite P
Riverside, CA 92507

Telephone (909) 697-6582
Fax (909) 697-4410

Administrative Agency

Inland Agency
Linda Dunn, Executive
Director

Executive Committee

Jan Green, Chair
San Bernardino Valley
College

Mary Price ,Vice Chair
Riverside County
Department of Community
Action

Shirley Bradley, Secretary
Riverside County
Department of Public
Health

Sandy Bradley
American Cancer Society

Carolyn Daniels
New Hope Missionary
Baptist Church/
Loma Linda University
Cancer Institute

Dorothy Ellis
Beaumont Soroptimist/
San Gorgonio Memorial
Hospital

Becky Foreman
YWCA of Riverside
County

Vivian Henderson
Riverside Community
Hospital

June Hibbard
San Bernardino County
Department of Public
Health

July 3, 2001

Dear Dr. Bretz,

On behalf of the Desert Sierra Breast Cancer Partnership, I would like to send our deepest appreciation for serving as a member of the Mini-grant Review Committee. The selection process went extremely well due to your efforts and input. We are pleased to announce the five community based organizations that will be funded for the 2001-2002 funding cycle. Please find an attached the mini-grant matrix reflecting the selection.

Again, thank you for your participation. We are fortunate to call you an active Partnership member, and even more fortunate to call you a team player in the fight against breast cancer! We look forward to working with you in the future. Your efforts truly help to ensure that

"Every Woman Count! Every Year!"

Sincerely,

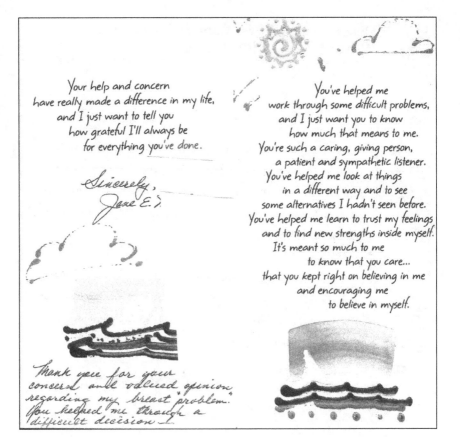

Your help and concern
have really made a difference in my life,
and I just want to tell you
how grateful I'll always be
for everything you've done.

Sincerely,
Jane E.

You've helped me
work through some difficult problems,
and I just want you to know
how much that means to me.
You're such a caring, giving person,
a patient and sympathetic listener.
You've helped me look at things
in a different way and to see
some alternatives I hadn't seen before.
You've helped me learn to trust my feelings
and to find new strengths inside myself.
It's meant so much to me
to know that you care...
that you kept right on believing in me
and encouraging me
to believe in myself.

Thank you for your
concern and valued opinion
regarding my breast "problem."
You helped me through a
difficult decision.

Thank you for your life giving help this last year, again you saved my foot! So much has happened for us that has been good because of you.

We thank God for you. Keep you in our daily prayers for good health that you may continue to give your healing hands to so many who need your excellent wisdom and life saving care.

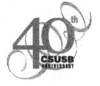

ALBERT K. KARNIG
President

October 24, 2005

Dr. Phillip Bretz, Director
Desert Breast and Osteoporosis Institute
35-280 Bob Hope Drive, Suite #103
Rancho Mirage, California 92270

Dear Dr. Bretz:

After reading in a recent edition of *The Desert Sun* that you participated in the "Tour of Hope" to raise money for cancer research, I wanted to send you a quick note to tell you that I admire your valuable efforts in increasing public knowledge about cancer, as well as your excellent work in developing innovative procedures to treat and to prevent this devastating disease, which, as you point out, claims an unacceptable number of lives every day.

Thanks for making a difference, both in the community and in people's lives, and best of luck in your diverse—and vitally important—responsibilities.

Sincerely,

Albert K. Karnig
President

HOLOGIC®

March 22, 2005

Phillip Bretz, MD
Desert Breast Osteoporosis Institute
35-280 Bob Hope Dr #103
Rancho Mirage, CA 92270
Tel 760-324-8323
Fax 760-324-8779

Dear Dr. Bretz,

It has been a pleasure talking to you and reading through your voluminous scientific history that you sent. We are very interested in further contact to discuss the possibility of your contributing to our tomosynthesis clinical trials. You would be a great addition to our team.

I have no current plans to be in your area, but perhaps you might be planning to be in Boston in the near future and if so we would invite you to our facility where we could show you our progress. If you are not planning such a trip, please advise and I will have some people local to you contact you and we can start our introductions.

Sincerely,

Andy Smith, Ph.D.
Principal Scientist
Hologic Inc

Desert Hot Springs, CA
May 12, 1989

Dear Dr. Welsh,

At last, someone has figured
out a way of making Mammography a
pleasant experience. When I walked in
to the "Desert Breast Institute" I couldn't
believe my eyes: the huge elegantly
furnished waiting room, the candy, the coffee
and the young, attractive, and friendly staff.
The radiologist was gentle. I appreciated
seeing and hearing the tape and having
the doctor showing and explaining my own films
It should be easy to return for checkups.

Gratefully, Edith E. Chrisman

12-8-97

Dear Dr. Brety,

I can't tell you how much I appreciated you calling me with the good news late Friday. Not only was I grateful for the news - I was equally grateful for your sensitivity to call me prior to the weekend. I wasn't expecting a call till Tuesday.

I think you and your staff are wonderful. From the first phone call to your office, I was treated with a friendly, compassionate and personal manner. This helped to ease the fear.

My best to all of you. With a grateful heart.

Annie T,

Words are not enough to express my appreciation
for your true dedication as a physician and
selfless benevolence as a fellow human being.
It's no wonder you are so well-respected and loved
by so many. I shall never forget your kindness.

Thank you very much.

Fondly,

Lisa

Lisa

Dear Dr. Bretz,

I don't know how you did it, but I am eternally grateful! We owe you big time. I foresee your honey implants as a reality in the near future...

Sincerely,

Yvonne E

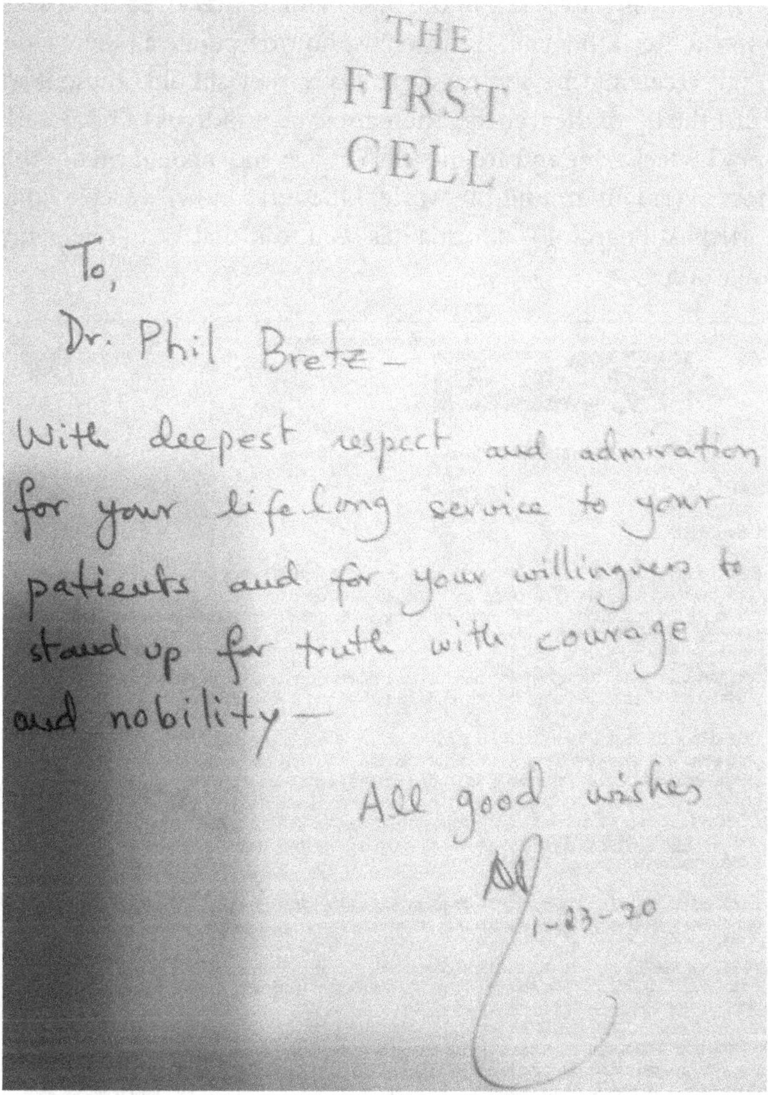

THE
FIRST
CELL

To,

Dr. Phil Bretz —

With deepest respect and admiration
for your life-long service to your
patients and for your willingness to
stand up for truth with courage
and nobility —

All good wishes

AV

1-23-20

The following are a few of the many emails I received from around the world. Read them all. It shows just how desperate all these women are, not receiving the compassionate care they should. These women are just the tip of the iceberg. There must be hundreds of thousands of them who feel alone and are shaken. Yes, Lavender could change things almost overnight around the world. Of course, now I receive none as the Medical Board of California has seen to it that I can't help any of those women.

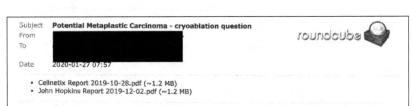

Dear Dr. Bretz,

By some miracle I stumbled upon your TED talk among the old files I've collected over the years, while my mom was fighting cancer; a battle that she had lost 3.5 years ago. The very painful memories of her suffering and the many wrong turns along the cold hallways of mainstream medicine are still very fresh in my mind.

And now I am facing the uncertainty and fear that cancer diagnosis brings, it's like staring into the abyss...I am 46 years old, a mother of two daughters 26 and 8 years old.

On October 25, 2019 I have had my first mammogram that followed a normal thermography and an ultrasound that showed a 6 mm lump. Right then the radiologist performed a needle biopsy that Seattle (████ lab ruled as normal "hyalinized fibroadenoma", but John Hopkins medical laboratory had a different opinion. I have learned from our experience with my mom's cancer, that sending samples to John Hopkins can be very informative, to say the least. So, I did request it this time as well. Dr.████████John Hopkins suspected it could be metaplastic carcinoma and suggested a conservative excision.

Just last week I had an appointment with a surgeon and inquired about cryoablation. I got a very dismissive answer, saying that it was still in clinical studies and that surgery would be preferred.

To say the least, I am very confused and concerned. All my life I've embraced natural intuitive living. I am a believer in conservative or natural methods of treatment whenever possible, surgery would be the absolutely last resort, in my opinion.

Finding your TED talk and Visionary Breast Center web site was a breath of fresh air, it felt right on par with my approach to life and health. I cried when you got emotional on stage: my God, you really care! I've met so many cold and unsympathetic doctors, when my mom refused chemo and used natural FDA-approved methods to support her with stage III ductal carcinoma for 9 years, doctors who butchered her breast and created more issues than solved, doctors who finally devastated last of her body resources at the operating table during unnecessary 8-hour surgery, 24 hours later my mom passed away. To be honest, I'm terrified to get back into this system of mainstream medicine that nukes the house to get rid of the cockroaches.

I am seeking an advice and would like to know if I might be the candidate for cryoablation, or if I should do the surgical biopsy first (which I remember left my mom with a hematoma larger than the original tumor and caused more issues down the road). What would my next steps be? Could I get a consultation at your Center?

Attached are two pathology reports. I wish I'm just overreacting, and it turns out to be benign, but I would like to know for sure, and if possible avoid surgery.

Subject	**Lavender Way. Lavender Procedure**	roundcube
From	▓▓▓▓▓▓▓▓▓▓▓▓▓▓▓▓▓▓▓▓▓	
To	▓▓▓▓▓▓▓▓▓▓▓▓▓▓▓▓▓▓▓▓▓	
Date	2020-11-24 09:34	

Dear Dr. Bretz,

I first listened to your interview with Dr. Alex Mostovoy few months ago, and again to your presentation during the Canadian Association of Clinical Thermography. Incredible presentation.

I live and practice integrative medicine here in Africa. I see quite a few cancer cases, especially those who would wan[t] to avoid the standard treatment.
Am not a surgeon, but a family physician.

I have a good office practice.

My question: is your Lavender Way something I can practice here in Africa. If yes, I very much would appreciate an opportunity to come learn from you.

I understand from your lecture that you are not doing anymore procedures at this time, but I could start with the basic theoretical first hand.

Kindly let me know how to proceed if you consider that I am eligible.

Many thanks.

7/22/2019   Roundcube Webmail :: DCIS

Subject	**DCIS**	roundcube
From	▓▓▓▓▓▓▓▓▓▓▓▓▓▓▓▓▓▓	
To	▓▓▓▓▓▓▓▓▓▓▓▓▓▓▓▓▓▓	
Date	2019-07-22 10:32	

Dear Dr. Bretz,

I live in the Netherlands. I am recently diagnosed with a cyst in my breast and something behind it. Doctors are not very sure about the diagnostic and said that it could be DCIS or it could be some invasive cancer. So, they offered me mastectomy.

I am wondering whether cryoablation therapy could be done in my situation.

I look forward to your reply,

With regards,

2/8/2021   Roundcube Webmail :: Seeking your guidance and treatment

Subject	**Seeking your guidance and treatment**	rou
From	▓▓▓▓▓▓▓▓▓▓▓▓▓▓▓▓▓▓	
To	▓▓▓▓▓▓▓▓▓▓▓▓▓▓▓▓▓▓	
Date	2020-01-19 05:10	

Dear Dr. Bretz,

I heard your ted talk yesterday and it gave me a ray of hope for my mother who was diagnosed with breast cancer. She is 68 years old and her appetite and energy levels are good.

I am based in India and I would like to look at any possibility of us consulting you as I am not keen on going with conventional treatments which might harm her health. I would like to know if there is any way I can consult you over the phone/skype or if there are any facilities outside United Stated where we can take the treatment.

I will be really obliged and thankful for any advice I can receive from you at this stage.

Regards,

Dear Dr Bretz,

I listened with great appreciation to your interview with Dr Mostovoy. https://www.youtube.com/watch?v=70VJ4g9DIj0. Thank you so much for that!

I was diagnosed in mid-August with invasive ductal carcinoma, ER+PR+HER2-. An MRI showed no additional tumors. They put a titanium marker in the lump during the needle biopsy procedure. The lump was the size of a peppercorn, under my left armpit. I have very small, "dense" breasts, and am quite underweight, so can easily feel the lump just under the skin.

I took hormone replacement therapy from age 50 to age 68 and quit on the day of the diagnosis.

Since the tumor is so small, I have been taking some time to research and learn about the best course of action. I understand that chemo and radiation are very damaging to the immune system, giving rise to recurrence of cancer.

Meanwhile, I have been trying to follow the ███████Therapy to build up my immune system (juicing, only whole plant foods, and coffee enemas to detox) and trying to figure out what to do next. I thought I was healthy because I have been on a whole plant food diet with plenty of exercise for four years. I did not know at the time that my tiny skin cancer (removed), colon polyps (benign), and uterine polyps (ablated) indicated a severe immune system deficiency.

The lump has gotten smaller and seems that now I am only feeling the titanium marker. However, the area from 3 o'clock to 6'oclock seems almost imperceptibly swollen, and I occasionally feel twinges, so I wonder what is going on there. I am considering going to the █████████████████ run by Dr. █████████ (who is now carrying the torch for the late ████████), to fix my immune system and rid my body of any cancer in my body to prevent metastasis.

I would like to get the Lavender procedure to remove the lump. Can it be done with the marker in place or would that be removed first? Are there any doctors in Rochester, NY who perform it? The surgeon I spoke with here insisted on lumpectomy with clear margins, removal of all sentinel lymph nodes, radiation, and chemo, so I declined in order to buy time to research. Interestingly, the site cancer.gov does not mention cryosurgery for breast cancer.

I would appreciate any recommendations you can provide.

---

pregnancy with HER2 tumor   Message 1 of 460

From   ████████████████████████████████████

To   ████████████████████████████████████

Date   **Today 14:16**

Dear Sir/Madam

we are from Israel.
My name is ██████, and i am writing on behalf of a family member.
a pregnant woman (week 24), she was diagnosed with a breast tumor, (HER2 2.5 centimeter, probably localized, 3 bumps in the armpit).
We wonder about alternatives to chemotherapy. and any other support or advice that your clinic can offer.
our assumption is that we don't have a clinic with a similar approach to yours, here in Israel

Many thanks,

Good day Dr,

My name is █████████████ and i am from Nigeria, my mum is diagnosed of breast cancer and the doctor has advised she undergo surgery to cut the breast so the cancer wont spread.
Please i will need your medical advise on the best treatment for my mum.

Regards,

Subject **Please help me?**
From
To
roundcube
Date 2020-10-17 19:48

Dear Dr. Bretz,

I am ███. I live in Vienna, Austria.

I have a very large breast tumour in my left breast. It is the size of a lemon and is clearly visible on the left side of my left breast. I have not had surgery, chemo, etc as I want to heal it without destroying me and my body. I have had it now for about 10 years. It started as a pea-sized lump and I healed it within weeks with the ████ Protocol. A simple meal of flax oil, flax seeds and cottage cheese to be taken daily. I also juiced daily and became vegetarian/vegan then. It worked.

I stopped the treatment too soon; after a few months. The lump returned after 2 years as I was going through a lot of stress. I kept putting off treating it because I'd lost the fear of cancer, assuming that it is easily healed with the ████ Protocol once I do it again. But I left it too long. It is now huge and is becoming painful, itchy, and refusing to leave, despite me doing all I can to heal it. I am using THC cannabis oil daily, juicing, ████ Protocol, meditation, Zhineng Qigong, trampolining, eating healthy, cancer destroying frequencies (youtube, where I found your Tedx talk video) etc, but it refuses to budge. I have not been to a Dr/Hospital again after the 1st diagnosis, as I know they will just freak out again and try again to force me to do the usual treatments, chemo & co, which I refuse to do.

But I need help now. I do not have much money, but I would appreciate any advice you could give me please? Is it too late for me? I am otherwise a young and healthy 60 yr old woman. I look like 40 (everyone around me says) and don't act old either. I still work fulltime as a receptionist, simply because I have to work for an income. Usually I am also really positive and happy, but right now I am scared out of my skull and despairing as it seems I have nowhere to turn and no-one to help me. I do not need the Drs/hospitals kind of "help." I want to live. Healthy & cancer free.

Can you please help me? Can the Lavender Procedure work for a tumour this size, or is it too big? Can you help me please?

God bless the work you do to save us.

Subject **Thank you!**
From
To
roundcube
Date 2020-10-15 15:22

Good afternoon Dr. Bretz,

I work with Alexander ███ by way of having an Infrared Clinic in ████████ Canada - out on the East Coast.

Today I watched the interview you and Alex did on what you do and I feel compelled to write to you and let you know how grateful and thankful I am for this opportunity to learn and for all you do!

Greatly appreciated and I will certainly buy your book(s) and just placed my order for Dr. Raza's book The First Cell.

Many Blessings to you & your Team!

The following are copies of my publications in various peer-reviewed journals.

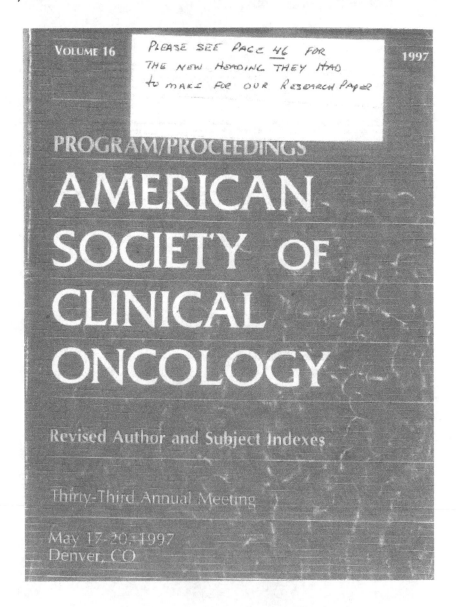

THEY MADE A
NEW CATEGORY
FOR US, ALSO SEE PG 48.

The Breast Journal

September/October 2000
Volume 6, Number 5

Official Journal of the American Society of Breast Disease,
The Senologic International Society,
and
The International Society of Breast Pathology

Now available on-line at www.blackwellscience.com

Blackwell
Science

Shahla Masood, MD, Editor

THE COMPASS TREATMENT, A NEW ERA OF TREATMENT IN BREAST CANCER NEOADJUVANT THERAPY AND RADIATION WITHOUT SURGERY

Bretz* P., Dreisbach, P., Desert Breast Institute, Palm Desert, CA, 92260
Bacus, S., Advanced Cellular Diagnostics, Inc, Elmhurst, IL, 60126

Key Words: core biopsy, strategic analysis, neoadjuvant chemotherapy, no surgery

An understanding of the natural history of invasive breast cancer coupled with effective chemotherapy opened the door for vast improvements in the care of breast cancer patients. Often, axillary node dissection was used as the major guide in recommending adjuvant chemotherapy. Over the past decade for the purpose of neoadjuvant chemotherapy, lymph node status has been supplanted by strategic analysis. This is based on core sample, tumor grade, size, lymphatic invasion, mammographic appearance, clinical exam, family history and extensive tumor analysis. This has identified aggressive invasive tumors that are likely to have already metastasized long before the patient is diagnosed. Since 1989 we have treated 96 patients ranging in age from 28 to 83 with neoadjuvant chemotheapy based on strategic analysis following core biopsy. Tumor size ranged from 1.2 cm to over 8cm. All patients have received at least four courses of CAF. Neoadjuvant therapy has identified "responders" who showed consistent tumor ablation to the point of total tumor dissolution based on clinical exam, mammogaphy and repeat core sampling. In the past five years we have continued chemotherapy including at times Taxol well past four courses, if mammographic evidence pointed to total tumor eradication.

Compass Treatment Results
5/96 (5.2%) had modified radical mastectomy
84/96 (87%) had lumpectomy and radiation
7/96 (7.3%) had no surgery, only chemotherapy and radiation
32/96 (33%) had no node dissection
18/96 (18%) had sentinel node biopsy
18/96 (18%) had no tumor removed
3/96 (3.1%) local/regional recurrence, none of the above eighteen patients
89/96 (92%)* have survived, followed from 2 to 10 years**
one patient died of myocardial infarction free of cancer*

Individualized treatment at a dedicated comprehensive breast institute following strategic analysis guidelines and response evaluation accounts for the above results. Our comprehensive team is active and in place before the diagnosis is made. These results point to patients doing better at a dedicated comprehensive center. We conclude implementation of Nationwide Networked Comprehensive Breast Centers is in order to achieve optimal patient care including lowering mortality and mastectomy rates. For those patients with no tumor found at surgery or for those with no tumor on repeat core biopsy and having no surgery, the classic paradigm of "clear margins for radiation" comes into question. We also conclude that it is possible to effectively treat some invasive breast cancer patients without surgery.

Supplement to

INTERNATIONAL JOURNAL OF

Radiation Oncology

BIOLOGY·PHYSICS

VOLUME 75, NUMBER 3, SUPPLEMENT

2009

PROCEEDINGS
OF THE
AMERICAN SOCIETY
FOR
RADIATION ONCOLOGY
51ST ANNUAL MEETING

ASTRO
TARGETING CANCER CARE

McCormick Place West
November 1–5, 2009
Chicago, Illinois

Official Journal of
ASTRO AMERICAN SOCIETY FOR RADIATION ONCOLOGY
PAEDIATRIC RADIATION ONCOLOGY SOCIETY

Affiliated with
LATIN AMERICAN ASSOCIATION OF THERAPEUTIC RADIATION AND ONCOLOGY

ELSEVIER

0360-3016(20091101)75:3S;1-2

2091 An Autologous Abdominal Free-fat Patch Surmounts the Problem of Skin Spacing during Accelerated Partial Breast Radiation (APBR)

P. Bretz[1], D. Mantik[2], T. Mesek[2], S. Ling[2], P. Dreisbach[3]

[1]*Desert Breast and Osteoporosis Institute, La Quinta, CA,* [2]*21st Century Oncology, Palm Desert, CA,* [3]*Eisenhower Medical Center, Rancho Mirage, CA*

Purpose/Objective(s): A problem in dosimetry planning using a partial breast radiation device is lack of skin spacing. As a consequence of this lack of skin spacing many after-loading catheters must be extracted without treatment. Each member of the comprehensive team must be aware of the surgical and radiation techniques that optimize individualized treatment. In order to solve this problem of skin overdosing, we have developed two techniques.

Material/Methods: APBR is used to treat the area most likely to develop a local recurrence, i.e., that centimeter around the original lumpectomy margin. If successful, high dose rate brachytherapy using Iridium-192 is administered in two sessions per day over five days for a total dose of 34 Gy. Instead of elliptically excising the tumor, often leaving little skin spacing and frequent skin indentation, the surgeon enters the breast through the areola. The initial incision is carried down for at least a centimeter and then cautery is used to divide the tissue until the tumor is reached. The tumor is excised (with clear margins) preferably in the shape of the balloon. This technique allows for a supportive wall of tissue. For cases that still have skin spacing problems an autologous abdominal free-fat patch transfer has been devised. The patch is removed through an appendectomy-like incision just medial to the left anterior superior iliac crest. The size varies and the thickness of the patch removed generally is at least 1 cm thick. The patch is trimmed and two stay sutures are used to tack the patch to the roof of the defect.

Results: Since having to abandon our very first attempt at balloon placement we have successfully implanted and radiated 35 patients using the above two techniques including the fat patch in 15 cases. Patients have been followed for 10 months up to seven years without any local recurrences. Three patients developed spider-like vein prominence and some firmness over the lumpectomy site but no long term severe effects have been encountered. In some cases the fat patch is visible on ultrasound and mammography. In our last patient we used a new type of multi-lumen catheter/balloon but could still not safely protect the skin. We, therefore, placed a patch the same day and used it that same day, a dramatic result visible on CT.

Conclusions: APBR remains an evolving art, especially with new devices steadily emerging. The art includes shaping the lumpectomy cavity to conform to the balloon options, as well as advances in radiation planning. All must dovetail harmoniously to achieve a superior outcome. Wherever this may lead, though, we conclude that the two techniques cited here can be employed immediately to reduce skin doses. If employed, these techniques will promptly permit more frequent use of after-loading catheters.

Author Disclosure: P. Bretz, None; D. Mantik, None; T. Mesek, None; S. Ling, None; P. Dreisbach, None.

JULY/AUGUST 1997
Volume Four, Number Four

CURRENT CLINICAL TRIALS ONCOLOGY™

NATIONAL CANCER INSTITUTE
PDQ®

SEE PAGE P-23 MARKED
WITH A PAPER CLIP FOR
OUR PARTICIPATION IN NCI
SPONSORED CLINICAL TRIALS

P-24 | Protocols

St. Michael's Hospital. Toronto, Ontario M5B 1W8 Canada. INVESTIGATOR: Jarley Koo. 416-864-5955.

Toronto Sunnybrook Regional Cancer Centre. Toronto, Ontario M4N 3M5 Canada. INVESTIGATOR: Kathleen I. Pritchard. 416-488-4616.

Women's College Hospital. Toronto, Ontario M5S 1B6 Canada. INVESTIGATOR: H. Lavina Lickley. 416-323-6225.

Hopital Laval. Ste-Foy. Quebec G1V 4G5 Canada. INVESTIGATOR: Martin Potvin. 418-656-4810.

Hopital Notre Dame. Montreal, Quebec H2L 4M1 Canada. INVESTIGATOR: Marc Poljicak. 514-277-4095.

Hotel Dieu de Levis. Levis, Quebec G6V 3Z1 Canada. INVESTIGATOR: Felix Couture. 418-835-7121.

Hotel Dieu de Montreal. Montreal, Quebec H2W 1T8 Canada. INVESTIGATOR: Andre Robidoux. 514-843-2697.

Hotel Dieu de Quebec. Quebec City, Quebec G1R 2J6 Canada. INVESTIGATOR: Antoine Kibrite. 418-691-5370.

Jewish General Hospital. Montreal, Quebec H3T 1E2 Canada. INVESTIGATOR: Richard G. Margolese. 514-342-3504.

Maisonneuve-Rosemont Hospital. Montreal, Quebec H1T 2M4 Canada. INVESTIGATOR: Yves Eugene Leclerc. 514-252-3822.

Montreal General Hospital. Montreal, Quebec H3G 1A4 Canada. INVESTIGATOR: Michael P. Thirlwell. 514-937-6011.

Royal Victoria Hospital. Montreal. Montreal, Quebec H3A 1A1 Canada. INVESTIGATOR: Henry R. Shibata. 514-843-1526.

St. Sacrement Hospital. Quebec City, Quebec G1S 4L8 Canada. INVESTIGATOR: Luc Deschenes. 418-682-7893.

Baptist Medical Center-Montclair. Birmingham, Alabama 35213 U.S.A. INVESTIGATOR: Thomas Allen Gaskin, III. 205-780-7150.

Hematology-Oncology Center, P.C. Mobile, Alabama 36640-0460 U.S.A. INVESTIGATOR: John E. Feldman. 334-433-2233.

Providence Hospital - Mobile AL. Mobile, Alabama 36685 U.S.A. INVESTIGATOR: Michael W. Meshad. 205-639-1661.

Greater Phoenix Community Clinical Oncology Program. Phoenix, Arizona 85006-2726 U.S.A. INVESTIGATOR: David Kyle King. 602-258-4875.

Lutheran Healthcare Network. Mesa, Arizona 85214 U.S.A. INVESTIGATOR: Michael M. Long. 602-926-6265.

Walter O. Boswell Memorial Hospital. Sun City, Arizona 85351 U.S.A. INVESTIGATOR: Teresita C. Barnett. 602-933-1337.

University of Arkansas for Medical Sciences. Little Rock, Arkansas 72205 U.S.A. INVESTIGATOR: John Ralph Broadwater, Jr. 501-686-5547.

Bay Area Tumor Institute Community Clinical Oncology Program. Oakland, California 94609 U.S.A. INVESTIGATOR: James H. Feusner. 510-428-3689.

Beckman Research Institute of the City of Hope. Duarte, California 91010 U.S.A. INVESTIGATOR: Lawrence David Wagman. 818-359-8111.

David Grant Medical Center. Travis Air Force Base, California 94535 U.S.A. INVESTIGATOR: Kevin P. Ryan. 707-423-7331.

Donald N. Sharp Memorial Community Hospital. San Diego, California 92123 U.S.A. INVESTIGATOR: Christine Anna White. 619-450-5998.

Eisenhower Medical Center. Rancho Mirage, California 92270 U.S.A. INVESTIGATOR: Philip D. Bretz. 619-568-3414.

Hoag Memorial Hospital Presbyterian. Newport Beach, California 92663 U.S.A. INVESTIGATOR: Robert O. Dillman. 714-760-2091.

Jonsson Comprehensive Cancer Center, UCLA. Los Angeles, California 90024 U.S.A. INVESTIGATOR: Susan M. Love. 310-230-1712.

Kaiser Permanente Medical Center - Vallejo. Vallejo, California 94589 U.S.A. INVESTIGATOR: Louis Fahrenbacher. 707-648-6335.

Loma Linda University Medical Center. Loma Linda, California 92354 U.S.A. INVESTIGATOR: Carlos A. Garberoglio. 909-824-4286.

Long Beach Community Medical Center. Long Beach, California 90814 U.S.A. INVESTIGATOR: Eknath A. Deo. 310-597-5501.

Providence-St. Joseph Medical Center - Burbank. Burbank, California 91505 U.S.A. INVESTIGATOR: Raul R. Mena. 818-840-0921.

San Diego Kaiser Permanente Community Clinical Oncology Program. San Diego, California 92120 U.S.A. INVESTIGATOR: Scott M. Browning. 619-528-2591.

San Gabriel Valley Medical Center. San Gabriel, California 91776 U.S.A. INVESTIGATOR: H. Rex Greene. 818-397-3737.

Scripps Memorial Hospitals-Stevens Cancer Center. Encinitas, California 92023 U.S.A. INVESTIGATOR: Joel Ian Bernstein. 619-453-9200.

St. Joseph Hospital - Orange. Orange, California 92613-5600 U.S.A. INVESTIGATOR: Robert T. Eagan. 714-771-8259.

St. Mary Medical Center. Long Beach, California 90813 U.S.A. INVESTIGATOR: N. Simon Tchekmedyian. 310-500-0345.

University of California Davis Medical Center. Sacramento, California 95817 U.S.A. INVESTIGATOR: Frederick James Meyers. 916-734-3772.

White Memorial Medical Center. Los Angeles, California 90033 U.S.A. INVESTIGATOR: Matthew Tan. 213-264-2633.

Colorado Cancer Research Program, Inc. Community Clinical Oncology Program. Denver, Colorado 80218 U.S.A. INVESTIGATOR: Robert F. Berris. 303 777 2663.

Memorial Hospital - Colorado Springs. Colorado Springs, Colorado 80909 U.S.A. INVESTIGATOR: David L. Headley. 719-634-4130.

University of Colorado Cancer Center. Denver, Colorado 80262 U.S.A. INVESTIGATOR: Douglas K. Rovira. 303-270-8801.

Hartford Hospital. Hartford, Connecticut 06102-5037 U.S.A. INVESTIGATOR: Patricia A. De Fusco. 860-246-6647.

George Washington University Medical Center. Washington, District of Columbia 20037 U.S.A. INVESTIGATOR: Theodore Tsangaris. 202-994-9995.

Baptist Regional Cancer Institute - Jacksonville. Jacksonville, Florida 32207 U.S.A. INVESTIGATOR: Neil Abramson. 904-202-7048.

Halifax Medical Center. Daytona Beach, Florida 32114 U.S.A. INVESTIGATOR: Harry H. Black. 904-252-4853.

Medical Center Clinic - Pensacola. Pensacola, Florida 32514 U.S.A. INVESTIGATOR: Philip M. Wade. 904-474-8413.

Mount Sinai Community Clinical Oncology Program. Miami Beach, Florida 33140 U.S.A. INVESTIGATOR: Enrique Davila. 305-535-3310.

Nemours Childrens Clinic. Orlando, Florida 32806 U.S.A. INVESTIGATOR: Clarence E. Brown, III. 407-648-3800.

Ocala Oncology Center. Ocala, Florida 32671 U.S.A. INVESTIGATOR: Thomas Howard Cartwright. 352-732-4032.

Sarasota Memorial Hospital. Sarasota, Florida 34239 U.S.A. INVESTIGATOR: Stephen H. Goldman. 941-957-1000.

Winter Park Cancer Care Center. Winter Park, Florida 32792 U.S.A. INVESTIGATOR: Steven G. Lester. 407-646-7777.

Atlanta Regional Community Clinical Oncology Program. Atlanta, Georgia 30342-1101 U.S.A. INVESTIGATOR: Ernest W. Franklin, III. 404-250-3600.

Dekalb Medical Center. Inc. Decatur, Georgia 30033 U.S.A. INVESTIGATOR: LaMar S. McGinnis, Jr. 404-292-2700.

University of Hawaii. Honolulu, Hawaii 96844 U.S.A. INVESTIGATOR: Robert H. Oishi. 808-548-8530.

Mountain States Tumor Institute. Boise, Idaho 83712 U.S.A. INVESTIGATOR: Thomas M. Beck. 208-381-2711.

St. Josephs Regional Medical Center - Lewiston. Lewiston, Idaho 83501 U.S.A. INVESTIGATOR: Malcolm William Winter. 208-743-7427.

Carle Cancer Center Community Clinical Oncology Program. Urbana, Illinois 61801 U.S.A. INVESTIGATOR: Alan K. Hatfield. 217-383-3010.

Central Illinois Community Clinical Oncology Program. Springfield, Illinois 62781-0001 U.S.A. INVESTIGATOR: James L. Wade, III. 217-876-6600.

Highland Park Hospital. Highland Park, Illinois U.S.A. INVESTIGATOR: Arthur Greene Miske. 312-641-1150.

Illinois Masonic Medical Center. Chicago, Illinois U.S.A. INVESTIGATOR: Yosef H. Pilch. 312-

Kellogg Cancer Care Center Community Clinical Program. Evanston, Illinois 60201 U.S.A. INVESTIGATOR: Janardan D. Khandekar. 708-

Michael Reese Hospital & Medical Center. Chicago, Illinois 60616-3390 U.S.A. INVESTIGATOR: Barbara 312-836-2860.

Northwestern University Robert H. Lurie Cancer Chicago, Illinois 60611 U.S.A. INVESTIGATOR: Bowen Benson, III. 312-908-9412.

Oncology Care Centers - Belleville. Belleville, Illinois 618-236-1011.

Rockford Clinic. Rockford, Illinois 61103 U.S.A. INVESTIGATOR: William R. Edwards. 815-

University of Illinois at Chicago Health Sciences Chicago, Illinois 60612 U.S.A. INVESTIGATOR: W. Boddie, Jr. 312-996-0490.

West Suburban Hospital Medical Center. Oak Park 60302 U.S.A. INVESTIGATOR: John L. Showel. 312-383-4814.

Community Hospitals of Indianapolis - Regional Center. Indianapolis, Indiana 46219 U.S.A. INVESTIGATOR: Shivaji K. Gunate. 317-355-

Memorial Hospital of South Bend. South Bend, 46601 U.S.A. INVESTIGATOR: Rafat H. Ansari. 219-234-5123.

Methodist Cancer Center - Indianapolis. Indianapolis, Indiana 46202 U.S.A. INVESTIGATOR: William Dugan, Jr. 317-927-5770.

St. Vincent Hospital and Health Care Center Department. Indianapolis, Indiana 46260 U.S.A. INVESTIGATOR: John A. Cavins.

Cedar Rapids Oncology Project Community Clinical Oncology Program. Cedar Rapids, Iowa 52403 U.S.A. INVESTIGATOR: Martin Wiesenfeld. 319-

University of Iowa Hospitals and Clinics. Iowa City 52242 U.S.A. INVESTIGATOR: Peter R. Jochimsen. 319-356-3584.

Columbia Wesley Medical Center. Wichita, Kansas U.S.A. INVESTIGATOR: John Loren Kiser. 316-

University of Kansas Medical Center. Kansas City, Kansas 66160-7357 U.S.A. INVESTIGATOR: William 913-588-6112.

Wichita Community Clinical Oncology Program. Wichita, Kansas 67214 U.S.A. INVESTIGATOR: Herry Hynes. 316-268-5784.

Baptist Hospital East. Louisville, Kentucky 40207 U.S.A. INVESTIGATOR: Manuel Grimaldi. 502-897-

Lexington Clinic, PSC. Lexington, Kentucky 40504 U.S.A. INVESTIGATOR: Thomas M. Wills. 606-254-4201.

Lucille Parker Markey Cancer Center, University of Kentucky. Lexington, Kentucky 40536-0093 U.S.A. INVESTIGATOR: Edward H. Romond. 606-323-

University of Louisville School of Medicine. Louisville, Kentucky 40292 U.S.A. INVESTIGATOR: John H. Hamm. 502-629-2500.

Ochsner Community Clinical Oncology Program. New Orleans, Louisiana 70121 U.S.A. INVESTIGATOR: G. Kardinal. 504-842-3910.

Tulane University School of Medicine. New Orleans, Louisiana 70112 U.S.A. INVESTIGATOR: Edward Sutherland. 504-588-5355.

Eastern Maine Medical Center. Bangor, Maine 04401 U.S.A. INVESTIGATOR: Philip L. Brooks. 207-

Franklin Square Hospital. Baltimore, Maryland 21237 U.S.A. INVESTIGATOR: E. George Elias. 410-

National Naval Medical Center. Bethesda, Maryland 20889-5000 U.S.A. INVESTIGATOR: James N. Frame. 301-496-0901.

Baystate Medical Center. Springfield, Massachusetts U.S.A. INVESTIGATOR: Donald J. Higby. 413-

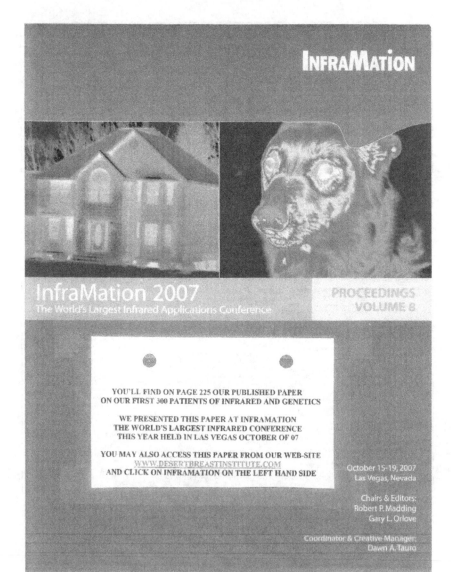

YOU'LL FIND ON PAGE 225 OUR PUBLISHED PAPER
ON OUR FIRST 300 PATIENTS OF INFRARED AND GENETICS

WE PRESENTED THIS PAPER AT INFRAMATION
THE WORLD'S LARGEST INFRARED CONFERENCE
THIS YEAR HELD IN LAS VEGAS OCTOBER OF 07

YOU MAY ALSO ACCESS THIS PAPER FROM OUR WEB-SITE
WWW.DESERTBREASTINSTITUTE.COM
AND CLICK ON INFRAMATION ON THE LEFT HAND SIDE

INFRAMATION

Melding Three Emerging Technologies: Pharmacogenomics, Digital Infrared and Argon Gas, to Eliminate Surgery, Chemotherapy and Radiation in Diagnosing and Treating Breast Cancer

Phillip Bretz M.D., Richard Lynch, D.O.
Infrared Institute of the Desert @
Dolores Ash Women's Center
Rancho Mirage, California

ABSTRACT

In America, breast cancer kills a woman every fifteen minutes. It is the biggest killer of women between the ages of 40 and 55 and is the most common cancer in women except lung cancer. There are approximately 240,000 new cases resulting in over 43,000 deaths annually. For over one hundred years, we believed the answer was in radical surgery, introduced in the 1800s, followed by mammography and chemotherapy in the late 1950s and more sophisticated forms of radiation like partial breast irradiation. Yet all these diagnostic and therapeutic modalities have not put breast cancer into the history books like polio.

This paper will serve as the primer for introducing a new paradigm shift in diagnosing and treating breast cancer. Accelerated advances in evolving technologies namely Pharmacogenomics, Digital Infrared and Argon Gas have opened up the possibility of diagnosing breast cancer at such an early stage (without mammography) that it will be possible to eliminate surgery, chemotherapy and radiation in diagnosing and treating this killer. While the data presented here is limited very early experience, the authors believe the data from these patients followed for the next five years will bring this triad of genetics/IR, and Argon into mainstream medicine.

INTRODUCTION

There are several reasons why the current breast cancer detection and treatment system in place in the United States is failing in its ability to serve all women in a way that is non-injurious and minimally invasive. First, radiation is cumulative and injurious, especially in younger breasts. Second, mammography has a false negative rate between 15% and 20%, highest in younger women with dense breast tissue where the more aggressive breast cancers originate. Third, only 60% of women with health insurance get annual mammography and without insurance, that number drops to a low of 12.5% in Texas. While radical surgery initially was thought to "get it all," surgery, no matter how minimally invasive, does nothing if the patient has metastatic (cancer that has spread) disease. Chemotherapy is toxic and very expensive, and may predispose patients to different cancers in the future. For stage four metastatic cancers, there are virtually no survivors. Radiation, either external beam or partial breast irradiation, is not without local and systemic adverse side effects, including lasting skin damage and pain and more distant problems such as coronary artery disease and pulmonary fibrosis. In addition, there are about 700,000 breast biopsies each year. 60 to 80 percent of these biopsies are negative, indicating a need for a modality that could reduce these negative surgeries.

PHARMACOGENOMICS

A one centimeter breast cancer contains on average 1 billion cancer cells and has been present for about ten years, growing from a single cell microns in diameter. A typical breast cancer begins to develop "neo-angiogenesis", the formation of new blood vessels, about 2-4 years after it is born. With the appearance of angiogenesis, that tumor has a way of spreading without going through the lymph nodes. That is, it can spread through the blood stream. Mammography and MRI can resolve targets down to about 3-4mm, however, the problem is that at that size angiogenesis may not as yet have taken place and the MRI will have a difficult time casting suspicion because it lacks the ability to assign a wash out curve.

If the tumor has neo-angiogenesis contrast medium goes into the tumor at a rate equal to the amount of blood vessels and it goes out again fast. So MRI predicts cancer on the bases of a curve, fast in and fast out. The detector in FLIR's A40 infrared camera with its spatial resolution should image the heat from a developing

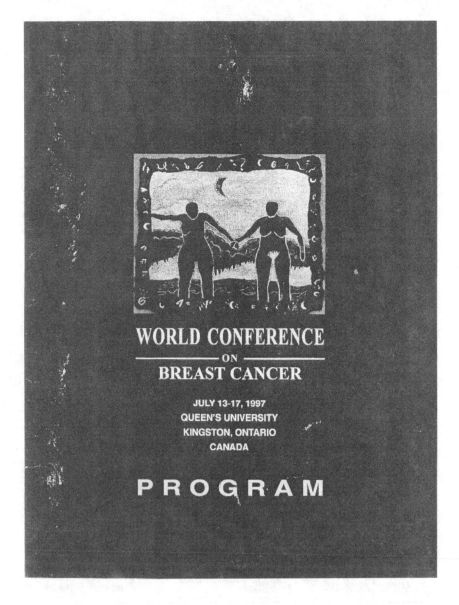

TIME	LOCATION	ACTIVITY
4:00 pm - 5:30 pm	Walter Light Hall Room 210	12. **Ethics and Breast Cancer: A Canadian Perspective** A. Ethics, Cancer and Feminism, *Dr. Susan Sherwin*, Canada B. Ethics and Risk Assessment in Breast Cancer, *Dr. Christy Simpson*, Canada C. Ethics, Feminist Principles & the Individual Woman with Breast Cancer, *Dr. Sandra Taylor*, Canada
	Goodwin Hall Room 254	13. **Male Breast Cancer** A. Male Breast Cancer: A Qualitative Study, *Gill Reilly*, Canada B. Male Breast Cancer from a Patient's Perspective, *Derek Rance*, Canada C. TBA
	Goodwin Hall Room 248	14. **Diagnosis, Treatment, and Outcomes in Chemotherapy** A. The Diagnosis Dilemma: How much? When? *Dr. David Ginsburg*, Canada B. High Dose Chemotherapy in Patients with Metastatic Breast Cancer: A Canadian Experience, *Dr. Stefan Glück*, Canada C. Using Primary Chemotherapy to Treat Breast Cancer without Demonstrable Metastases to Identify "Responders" and to Minimize or Avoid Surgery, *Dr. Phillip Bretz*, United States D. Depressive Symptoms in Cancer Patients on Chemotherapy, *Jose S. Garcia*, Philippines
	Walter Light Hall Room 205	15. **Problems In Delivery of Health Care for Breast Cancer Patients** A. A Strategy for Improved Delivery of Health Care to Black South African Breast Cancer Patients, *Dr. Virginia Mullin*, United States B. Problems with Delivery of Services in Vietnam, *Dr. Thi Hoai Duc Nguyen*, Vietnam C. Social Taboos and Unnamed Disease, *Dr. Razia Sultana*, Bangladesh D. Northeastern Ontario: Challenges for Breast Cancer Care, *Margaux Lachance*, Canada
	Dunning Hall Room 14	16. **Genetics, Markers and Breast Cancer Risk** A.. Prognostic Markers for Node Negative Breast Cancer, *Dr. Irene Andrulis*, Canada B. Serum CA 15-3: Its Utility in Monitoring the Clinical Course of Patients with Breast Carcinoma, *Felina R. Masadao*, Philippines (invited)

This Society of Photo-Optical Instrumentation Engineers (SPIE) (invited paper for oral presentation) has a little story attached to it. I was in the office working and all of a sudden two men came in who identified themselves as CIA. They said they were interested in my work with modified military infrared because the military had used infrared to kill people and I was using a version of it to help cure breast cancer. They had read the presentation from InfraMation Thermography Conference, FLIR's yearly conference One thing led to another and I found myself presentating at the SPIE Defense and Security Conference.

Breast Conservation Therapy in a Community Hospital, Influence of Multidisciplinary Team Approach

Osborne D, Szably D, Bryant T, Umstot R, Carman B, Hershey R, Stah MK, White C, & Vann S.

Marietta Memorial Hospital, Marietta, Ohio 45750

Introduction: Time-tested scientific studies have established breast conservation therapy (BCT) as equal to mastectomy for early stage breast cancer. 1990 NIH consensus conference recommended BCT as the preferred treatment for Stage I & Stage II breast cancer. Pattern of care studies has shown marked geographical variation and gross under utilization of BCT in community level. Physician bias, complex multidisciplinary nature of BCT and concern of not being able to obtain the survival results published by academic centers are often cited as the reasons.

Our hospital's community hospital serving 60,000 population. 50 – 60 breast cancers are seen yearly. In 1992 a multidisciplinary cancer center was established to meet the growing needs of the community. Since then we have seen a steady increase in BCT. We wish to report our changing practice pattern of BCT utilization, clinico pathologic features, 5-year survival, local control, and cosmetic results.

Material & Method: Between 1993 and 1998 our multidisciplinary group evaluated 263 women with Stage I & Stage II breast cancer. Cases were prospectively discussed in a multidisciplinary tumor conference. Women were encouraged to make a choice based on treatment recommendation and their personal preference. 155 women (61%) chose BCT, and 99 (39%) chose mastectomy. Median age, age range and age <50 for BCT and mastectomy group were 56, 29-90, 32% and 62, 31-88, 25% respectively.

Women undergoing BCT were subjected to re-excision (28%) when margins were positive. Residual tumor was noted in 28 %. 15 women with T1a and T1b tumors were treated without axillary node sampling. Level I & II axillary node sampling was performed in 140 women. Women needing mastectomy were subjected to standard modified radical mastectomy. Radiation therapy was administered to all except 2 patients. Breast was treated to 5040 Cgy with 6mv Linear accelerator. In 140 (92%) women the tumor bed was boosted with electron to a total dose of 6300 Cgy. Regional nodal radiation was used in all with positive nodes and those who did not have axillary node sampling. Systemic adjuvant therapy consisted of Chemotherapy alone 13% , Chemotherapy & Tamoxifen 20% , or Tamoxifen alone 43% in BCT group. Mastectomy patients received Chemotherapy alone in 19%, Chemotherapy & Tamoxifen in 18% and Tamoxifen alone in 43%.

Results: Patients were followed in the oncology clinics and by referring physicians. All patients were tracked through Tumor Registry. 9 patients were lost for follow-up. Local recurrence was documented in 4 patients undergoing BCT. 3 patients in the mastectomy group developed chest wall recurrence. When the multidisciplinary program was introduced in 1993 only 27% underwent BCT. Mastectomy was performed in 73%. This practice pattern gradually changed. In 1999, BCT was used in 90% of women and mastectomy only in 10%. Five-year survival results for BCT and Mastectomy are outlined in Table 1.

Table 1.

	Stage I	Stage II	Stage II, Node +	Stage II, Node -
BCT (%)	93	85	83	87
Mastectomy (%)	94	80	75	85

Conclusion: In a small community hospital with multidisciplinary team approach we have optimized the utilization to have achieved local control and 5 year survival results that are comparable to the published results from the randomized trials. We will report detailed clinical and pathological features, 5-year survival and cosmetic results.

THE COMPASS TREATMENT, A NEW ERA OF TREATMENT IN BREAST CANCER NEOADJUVANT THERAPY AND RADIATION WITHOUT SURGERY

Brutz* P., Dreisbach, P., Desert Breast Institute, Palm Desert, CA, 92260

Bacus, S., Advanced Cellular Diagnostics, Inc, Elmhurst, IL, 60126

Key Words: core biopsy, strategic analysis, neoadjuvant chemotherapy, no surgery

An understanding of the natural history of invasive breast cancer coupled with effective chemotherapy opened the door for vast improvements in the care of breast cancer patients. Often, axillary node dissection was used as the major guide in recommending adjuvant chemotherapy. Over the past decade for the purpose of neoadjuvant chemotherapy, lymph node status has been supplanted by strategic analysis. This is based on core sample, tumor grade, size, lymphatic invasion, mammographic appearance, clinical exam, family history and extensive tumor analysis. This has identified aggressive invasive tumors that are likely to have already metastasized long before the patient is diagnosed. Since 1989 we have treated 96 patients ranging in age from 28 to 83 with neoadjuvant chemotherapy based on strategic analysis following core biopsy. Tumor size ranged from 1.2 cm to over 8cm. All patients have received at least four courses of CAF. Neoadjuvant therapy has identified "responders" who showed consistent tumor ablation to the point every five years we have continued chemotherapy including at times Taxol with past four courses, if mammographic evidence pointed to total tumor eradication.

Compass Treatment Results

5/96 (5.2%) had modified radical mastectomy

84/96 (87%) had lumpectomy and radiation

7/96 (7.3%) had no surgery, only chemotherapy and radiation

32/96 (33%) had no node dissection

18/96 (18%) had sentinel node biopsy

18/96 (18%) had no tumor removed

3/96 (3.1%) local/regional recurrence, none of the above eighteen patients

89/96 (92%)* have survived, followed from 2 to 10 years**

one patient died of myocardial infarction free of cancer*

Individualized treatment at a dedicated comprehensive breast institute following strategic analysis guidelines and response evaluation accounts for the above results. Our comprehensive team is active and in place before the diagnosis is made. These results point to patients doing better at a dedicated comprehensive center. We conclude implementation of Nationwide Networked Comprehensive Breast Centers is in order to achieve optimal patient care including lowering mortality and mammography rates. For those patients with no tumor found at surgery or for those with no tumor on repeat core biopsy and having no surgery, the classic paradigm of "clear margins for radiation" comes into question. We also conclude that it is possible to effectively treat some invasive breast cancer patients without surgery.

LABORATORY ASSESSMENT OF THE STATUS OF HER-2/NEU PROTEIN AND ONCOGENE IN BREAST CANCER SPECIMENS.

Ashfaq R*, Wang S, Saboorian MH, Gokaslan ST, and Frenkel E. University of Texas Southwestern Medical Center, Dallas, Texas 75235-9073.

AIM: To evaluate clinical utility of three commercially available assays for Her-2/neu oncogene and protein levels. Her-2/neu protein is overexpressed, mostly due to gene amplification, in 20-30% of human breast cancers and shown to have prognostic and predictive values, such as for Herceptin, a new monoclonal antibody therapy in treatment of breast cancers.

METHODS: One immunohistochemistry (IHC) assay using the Dako polyclonal antibody A0485 which measures Her-2/neu protein levels were compared with two new, high sensitivity (FISH) assays, i.e., INFORM™ and Path Vysion™, in a cohort of 52 formalin-fixed and paraffin-embedded breast tissues. These tissues were randomly selected from 84 consecutive infiltrating breast cancer specimens, which were first stratified based on the Her-2/neu protein levels by IHC.

RESULTS: The two FISH assays achieved 98% concordance rate, i.e., 14 specimens (27%) with Her-2/neu gene amplification and 37 specimens (71%) without gene amplification, with the Path Vysion™ assay having certain advantages over the INFORM™ assay. In contrast, the IHC assay detected Her-2/neu overexpression in a high percentage of cases, including 13 high positive specimens (25%) and 13 medium positive specimens (25%). Although 10 of these 13 IHC high positive specimens showed gene amplification by FISH, 9 of 13 IHC medium positive specimens showed no gene amplification. Statistical analyses also suggest that the difference between IHC and FISH assays are primarily in the cases with medium positive IHC, but negative FISH results.

CONCLUSION: As the role of Her-2/neu oncogene and protein has gained increasing importance in clinical management of breast cancer patients, it is crucial to evaluate accurately and conveniently the Her-2/neu status in a clinical laboratory. This study indicates that the best approach at present time is to use the IHC assay as a triage step, followed by Path Vysion™ FISH assay to further analyze the IHC medium and high positive cases.

DOES GENETIC COUNSELING IMPACT DECISION FOR PROPHYLACTIC SURGERY IN PATIENTS PERCEIVED TO BE AT HIGH RISK FOR BREAST CANCER?

Morris KT*, Johnson N, Krasikov N, Allen, M

Oregon Health Sciences University; Legacy Cancer Services

Portland, OR 97201

This study evaluates the impact that a comprehensive genetic risk assessment program has on patients considering prophylactic surgery based on perception of high risk from family history.

Sixty patients underwent in depth family history evaluation and were given estimation of risk. Recommendations were made for and against testing. Ramifications of testing, including job and genetic discrimination, familial dynamics, and the ethical responsibility for sharing information with relatives were covered. The average age was 45 (range 20 - 83). Twenty-four women (40%) were considering prophylactic surgery believing themselves to be at high risk. Of these, 17/24 were felt to be high risk by the genetic counselors and had testing recommended. Four (16%) had a known family mutation. Five patients proceeded with prophylactic surgery based solely on high risk assessment, citing concerns over genetic privacy as reasons forgo testing. Seven patients were tested; three were positive. Two patients proceeded with mastectomy despite a negative test. One decided against mastectomy despite a positive test. In all, after counseling, prophylactic surgery was carried out in less than half the initial candidates.

Breast cancer risk estimation and genetic evaluation can be quite complex. Comprehensive genetic risk assessment programs can play a significant role in the management of patients considering prophylactic surgery for perceived high risk.

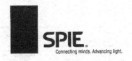

2012
Defense
Security+Sensing
23–27 April 2012

Technical Program
spie.org/dss

Location
Baltimore Convention Center
Baltimore, Maryland, USA

Conferences and Courses
23–27 April 2012

Exhibition
24–26 April 2012

spie.org/mobileapps

Conference 8354 · Room: Conv. Ctr. 302

9:50 pm: **Sportswear textiles emissivity measurement: comparison of IR thermography and emissometry techniques**, Paolo Bison, Ermanno G. Grinzato, Consiglio Nazionale delle Ricerche (Italy); Antonio Libbra, Alberto Muscio, Univ. degli Studi di Modena e Reggio Emilia (Italy) . . . . [8354-25]

Coffee Break . . . . 10:10 to 11:00 am

SESSION 6
Room: Conv. Ctr. 302 . . . . Wed. 11:00 am to 12:00 pm

Security and Surveillance

Session Chairs: Gregory R. Stockton, Stockton Infrared Thermographic Services, Inc. (USA); Andrés E. Rozlosnik, SI Termografía Infrarroja (Argentina)

11:00 am: **Real-time object detection and tracking for night vision systems based on information fusion**, Nikos Fragoulis, Christos Theoharatos, Vassilis Tsagaris, IRIDA Labs. (Greece) . . . . [8354-27]

11:20 am: **Achieving thermography with a thermal security camera using uncooled amorphous silicon microbolometer image sensors**, Yu-Wei Wang, Curtis Tesdahl, James Owens, David Dorn, Pelco by Schneider Electric (USA) . . . . [8354-28]

11:40 am: **Using aerial infrared thermography to detect utility theft of service**, Gregory R. Stockton, RecoverIR, Inc. (USA) and United Infrared, Inc. (USA) and Stockton Infrared Thermographic Services, Inc. (USA); R. Gillem Lucas, RecoverIR, Inc. (USA) . . . . [8354-29]

Lunch/Exhibition Break . . . . 12:00 to 1:00 am

SESSION 7
Room: Conv. Ctr. 302 . . . . Wed. 1:00 to 2:50 pm

Biological Applications

Session Chairs: Morteza Safai, The Boeing Co. (USA); Piotr Pregowski, Pregowski Infrared Services (Poland)

1:00 pm: **Development and validation of experimental models for hyperemic thermal response using IR imaging**, Eulalia Moreno, Boston Univ. (USA); Jose Benjamin Giron Palomares, Sheng-Jen Hsieh, Texas A&M Univ. (USA) . . [8354-30]

1:20 pm: **Breast cancer in tough economic times, new paradigms emerging** *(Invited Paper)*, Phillip Bretz, Desert Breast and Osteoporosis Institute (USA) and Desert Breast Foundation (USA); Richard Lynch, Desert Breast and Osteoporosis Institute (USA) . . . . [8354-31]

1:50 pm: **Investigation of thermal effects caused by interaction of laser radiation with soft tissues**, Mariusz Kastek, Andrzej Zając, Henryk Polakowski, Tadeusz Piatkowski, Jan Kasprzak, Military Univ. of Technology (Poland)[8354-33]

2:10 pm: **Human and detection in the thermal infrared spectrum**, Ayman A. Abaza, West Virginia High Technology Consortium Foundation (USA); Thirimachos Bourlai, West Virginia Univ. (USA) . . . . [8354-34]

2:30 pm: **Infrared imaging for prediction of chicken embryo developmental stages**, Rebecca A. Frederick, Tulane Univ. (USA); Sheng-Jen Hsieh, Jose Benjamin Giron Palomares, Texas A&M Univ. (USA) . . . . [8354-35]

SESSION 8
Room: Conv. Ctr. 302 . . . . Wed. 2:50 to 3:30 pm

Research and Development Topics I

Session Chairs: Ralph B. Dinwiddie, Oak Ridge National Lab. (USA); Gary L. Orlove, FLIR Systems, Inc. (USA)

2:50 pm: **Accurate thermal imaging of low-emissivity surfaces using approximate blackbody cavities**, Fiona Turner, Stuart Metcalfe, Jon Willmott, Peter Drögmöller, Land Instruments International (United Kingdom) . . . . [8354-37]

3:10 pm: **Microscale thermal analysis with cooled and uncooled infrared cameras**, Junko Morikawa, Tokyo Institute of Technology (Japan); Eita Hayakawa, ai-Phase Co., Ltd. (Japan); Toshimasa Hashimoto, Tokyo Institute of Technology (Japan) . . . . [8354-38]

Thursday 26 April

SESSION 9
Room: Conv. Ctr. 302 . . . . Thurs. 8:00 to 9:50 am

Research and Development Topics II

Session Chairs: Ralph B. Dinwiddie, Oak Ridge National Lab. (USA); Gary L. Orlove, FLIR Systems, Inc. (USA)

8:00 am: **On the thermal-offset in NIR hyperspectral cameras**, Francisca I. Parra, Jorge E. Pezoa, Pablo F. Meza, Sergio N. Torres, Univ. de Concepción (Chile) . . . . [8354-39]

8:30 am: **Variable filter array spectrometer of VPD PbSe**, Rodrigo Linares-Herrero, German Vergara, Teresa Montojo, Raul Gutierrez, Carlos Fernandez-Montojo, Arturo Baldasano, New Infrared Technologies, Ltd. (Spain) . . . [8354-40]

8:50 am: **Radiance and atmosphere propagation-based method for the target range estimation**, Hoonkyung Cho, Joohwan Chun, KAIST (Korea, Republic of) . . . . [8354-42]

9:10 am: **Spatial concentration distribution model for short-range continuous gas leakage of small amount**, Meirong Wang, Lingxue Wang, Jiakun Li, Yunting Long, Yue Gao, Beijing Institute of Technology (China) . . . . [8354-43]

9:30 am: **Gas imaging detectivity model combining leakeage spot size and range**, Jiakun Li, Lingxue Wang, Meirong Wang, Yue Gao, Tingfa Xu, Beijing Institute of Technology (China) . . . . [8354-44]

POSTERS–THURSDAY
Room: Conv. Ctr. Hall A . . . . Thurs. 6:00 to 7:30 pm

All symposium attendees are invited to attend the poster sessions. Come view the high-quality papers that are presented in this alternative format, and interact with the poster author who will be available for discussion. Enjoy light refreshments while networking with colleagues in your field. Attendees are required to wear their conference registration badges to the poster sessions.

Authors may set-up their posters between 10:00 am and 5:00 pm the day of their poster. Posters that are not set-up by the 5:00 pm cut-off time will be considered no-shows and their manuscripts may not be published. Poster authors should be at their papers from 6:00 pm to 7:30 pm to answer questions from attendees. All posters and other materials must be removed no later than 8:00 pm. Any papers left on the boards at the close of the poster session will be considered unwanted and will be discarded. SPIE assumes no responsibility for posters left up after the end of each poster session.

A method for infrared video mosaic based on SURF, Yunjin Chen, National Univ. of Defense Technology (China) and Graz Univ. of Technology (Austria); Ying Feng, Yu Cao, National Univ. of Defense Technology (China) . . . . . [8354-41]

This is a critique of my talk at the SPIE conference from an independent observer.

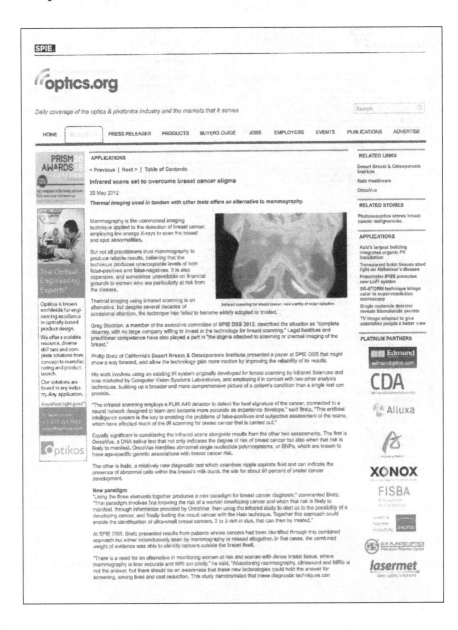

5th ANNUAL MULTIDISCIPLINARY SYMPOSIUM on BREAST DISEASE

February 13-16, 2000

Cavalieri Hilton Hotel
Rome, Italy

SYLLABUS

A PROGRAM OF

The University of Florida
Health Science Center/*Jacksonville*

CO-SPONSORED BY

Catholic University/*Rome, Italy*
and The Susan G. Komen
Breast Cancer Foundation
Dallas, Texas

IN COOPERATION WITH

The World Society for Breast Health,
The Italian Society of Medical Radiology (Senologic Section),
The Italian Society of Senology,
The University of Florida Shands Cancer Center,
and The Breast Journal

COURSE DIRECTOR
Shahla MASOOD

CO-DIRECTORS
Aurelio PICCIOCCHI
Vincenzio LATTANZIO

GENERAL SECRETARY
Riccardo MASETTI

569

Using primary chemotherapy to treat invasive breast cancer without demonstrable metastases, to identify "responders" in order to minimize or avoid surgery. *P.D. Bretz, P.B. Dreisbach, Desert Breast Institute, Rancho Mirage CA.*

An understanding of the natural history of invasive breast cancer coupled with effective chemotherapeutic drugs opened the door for vast improvements in the care of breast cancer patients. Often, auxillary lymph node dissection was used as the major guide in recommending adjuvant chemotherapy. Tumor analysis and pathology based on core sample has helped make possible the identification of invasive tumors for which primary or pre-op chemotherapy has been given. Since 1989, we have treated 55 invasive breast cancer patients ranging in age from 28 to 83 with primary chemotherapy. All patients received at least four courses of adriamycin, cyclophosphamide and 5-FU, unless tumor growth was observed. More than four cycles were given in patients who showed continued tumor dissolution. Primary chemotherapy has identified "responders" who showed consistent tumor ablation to the point of total tumor dissolution based on clinical exam, mammography and repeat core sampling. Tumor size has ranged from 1.2 cm to over 8 cm. Six patients had no demonstrable tumor at surgery. Four patients had mastectomy and forty-nine had lumpectomy. Nineteen of the forty-nine had no lymph node dissection and three did not have radiation therapy. Two patients had no demonstrable tumor after primary chemotherapy and did not have surgery. Tumor analysis was done on all patients. Tumor disappearance did not always correspond with the predicted tumor response based on the analysis. In the past three years, we have continued primary chemotherapy past four cycles if the clinical mammographic evidence pointed to total tumor eradication in the breast. For those patients with no cancer on repeat core sample the classic paradigm of "clear margins for radiation" comes into question. We have had no local recurrences, however, four deaths have been recorded excluding the patient with the 8 cm tumor. We recommend individualized treatment to obtain maximum local control including minimizing or avoiding surgery. Omitting surgery and/or radiation therapy in a subset of patients where no tumor is found should be studied.

CHAPTER 12

A PEEK AT SACRIFICING AMERICA'S WOMEN II

I HESITATED INCLUDING THESE next few pages as they are really part of the story of *Sacrificing America's Women II*, and it's a little far afield of the point of *Sacrificing America's Women I*. However, I decided to give a little teaser as to what happens to a lone wolf when you are up against the powers that be. Maybe you'll see a pattern here?

As you will read, the FDA declared that my protocol (the first-ever authored to actually prevent breast cancer with a pill) was "flawed." No problem. As you will read, the FDA actually asssigned to me my own personal doctor to make the protocol perfect in their eyes. You need to know just how unprecedented and how far outside the box my thinking was back then to propound such an idea. And I want you to see the outpouring of support from other researchers around the country praising my protocol. So, on one hand, I had wide support for my innovative protocol and on the other hand, a small band of about six (old guard advisory committee) declared my study "flawed." In my opinion, it's these types of leaps of faith studies that produce real results. As you will come to know, while I received a lot of push back from all corners, the fact is that when the study was finally done after being ursurped from me, Tamoxifen reduced the risk of breast cancer by 45-50% in high-risk women. Then that trial was followed up with the Study of Tamoxifen and Raloxifene (STAR) trial, and Evista also reduced breast cancer risk by 45-50%, while at the same time, helping prevent osteoporosis. As a consequence of that, women in effect get a double hit off of Evista reducing breast cancer risk and helping prevent osteoporosis. All that started with me, while every other researcher in the country wasn't seeing the opportunity, or they were afraid of ridicule and putting an end to career advancement for these adacemic researchers who can't really step out of line or one-up their superiors.

At DBI I didn't have a boss so when I wanted to do something, I just did it forthwith, like I wrote the original prevention trial in one day and sent it into the FDA. That's how you get things done; but that kind of opportunity is closed off (which is problemic of our system) to most researchers. First, we'll read the FDA advisory committee's recommendation that my trial was "flawed." I must say, though, the FDA itself always treated me with diginity and acted swiftly, working with me to refine the protocol. It was the outside people (old guard researchers) that voted against. In fact, after the open hearing, the FDA contacted me and said I could still do my trial, I just needed the money.

By the time the open FDA hearing came up, we had been to the USSR and Washington multiple times and I began to call my team, "SHOWTIME." That was the name given the the LA Lakers basketball team when they were winning championships. All this happend in about six months from the time I submitted the first draft. That in itself was pretty unheard of, making the government move off the dime, as it were. After my study was rejected, it took the NSABP many months to get their version through. More time wasted.

Later on, when the Director of Cancer Prevention of the National Cancer Institute was forced to appear in Dr. Frank Young's office (Deputy Director of US Department of Health and Human Services (HHS)), I was told that the proposed study with the Soviets was just too big a vision. What the hell? Unbridled bold vision in my opinion is what is needed to beat breast cancer.

We'll start with the opening page of the FDA open hearing stating that the sponsor (usually a major institution or group like NSABP or Eastern Cooperative Oncology Group (ECOG)) was just me. While the story in *Sacrificing America's Women II* encompasses a wide adventerous tale from the US to the USSR, to the White House and FDA, here I'll just present the opening page and then the FDA advisory committee and then to the support letters from major people. Like I said, maybe you'll see a pattern that goes against the true American spirit. At one point in this adventure, our study was called "first and dirty" by the head of one of the major groups who just didn't think of it ahead of me or was caught up in a quagmire of bureaucracy that functionaries developed and couldn't get it done. We'll just be scratching the surface of this American adventure here. That's my IND 34,223 below.

```
                              AGENDA
            FDA ONCOLOGY DRUGS ADVISORY COMMITTEE MEETING
                      CROWN PLAZA HOLIDAY INN
               1750 ROCKVILLE PIKE, ROCKVILLE, MD.
                         JUNE 29, 1990

                        ALL SESSIONS OPEN


    IND·34223    Proposal For " A Clinical Trial To
                 Determine The Worth Of Tamoxifen In The
                 Prevention Of Breast Cancer "


    SPONSOR      Phillip D. Bretz, M.D.
                 Desert Breast Institute
                 Rancho Mirage, Calif.



    Speakers Should Time Their Presentations To Allow 10
    Minutes Of Questions And Discussion After The Presentation


    800-810AM    Announcements                   Dr. Hascall
                                                 Executive Sec.


    810-845AM    ICI Pharm. Presentation         Dr. Patterson
                 Animal Carcinogenicity Studies  Dr. Topham
                 Second Tumors In Adjuvant       Dr. Plourde
                 Clinical Trials                 ICI Pharm.
                 Clinical Side Effects
                 Eye Effects


    845-920AM    Rationale. Results Of Pilot     Dr. Love
                 Study At U. Wisc., Mad.         U. Wisc., Mad.


    920-950AM    Results Of Pilot Study.         Dr. Powles
                 Status Of Prevention Study      Royal Marsden H.
                 In The U.K.                     London, U.K.


    950-1005AM   BREAK


    1005-1045AM  Proposed Breast Cancer          Dr. Bretz
                 Prevention Study                Desert Breast
                                                 Institute
```

Food and Drug Administration
Rockville, MD 20857

IND 34,223   Date   JAN 1 9 1990

Phillip Bretz, M.D.
39000 Bob HoperDrive, Suite C
Rancho Mirage, California 92270

Dear Sir or Madam:

We acknowledge receipt of your Investigational New Drug Application (IND) submitted pursuant to Section 505(i) of the Federal Food, Drug, and Cosmetic Act. Please note the following identifying data:

     IND Number Assigned: **34,223**

     Sponsor: Phillip Bretz, M.D.

     Name of Drug: Tamoxifen

     Date of Submission: January 12, 1990

     Date of Receipt: January 16, 1990

Studies in humans may not be initiated until 30 days after the date of receipt shown above. If, within the 30-day waiting period, we identify deficiencies in the IND that require correction before human studies begin or that require restriction of human studies until correction, we will notify you immediately that the study may not be initiated ("clinical hold") or that certain restrictions must be placed on it. In the event of such notification, you must continue to withhold, or to restrict, such studies until you have submitted material to correct the deficiencies, and we have notified you that the material you submitted is satisfactory.

It has not been our policy to object to a sponsor, upon receipt of this acknowledgement letter, either obtaining supplies of the investigational drug or shipping it to investigators listed in the IND. However, if drug is shipped to investigators, they should be reminded that studies may not begin under the IND until 30 days after the IND receipt date or later if the IND is placed on clinical hold.

LOS ANGELES TIMES   SATURDAY, JUNE 30, 1990

Panel Objects to Proposed Study of Breast Cancer Drug

■ Health: The project would have involved 20,000 U.S. and Soviet women. Backers plan to redesign it and seek approval again.

By MARLENE CIMONS
TIMES STAFF WRITER L-30-1990

WASHINGTON—A federal advisory panel recommended Friday that the Food and Drug Administration reject a proposal to undertake a ground-breaking U.S.-Soviet study of 20,000 women to determine whether a hormonal drug can prevent breast cancer.

The FDA's Oncology Drugs Advisory Committee agreed that a long-term study should be conducted to determine the effect of the hormonal drug tamoxifen in preventing breast cancer and other cancers in healthy women.

But the panel said that its members had concluded that the design of the proposed 10-year, $100-million study of women in the United States and the Soviet Union was flawed. The committee said that it would recommend ways to correct the deficiencies.

"I'm disappointed for the women of the country," said Phillip D. Bretz, director of the Desert Breast Institute in Rancho Mirage and one of the proposed study's backers. "I felt it was time to do it. None of these answers are going to be resolved until this study is done."

Although the recommendation of an FDA advisory committee is not binding, it typically wields considerable weight in agency decision-making. The FDA must approve the U.S. segment of the study before it can begin.

The committee said there was insufficient information on how the study would be conducted, including recruitment of patients and handling of data. Some members also expressed concern that the volunteers would not be at high enough risk for breast cancer.

Bretz, however, said that the study was rejected because he did not have the academic ties of traditional researchers. He said that he would revise his study proposal in an effort to satisfy the committee's demands.

The proposed study, endorsed by American and Soviet cancer specialists in March, would involve administration of tamoxifen, an anti-estrogen drug already widely used in post-surgical breast cancer therapy, to women considered at high risk for breast cancer.

It would be the first large-scale study undertaken jointly in the United States and Soviet Union, its sponsors said. The pool of participants, about 10,000 from each country, would consist primarily of daughters, sisters or mothers of women who have had breast cancer and who are considered at high risk of developing the disease themselves. Half of the women would be given a medically worthless placebo for comparison purposes.

The researchers had predicted a 25% reduction in the incidence of breast cancer among the women who were given the drug.

The study would be coordinated by Bretz; Dr. Philip B. Dreisbach, of the Eisenhower Medical Center in Rancho Mirage, and Dr. David Zaridze, deputy director of the All-Union Cancer Research Institute in Moscow.

The study was opposed by some women's health advocacy groups, who said it is dangerous to experiment with drugs on healthy women.

"This is a drug that is not risk-free," said Cindy Pearson, program director of the National Women's Health Network. "It's a fine drug for a breast cancer patient—a woman facing the possibility of death is more than willing to take a drug that has some risk. But to jump from a drug that's effective in a group with a life-threatening disease to a huge trial in healthy women is crazy."

But Dr. Wendy Schain, a psychologist with Memorial Cancer Institute in Long Beach and a former breast cancer patient, recommended approval of the study. "This is the best we've got," she said. "We need to get these answers. We have no better way to get them."

Tamoxifen causes cancer in animals and has been linked to stroke, heart disease and endometrial cancer in women, according to the FDA. Sponsors of the proposed study, however, maintain that tamoxifen has minimal negative side effects and often reduces cholesterol and eases cardiovascular problems.

FDA officials said that a large study of a drug in healthy women was "a little unusual," but not unprecedented. "Any time you do a study on a drug for prophylaxis [prevention], you're going to use

healthy people," said Dr. Robert Temple, the FDA's director of new drug evaluation.

Tamoxifen, manufactured by the British firm Imperial Chemical Industries and sold under the brand name Nolvadex, has been used for more than a decade to prevent the recurrence of tumors in women whose cancer had spread to the underarm lymph nodes.

Recently, the FDA approved its use in the post-surgical treatment of early breast cancer in women who do not have node involvement. In this country, it is produced and marketed by ICI Pharmaceuticals of Wilmington, Del.

Tamoxifen works by blocking so-called estrogen receptors—areas on the surface of cells to which the hormone binds to exert its effects. In that way, it blocks the effects of estrogen, which is believed to play a role in the stimulation of tumor growth in breast cancer.

Breast cancer is the most common malignancy among women in the United States and the second leading cause of cancer death among women, after lung cancer. An estimated 150,000 new cases will be diagnosed this year.

May 9, 1990

Phil D. Bretz, M.D.
39-800 Bob Hope Drive
Suite C
Rancho Mirage, CA 92270

Dear Phil:

I enjoyed visiting with you about your interesting tomoxifen project. Linda Cadigan
and I are both very interested in helping you to move this forward.   There are many
ways that we can assist in increasing awareness both now and if the study is carried
out.

It would be so helpful to so many women to fund significant data supported answers to
the important questions you have posed.

It is imperative that the breast cancer research community accept this project as a
credible one. We cannot have another diet FIT on our hands. Both the players in the
United States and the Soviet Union must have the ability to carry out the work
accurately and well. It will be showcased and the eyes and the opinions of the
experts will be upon us.

I hope you will continue to keep us informed and let us know when you need our help.
We will be happy to attend the FDA hearing. Please give us the details and of course,
as I said to you, we would also be willing to work with you on your site visits.

We hope you will meet with success as you venture forth.

Sincerely,

Nancy Brinker   *Linda R. Cadigan*

Nancy Brinker   Linda R. Cadigan
Founding Chairman   President

NB/LRC:ecr

cc: Dr. Bernard Fisher
     Dr. Sam Broder

Now let's look at the letters of support (again just a spattering) I received from National Cancer Institute appointed Principal Investigators AFTER they had received my protocol. So, either everyone of these investigators was delelect in their support of my protocol, or what? Yes, what went on here? I ask this question a lot, don't I?

DAYTON CLINICAL ONCOLOGY PROGRAM

3525 Southern Boulevard □ Kettering, Ohio 45429 □ 513-299-7204

June 21, 1990

Phillip D. Bretz, M.D.
Desert Breast Institute
39-800 Bob Hope Drive
Suite C
Rancho Merage, CA   92270

Dear Dr. Bretz:

We at the Dayton CCOP have reviewed your proposed protocol and find some very exciting ideas and objectives that are well worth the effort to carry out. As a CCOP whose funding is provided by N.C.I., we would be most interested in having Cancer Control credits assigned to this protocol, thereby helping us meet one of our objectives.

Our CCOP is a consortium of eight hospitals, covering our entire region of southwestern Ohio. We have over 5,000 newly diagnosed cancer cases yearly and have exceeded our cancer control objectives the past two years.

After talking with the Principal Investigator of our CCOP, Howard M. Gross, M.D., we both feel that this is a much needed study, not only to answer the question posed regarding breast cancer, but also as it covers many areas related to the current health issues of American women.

Please let us know if we can help in anyway.

Sincerely,

Nancy G. Hines R.N., B.S.

Nancy A. Hines, R.N., B.S.
Executive Director

The Regional Cancer Center
Memorial Medical Center

J. Gale Katterhagen, M.D.   Research Division   Cancer Data System
Executive Director   Administrative Direct   788-2544   (217) 788-3580
(217) 788-4055   788-4054

Sent via FAX 6-8-90

June 8, 1990

Phillip D. Bretz, M.D.
Project Chairman
Desert Breast Institute
39-800 Bob Hope Drive, Suite C
Rancho Mirage, California 92270

Dear Dr. Bretz:

Thank you for your letter of May 25 concerning the breast
cancer prevention project using Tamoxifen.

We have reviewed the protocol and other materials you kindly
provided, and we would like to indicate to you our support.

We find this a very interesting study with possible
significant ramifications in the area of chemo prevention.

Again, we are extremely interested. Please, at your earliest
convenience, either call or write with further information.

With best regards,

Edward L. Braud, M.D.   J. Gale Katterhagen, M.D.
Co-Principal Investigator   Principal Investigator
Central Illinois CCOP   Central Illinois CCOP

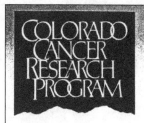

Colorado Cancer Research Program, Inc. · 3955 East Exposition · Suite 104 · Denver, CO 80206 · (303) 777-2663

June 13, 1990

Phillip Brétz, M.D.
39-800 Bob Hope Drive, #C
Rancho Mirage, CA 92270

Dear Doctor Brétz:

Thank you for your letter of June 8, 1990

The Colorado Cancer Research Program would be very interested in participating in the Tamoxifen breast cancer prevention trial. We are currently six participating hospitals as indicated on our letter-head. We may well have more in the future.

Certainly, all indications are that this should prove to be a fruitful investigation which we would be happy to help you do.

Yours truly,

Robert F. Berris, M.D.
Principal Investigator

/sb

ALTON OCHSNER
MEDICAL FOUNDATION
1516 Jefferson Highway
New Orleans, Louisiana 70121
Phone: 504/838-3000
Cable Address: OCHSCLINIC

June 6, 1990

Phillip D. Bertz, M.D.
Desert Press Institute
39-800 Bob Hope Dr.
Suite C
Rancho Mariage, CA 92270

Dear Dr. Bertz:

I have had the opportunity to review DBI protocol #B-1 entitled "A Clinical Trial to Determine the Worth of Tamoxifen in the Prevention of Breast Cancer." This is a very important study, particularly since it appears that Tamoxifen may be of value in the prevention of breast cancer in high risk individuals. A major chemo prevention trial such as this one should confirm the efficacy of Tamoxifen. It should also confirm Tamoxifen's possible protective effect in cardiovascular disease as well as osteoporosis.

The Ochsner Community Clinical Oncology Program would be interested in participating in this study once the study has been approved by the FDA and by the National Cancer Institute for CCOP credit.

Unfortunately, I will be unable to attend the June 29 meeting when the protocol is presented to the FDA. We sincerely hope this review goes well and look forward to working with you on this study in the future.

Sincerely,

Carl G. Kardinal, M.D.
Principal Investigator
Ochsner CCOP

PETER W. WRIGHT, M.D.
Oncology
Hematology
Internal Medicine

June 14, 1990

Phillip D. Bretz, M.D.
Desert Breast Institute
39-800 Bob Hope Dr, Suite C
Rancho Mirage, CA 92270

Dear Dr. Bretz:

Thank you for sending me a copy of your proposed breast cancer prevention trial, "A Clinical Trial to Determine the Worth of Tamoxifen in the Prevention of Breast Cancer" (DBI protocol #B-1).

The study is of great interest to me. Your protocol appears to be thoroughly researched and carefully drafted. I would be happy to support it.

I am currently principal investigator for the NSABP in the Seattle area and a member of the Breast Committee of the Puget Sound Oncology Consortium (PSOC).

It is my intention to submit the protocol for approval to the Human Subjects Review Committee at the Fred Hutchinson Cancer Research Center, the University of Washington, and it's affiliated hospitals in the Seattle area.

If this can be accomplished, then I would anticipate a broad interest and hopefully a broad participation among oncologists in the Pacific Northwest.

Please keep me advised of the status of your IND approval process.

Sincerely,

PETER W. WRIGHT, M.D.

kht/4392

c: Phillip D. Dreisbach, M.D.

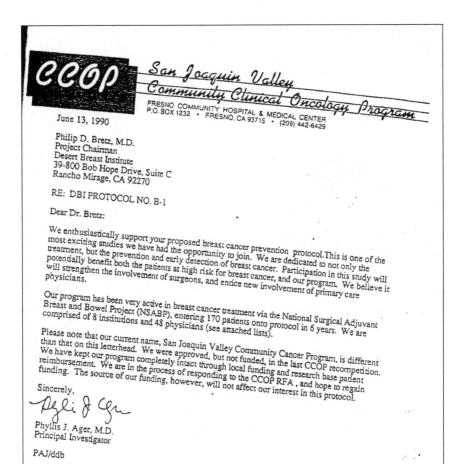

CCOP   *San Joaquin Valley Community Clinical Oncology Program*

FRESNO COMMUNITY HOSPITAL & MEDICAL CENTER
P.O. BOX 1232 • FRESNO, CA 93715 • (209) 442-6429

June 13, 1990

Philip D. Bretz, M.D.
Project Chairman
Desert Breast Institute
39-800 Bob Hope Drive, Suite C
Rancho Mirage, CA 92270

RE: DBI PROTOCOL NO. B-1

Dear Dr. Bretz:

We enthusiastically support your proposed breast cancer prevention protocol. This is one of the most exciting studies we have had the opportunity to join. We are dedicated to not only the treatment, but the prevention and early detection of breast cancer. Participation in this study will potentially benefit both the patients at high risk for breast cancer, and our program. We believe it will strengthen the involvement of surgeons, and entice new involvement of primary care physicians.

Our program has been very active in breast cancer treatment via the National Surgical Adjuvant Breast and Bowel Project (NSABP), entering 170 patients onto protocol in 6 years. We are comprised of 8 institutions and 48 physicians (see attached lists).

Please note that our current name, San Joaquin Valley Community Cancer Program, is different than that on this letterhead. We were approved, but not funded, in the last CCOP recompetition. We have kept our program completely intact through local funding and research base patient reimbursement. We are in the process of responding to the CCOP RFA, and hope to regain funding. The source of our funding, however, will not affect our interest in this protocol.

Sincerely,

Phyllis J. Ager, M.D.
Principal Investigator

PAJ/ddb

enc:

I read this letter from the CCOP twice. Wow. And, I quote, "This is one of the most exciting studies we have had the opportunity to join. We believe it will strengthen the involvement of surgeons, and entice new involvement of primary care physicians." These people really got it. As I envisioned, my protocol would reach out to all groups including the OB/GYN and primary care.

I knew if the edict came down from a surgeon looking down his nose at people telling them what to do, this concept was going nowhere and would waste $68 million. Even in 2021, if you're a woman with a first-degree relative with breast cancer and you're post-menopausal, (there are at least two FDA-approved drugs now to reduce the risk by 45-50%) ask yourself this: Has my primary care physician or OB/GYN ever broached the subject of active prevention with Tamoxifen or Evista? If the answer is no, then my premise years ago turned out to be right, that in spite of the positive results of the breast cancer prevention trial, it would not reach women like I intended. And if you are a high-risk woman and you develop breast cancer and your doctor hasn't discussed active prevention, that is negligence at this point. With approval letters like these, how could the FDA advisory panel say my protocol was "flawed?" Easy, Dr. Jordan had a saying, there were two kinds of people in research, those pissing on the tent and those pissing out of the tent. It was better to be in the tent. Apparently, I was never in the tent.

When reading these letters from all over the world like Sofia, Bulgaria, I knew I had done something really neat that would change things on a global level. It's hard to come up with global change. It's the same feeling I got during the first Lavender Procedure when I realized that if I can help cure breast cancer with these methods (finding small cancers before they can spread), and kill them in the office in about twenty minutes (patients resume normal activity immediately), this method would also change things globally for all women. I still have that feeling, in spite of any verdict by the Medical Board.

Now there's only two things in play here. One is the FDA advisory panel rejected my study because in truth it was somehow flawed or there was something else afoot. Let's look at two things totally ignored which never surfaced. One is the FDA itself made sure my protocol was exactly in line with what they wanted by assigning Dr. Justice to help me revise it multiple times. So, for the advisory panel to find "flaws," they found "flaws" within the FDA itself. In other words, I just didn't type out something helter-skelter in my garage and send it in. Second, you have had a chance (above) to read the letters of support from just a spattering of those I received. The folks at Dayton found my protocol to be, "very exciting ideas and objectives that are well worth the effort to carry out." And from Dr. Peter Wright (himself, a principal investigator with the NSABP), he says, "The study is of great interest to me. Your protocol appears to be thoroughly researched and CAREFULLY crafted." So, either all these clinical trial investigators (who had seen many protocols over the years), are all wrong about the merits of my revolutionary protocol and can't interpret protocols well (but all these people carry a Principal Investigator number given by the National Cancer Institute just like me), or the NCI had given incompetent people an investigator number? I hardly think so, do you?

Or again, there was something else going on. Was the fix in? The fix of getting rid of me and usurping my protocol to the NSABP To my way of thinking, all Bernie had to do (Bernard Fisher, MD, at the time Director of the NSABP) to cast an endearing light on himself was to say, "Look what my boys did!" I was a Principal Investigator with the NSABP then. But no, there was a move behind closed doors to push me out and garner the accolades and money themselves. If they had let me participate in the trial when their protocol came out many months after mine was ready to go, I could have lived with that, since the protocol would be moving forward and it was my idea. I moved this country toward prevention when no one else had the vision. They were all trying to play catch-up.

But they excluded me from participating. You can draw your own conclusions. This entire matter is dealt with meticulously in *Sacrificing America's Women II*. They could make a movie about all this. Let's continue with this "peek" into *Sacrificing America's Women II*.

Going back to the initial sending of my protocol to the FDA, remember I actually typed that thing out in one day. It took learned people at the NSABP months to get their version straight (after mine was rejected), and somehow many of the safety factors were magically removed in theirs. How's that? The FDA insisted on those very safety factors in my protocol. Back when we were working on the revisions, Dr. V. Craig Jordan flew out from the University of Wisconsin (where he was at the time). He is, without a doubt, the world's authority on Tamoxifen. He advised us on many things to make my protocol as good as it should be. I owe him a debt of gratitude for that. When the

NSABP's protocol came out with much hoopla, a number of the safety factors were removed and no one ever fessed up. Even with Dr. Jordan's help dissecting my protocol ten ways from Sunday, it was going to cost $100 million USD. The protocol from the NSABP called for only $68 MILLION and I wondered why, until I was relayed a copy and the safety factors, especially the uterine biopsies, were out. So, they were just trying to save money you say? The so-what is, if memory serves, two women died on that trial of uterine cancer. Could those deaths have been avoided? And if the safety factor of uterine biopsies were removed including appropriate follow-up and people knew before the trial was launched, there might be a problem without including these biopsies and people died possibly because of that exclusion, is that a problem?

Among other things, that's why there was a Congressional Hearing into malfeasance. I had met with Dennis Ross at the White House at their invitation (achieved through Congressman Dornan) and we discussed these problems with him and called for a halt to the trial until such time as these issues were dealt with and women were safe who enrolled. Going back to the start, I waited for the reply from the FDA after sending the initial draft of my protocol. When it came (you saw the IND) the FDA assigned me my own doctor advisor to help refine the protocol into exactly what the FDA had in mind, like many of the safeguards that, until my protocol came along, were not necessary, but necessary now to ensure safety of otherwise healthy women. In fact, they said my initial protocol was "globally deficient." No problem, I thought, let's get it right, but let's get it done. This is all detailed in *Sacrificing America's Women II.*

In any case, we went through about four revisions including such safeguards as "UTERINE BIOPSIES," as we wanted to make sure we weren't substituting one cancer for another. Another one was an ophthalmology check by an ophthalmologist (MD) of each participant's eyes BEFORE they entered the trial and yearly after and as often as necessary. We were concerned about possible cataracts developing. Every time we included safety checks like those, it raised the cost of the trial substantially. If you were going to have each woman undergo a uterine biopsy to exclude them having an occult uterine cancer upon entering the trial, and yearly checks after for 16,000-20,000 participants over a more than ten-year period, the added cost was $10 million. That was true of the eye, heart and other issues. That was all fine with me and I felt just added to the credibility of the protocol. But something happened to all this behind closed doors.

Let's look at some newspaper clippings of these events. Oh hell, let's look at the front pages of my protocol and the protocol of the NSABP. See any similarities? Yes, the NSABP had a copy of my protocol before the June open hearing when we met Bernie at the annual meeting. You'll have to read the whole story.

DBI PROTOCOL NO. B-1

A CLINICAL TRIAL TO DETERMINE THE WORTH OF TAMOXIFEN
IN THE PREVENTION OF BREAST CANCER

FROM: DESERT BREAST INSTITUTE OPERATIONS OFFICE
         39800 Bob Hope Drive
         Rancho Mirage, CA 92270
         619-568-3414

DIRECTOR OF CLINICAL AFFAIRS

Phillip D. Bretz, M.D.

CO-DIRECTORS OF CLINICAL AFFAIRS

Douglas A. Bacon, M.D.
Philip B. Dreisbach, M.D.
Edward H. Gilbert, M.D.
Susan L. B. Groshen, Ph.D.
Adeline J. Hackett, Ph.D.
David B. Kaminsky, M.D.
John M. Kells
Malcolm C. Pike, Ph.D.
Linda F. Roger, R.N.
Wendy Schain, Ph.D.

DRAFT *CONFIDENTIAL*

NSABP PROTOCOL P-1

A CLINICAL TRIAL TO DETERMINE THE WORTH OF TAMOXIFEN
FOR PREVENTING BREAST CANCER

NATIONAL SURGICAL ADJUVANT BREAST AND BOWEL PROJECT (NSABP)

OPERATIONS CENTER
Room 914 Scaife Hall
University of Pittsburgh
3550 Terrace Street
Pittsburgh, PA 15261

TELEPHONE: 412-648-9720
FAX: 412-648-1912

BIOSTATISTICAL CENTER
230 McKee Place
Suite 600
Pittsburgh, PA 15213

TELEPHONE: 412-624-2666
FAX: 412-624-1082

NSABP Chairman: Bernard Fisher, M.D.
Director, NSABP Biostatistical Center: Carol K. Redmond, Sc.D.

Version as of January 24, 1992 (PLEASE DESTROY ALL OTHER VERSIONS)

Read the titles of the two protocols. Do they sound similar? Is there a name for that, it escapes me?

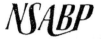

NATIONAL SURGICAL ADJUVANT
BREAST AND BOWEL PROJECT

3550 Terrace Street • Room 914
Pittsburgh, PA 15261
412/648-9720
FAX 412/648-1912

Bernard Fisher, M.D.
Chairman

OPERATIONS OFFICE
Bernard Fisher, M.D.
Director
Norman Wolmark, M.D.
Deputy Director, Medical
D. Lawrence Wickerham, M.D.
Deputy Director, Administration
Joan C. Dash, M.A.
Assistant Dir., Fiscal Affairs
Mary Ketner, R.N.
Assistant Dir., Clinical Affairs

August 7, 1991

Phillip D. Bretz, M.D.
Founder-Director
Desert Breast Institute
39-800 Bob Hope Drive, Suite 3
Rancho Mirage, CA 92270

Dear Phil:

Please accept my apology for not replying sooner to your inquiry about your possible participation in the NSABP Breast Cancer Prevention Trial. At the time I received your letter, I did not yet have all the information necessary to formulate a response.

Much, if not most, of the interest that has been generated regarding the implementation of a prevention trial came from your groundbreaking efforts, and I think you are to be commended for what you have attempted to do.

During the last year we have been actively engaged in the development of what I hope will be considered an appropriate study. We have not yet received final approval, but we are hoping to do so in the near future.

We will soon be sending out an RFA, and I hope your proposal will be acceptable to the selection committee. They will be interested primarily in those institutions that are willing to make a commitment to NSABP activities in general, as well as to the prevention trial. For further procedural information, please call Gladys Hurst at (412) 648-2066 or, for medical information, Mary Ketner at (412) 648-9597.

I hope you will keep in touch with me and that, from time to time, we may discuss further our mutual interest in this endeavor.

Sincerely,

Bernard Fisher, M.D.

BF:gdh

NSABP

NATIONAL SURGICAL ADJUVANT
BREAST AND BOWEL PROJECT

3550 Terrace Street · Room 914
Pittsburgh, PA 15261
412/648-9720
FAX 412/648-1912

Bernard Fisher, M.D.
Chairman

OPERATIONS OFFICE
Bernard Fisher, M.D.
Director
Norman Wolmark, M.D.
Deputy Director, Medical
O. Lawrence Wickerham, M.D.
Deputy Director, Administration
Joan C. Oash, M.A.
Assistant Dir., Fiscal Affairs
Mary Ketner, R.N.
Assistant Dir., Clinical Affairs

December 11, 1991

Phillip Bretz, M.D.
Eisenhower Medical Center
39000 Bob Hope Drive
Rancho Mirage, CA 92270

Dear Dr. Bretz:

The Steering Committee of the NSABP Breast Cancer Prevention Trial (BCPT) regrets to inform you that your center's proposal has not been selected for participation at this time. The NSABP received 182 proposals, but logistical constraints and funding restrictions necessitated that the number of approved centers be limited. Every proposal underwent three independent reviews; each reviewer scored the proposals in the areas of prior experiences, personnel, resources and recruitment, compliance and data management plans. Results were reviewed and approved by the BCPT Steering Committee.

The NSABP will keep your proposal on file. In the event that, individually or collectively, the selected centers cannot meet the recruitment goals of the trial, your proposal will be reconsidered. If you so desire, additional information regarding the review results can be made available through written request to: Mrs. Gladys Hurst, NSABP, 3550 Terrace Street, Room 914, Pittsburgh, PA 15261.

I hope that this decision will not affect your participation in other NSABP trials. We consider you to be a valuable member and in the future will do whatever possible to ensure your involvement.

Sincerely,

Bernard Fisher, M.D.
Chair of BCPT Steering Committee

BF/tro

These two letters came from Bernard Fisher, MD, then the Director of the NSABP. Read the second paragraph of the first letter. I was to be commended for what I had done. Then, read the next letter after we filled out their multi-page form to be a designated center. He at least scratched Phillip and hand-wrote Phil. Do you find it a little strange that I was a member in good standing of the NSABP, that I'm totally

excluded from even participating having thought the trial up? There
was something very wrong going on here.

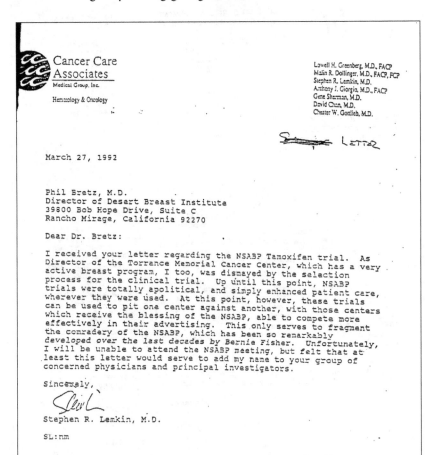

Cancer Care
Associates
Medical Group, Inc.

Hematology & Oncology

Lowell H. Greenberg, M.D., FACP
Malin R. Dollinger, M.D., FACP, FCP
Stephen R. Lemkin, M.D.
Anthony J. Giorgio, M.D., FACP
Gene Sherman, M.D.
David Chen, M.D.
Chester W. Gottlieb, M.D.

March 27, 1992

Phil Bretz, M.D.
Director of Desert Breast Institute
39800 Bob Hope Drive, Suite C
Rancho Mirage, California 92270

Dear Dr. Bretz:

I received your letter regarding the NSABP Tamoxifen trial. As
Director of the Torrance Memorial Cancer Center, which has a very
active breast program, I too, was dismayed by the selection
process for the clinical trial. Up until this point, NSABP
trials were totally apolitical, and simply enhanced patient care,
wherever they were used. At this point, however, these trials
can be used to pit one center against another, with those centers
which receive the blessing of the NSABP, able to compete more
effectively in their advertising. This only serves to fragment
the comradery of the NSABP, which has been so remarkably
developed over the last decades by Bernie Fisher. Unfortunately,
I will be unable to attend the NSABP meeting, but felt that at
least this letter would serve to add my name to your group of
concerned physicians and principal investigators.

Sincerely,

Stephen R. Lemkin, M.D.

SL:nm

Eisenhower and DBI were rejected because, I guess, we just didn't
measure up. I called Bernie. I told him I joined the NSABP because it
was pure science, but his treatment of me was pure bullshit. He said
something like *I'll look into it*, but never heard another word from him.
On reading the above letter from Dr. Lemkin, you'll see that he was
"dismayed" at the selection process the NSABP used for the prevention
trial. In the past, if you were a member, all the protocols were open to
you. Now, as Dr. Lemkin points out, this process only served to pit one

center against another. To wit: if there are two research centers in the same city and center (A) has the magic pill (Tamoxifen) and center (B) doesn't, what center are you going to go to? And this was for about a six-to-ten-year period where one center would have a leg up. It wasn't only that, but I'm sure Dr. Lemkin would have been VERY interested to learn after years of hard work for the NSABP, the NSABP allowed centers who weren't a member to do the trial. I think I stopped counting at six. Were they friends of Bernie's? Just what kind of shenanigans went on here? Oh, one last item to put the frosting on their cake having successfully disposed of me. Check out the chest pounding, like they thought it up, pure horseshit. And no one in the press picked up on my earlier efforts like the piece in the *LA Times*.

Friday, March 1, 1991   NCU   The San Diego Union   A-7

High hopes expressed for breast cancer drug

Study of its role in prevention is announced here

By Leigh Fenly
Staff Writer

An upcoming study using the synthetic hormone tamoxifen may show a 50 percent reduction in the incidence of breast cancer and a substantial decrease in coronary heart disease among post-menopausal women, according to researchers involved in the project.

The major nationwide breast cancer prevention trial, announced in San Diego this week, will include 16,000 post-menopausal women at high risk for breast cancer and will take five years to complete.

Researchers are also hopeful the study will show that tamoxifen has a role in preventing the bone disease osteoporosis, a bone-thinning condi-

tion common among post-menopausal women.

Funded by the National Cancer Institute (NCI), the study will be directed by the National Surgical Adjuvant Breast and Bowel Project (NSABP), a national cooperative of oncologists and nurses based in Pittsburgh.

"Some of us are already calling this the placebo vs. panacea trial," NSABP director Dr. Bernard Fisher said at the group's semiannual meeting here this week. Fisher declined to be interviewed.

In Bethesda, Md., NCI officials would not discuss the cost of the trial, although earlier estimates for such a study reached about $65 million.

Participants in the study will be recruited beginning this fall, at about 70 as yet undetermined cancer centers throughout the country.

NSABP has not completely determined what it considers "high risk."

See Cancer on Page A-7

I hope you can feel my level of frustration, disappointment, and how incredulous this whole thing was. The story is more involved with twists and turns that I detail in *Sacrificing America's Women II*. I also hope you can imagine the level of commitment I had and have for all women and the energy it took to get this prevention thing done, and, oh by the way, try and make the world a little safer by working with the Soviets. For some people in charge as you recall, that vision was just too big.

Going back before the FDA open hearing, my team and I went to the NSABP annual meeting. In those days Bernie was at the height of his career and about to get higher with my (unacknowledged) help. He was not really accessible to the nearly 1,000 minions in attendance. The only time you really saw him was during his presentation on stage. But we concocted a plan to intercept him as he had to make a showing at the party Imperial Chemical Industry (ICI), now Astra-Zeneca, threw. Once we confronted him, I introduced myself and said I didn't know if he knew what I was trying to do (you bet he did).

But his words were exactly (in his southern brawl), "I don't think it's time to do a prevention trial and besides what do you think I am, an entrepreneur?" He was handed the protocol. Only two things could have happened after with the NSABP having my protocol (basically revamped by the FDA themselves with Dr. Justice's help): (A) Somebody at the NSABP looked at my protocol and dismissed it as garbage, shredded it and they decided to do their own from scratch. Or (B) they went over it with a fine-tooth comb and used it to construct their own. Did Bernie actually read it? I have no idea but it would seem to me likely. It proved more likely when the FDA advisory committee voted the United States should do the $100 million prevention trial but in the next vote, cut me out totally. That meant I had got a major body of the government to approve my idea but now there was no one to carry it out. So, it was $100 million up for grabs. What should have happened was the NSABP or like group should have immediately stepped forward and said here is our protocol ready to go. For that matter, I should have received a letter (when I first sent in my protocol) from the FDA that they appreciate my wanting to do a prevention trial but they already have a protocol from whatever research group. There was nothing from anybody. Nothing from any major group or the NCI. I wasn't getting paid to know where this country was with breast cancer research or where it needed to be ten years from now. Remember, I thought of doing the prevention trial immediately after reviewing the NSABP protocols and there was nothing on prevention, just slash-poison-burn as Dr. Raza would put it. Check out the fax I received from the NSABP I received it not because of who I was (the originator of the idea) but because I was a member in good standing. This is after Bernie told me in person, it wasn't time to do a prevention trial.

BY:XEROX TELECOPIER 7010 : 8-12-14   7:55AM ;412 648 1912   #1401;# 1
JUL 16 '90 10:49   FROM NSABP HQDRS-PITT   PAGE.001

NATIONAL SURGICAL ADJUVANT PROJECT
FOR BREAST AND BOWEL CANCERS

OPERATIONS OFFICE
3550 Terrace Street • Room 914
Pittsburgh, Pennsylvania 15261
412/648-9720   FAX: 412/648-1912

Bernard Fisher, M.D.
Project Chairman

BIOSTATISTICAL CENTER
230 McKee Place • Suite 600
Pittsburgh, Pennsylvania 15213
412/624-2666 FAX: 412/624-1082

Carol Redmond, Sc.D.
Director, Biostatistical Center

DATE: July 16, 1990

ORGANIZATION NAME: _ELSENHOWER MED CNTR_

FAX NO.: _619 773 1286_

ATTENTION: _PHILIP BRETZ, MD_

SENDER: DR. BERNARD FISHER
                                    (2 pages)

IMPORTANT MESSAGE! URGENT REPLY REQUESTED!

The NSABP is planning a double-blinded
clinical trial of tamoxifen vs. placebo
(similar in concept, design and conduct
to Protocol B-14) for the prevention of
breast cancer in a normal and/or high-
risk population of post-menopausal women.

Your urgent (preferably within one day)
response to the enclosed survey will enable us to proceed with plans. Your responses will be considered approximate,
confidential and non-binding.

I would be interested in any other comments
you might have regarding this matter. If
you have questions regarding the planned
study, please contact Mr. Walter Cronin
at 412/624-2666 or Dr. Lawrence Wickerham
at 412/648-9720.

When I got that fax from the NSABP about how I should respond in twenty-four hours, what the hell was that? Bernie himself said just a few months prior it wasn't time to do a prevention project. Don't kid yourself, the midnight oil was burning at the NSABP to get a prevention protocol out there and get the money. I'd actually like to know if the NCI reviewed any protocols from any other group (like ECOG in Wisconsin), or was that fix in also? The cabal won out. I would think Bernie would have used all his clout. I would have loved to be a fly on the wall at the NSABP during those times.

Then later on, to be told by the Director of Cancer Prevention of the NCI when he had to appear at the HHS, when I had the Deputy Director of HHS (Frank Young) and two congressmen with me and others, that my vision of working with the Soviets was just too big. Wow, who appoints these people who remain in charge for decades? The vision necessary to defeat cancer needs to extend beyond our galaxy to the next. Or did anyone have any vision or did they just want another Cold War and billions spent on military weaponry to kill everyone on Earth ten times over? Further, what the Director of Cancer Prevention of the NCI said when I said at the HHS meeting loud enough for everyone in the room to hear (he was seated right next to me), was unbelievable and disheartening. I said, "Do you understand that all the money we are spending on clinical trials is not translating into optimal patient care?" Without a moment's hesitation he replied, "Phil, that's not my problem, it's my job to do sound scientific trials and it's your job to go to the library and read the results." And these are the people you pay with your tax dollars who are in charge for decades on end, good luck.

After you read these clippings, we will move away from *Sacrificing America's Women II*. I just wanted to give you an inkling of what is in store revelation-wise in *Sacrificing America's Women II*. There seems to be a hidden agenda for me everywhere I turn. And I'm only trying to help. Below is a photo of our first meeting at the Soviet Embassy on January 7, 1990. That's me talking to Yevgeniy G. Kutovoy, the Minister of the Embassy. Next to him is Terry McNight, our attorney (RIP), and Dr. David Kaminsky, partially cut off.

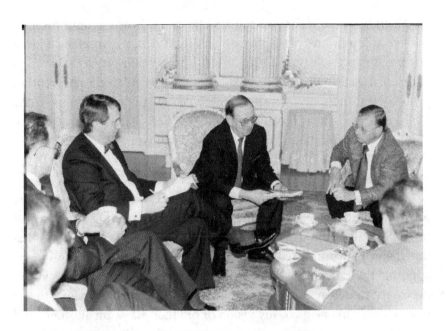

Here is the face sheet of our presentation to the Soviets.

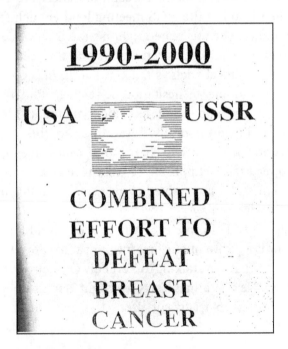

JOHN T. MYERS
7TH DISTRICT, INDIANA

OFFICES:
2372 RAYBURN BUILDING
WASHINGTON, DC 20515
TELEPHONE: 202-225-5805

107 FEDERAL BUILDING
TERRE HAUTE, IN 47808
TELEPHONE: 812-238-1619

107 HALLECK BUILDING
LAFAYETTE, IN 47901
TELEPHONE: 317-423-1661

Congress of the United States
House of Representatives
Washington, DC 20515

June 28, 1990

COMMITTEE ON APPROPRIATIONS

RANKING MINORITY MEMBER,
SUBCOMMITTEE ON ENERGY AND
WATER DEVELOPMENT

SUBCOMMITTEE ON AGRICULTURE
AND RURAL DEVELOPMENT

COMMITTEE ON POST OFFICE
AND CIVIL SERVICE

RANKING MINORITY MEMBER,
SUBCOMMITTEE ON COMPENSATION
AND EMPLOYEE BENEFITS

COMMITTEE ON STANDARDS
OF OFFICIAL CONDUCT

RANKING MINORITY MEMBER

Dr. John Johnson
Oncology Drug Products
Food and Drug Administration
5600 Fishers Lane
Rockville, Maryland 20857

Dear Dr. Johnson:

I am writing in support of the proposed Breast Cancer Prevention
Study (Women's Health Trial) which is under review by the Food
and Drug Administration.

Since January of this year when my wife was diagnosed with breast
cancer, I have become quite familiar with breast cancer care in
this country. My wife is currently being treated with tamoxifen
which will be used with the Breast Cancer Prevention Study and I
am convinced a study of this magnitude is what is needed to
advance a cure.

With one out of ten American women expected to be diagnosed with
breast cancer this year, it is critical that additional research
methods be explored. I have personally reviewed and discussed
the proposed Breast Cancer Prevention Study with other Members of
Congress and we feel the time is right to proceed with such a
project.

Sincerely,

John Myers

John Myers

JTM:sd

Here is an article of a Soviet doctor visiting us and saying that it's a good thing that we are starting to work together. Alas, that dream would not happen because that vision was too big.

Soviet, valley scientists praise joint cancer project

By SHELLEE NUNLEY
The Desert Sun

RANCHO MIRAGE — A U.S.-Soviet study that would allow women to take an experimental hormone believed to prevent breast cancer is likely to get federal approval this month, said a desert breast surgeon.

Dr. Phillip Bretz, director of the Desert Breast Institute, said the $100 million, 10-year study would be the most ambitious medical venture ever shared between the two nations.

Involving about 15,000 women from each country, the study would test the ability of tamoxifen, an anti-estrogen drug, to prevent breast cancer in high-risk but healthy women.

Bretz said one out of 10 American women gets breast cancer, which causes 44,000 deaths a year.

Dr. Boris Chivashvily, a breast surgeon from Moscow who will be involved in the study, said the incidence in the Soviet Union is unknown but it's the most common type of cancer among women.

He said, if approved, the study would later include women heavily exposed to radiation in the 1986 Chernobyl nuclear accident.

Chivashvily expressed gratitude for political changes that made the joint project possible.

"Five years ago, it was impossible. It seems to me only the beginning of this process," said Chivashvily, who is in the Coachella Valley visiting members of the research team, all affiliated with Eisenhower Medical Center but working independently on the study.

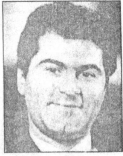

BORIS CHIVASHVILY
Hopes to help Chernobyl victims

Bretz said the U.S. Food and Drug Administration has until Friday to respond to the medical team's latest application.

Though the drug has been used to inhibit the return of breast cancer in women who've already had surgery, it has never been used to prevent the first incidence of cancer.

"This is the first time in over 40 years that anyone at the FDA has dared to utter the P word — prevention," Bretz said.

Other local experts involved in the project are oncologist Dr. Philip Dreisbach, pathologists Dr. David Kaminsky and Dr. Douglas Bacon, radiation oncologist Dr. Edward Gilbert, and Linda Roger, president of the Southwest Institute of Clinical Research in Rancho Mirage.

The study team visited the Soviet Union last winter.

TUESDAY, December 4, 1990

Just a quick story: We were in Moscow the night their first McDonald's opened up. It was a driving blizzard, yet probably more than 1,000 people lined up. They had four armed Soviet soldiers at the entrance controlling things. They let about fifty people in at one time and there was a whole bank of cash registers. We stood in line for a taste of home. Upon entering, it smelled just like home. I ordered a Big Macski (ha). At the time it was probably the largest McDonald's and they had different rooms dedicated to different countries with murals on the walls. I had my Raiders jacket on and a big video camera. No one would look at me. There was a guy who had bought three sundaes, chocolate, strawberry, and butterscotch, and he was just watching them melt. He had never seen one. A lady came by and said she was a teacher and had to talk quick because the KGB was there and didn't want anyone speaking to Americans. She asked me if I would tell my President that their children had no food and no shoes. I said I would. Below is the menu from the Moscow McDonald's.

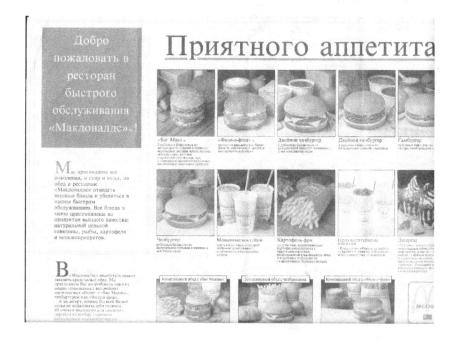

The following invitation was a cool reception we attended. It's where I met Luis Sullivan, then Director of HHS. It probably cemented in my mind the idea of running for Congress, which I did in 1994. I learned quickly that in those hallowed halls of Congress and behind closed doors was where everything was put into motion.

I also realized that in all these Congressional Hearings, no matter how passionate the speaker is, they all know that when the hearing is over that person has to get back on a plane and go home and things settle back down to normal. But as a Congressman I could have been in their faces every day until I got things straightened out about how to diagnose and treat breast cancer. I tried. It's a shame how people running for any public office are just crucified for some statement they made twenty years ago. Ask yourself if you would want your dirty laundry aired before the public? I would run again if there was a ground swell.

06/15/1990 16:30   FACSIMILE WASH. USA.   202 347 5028   P.01

DR Phillip Bretz, M.D.
Director, Desert Breast Institute
39-800 Bob Hope Dr Suite C
Rancho Mirage, CA 92270
Fax: 619-773-4867

June 15, 1990

Dear Dr. Bretz:

On the occasion of the Tenth Session of the USSR-US. Joint Health Committee The Minister of Health of the USSR request the pleasure of your and your wife company at a reception on Monday, the eighteenth of June from six until eight o'clock.

Soviet Embassy
1125 16th street N.W. Washington D.C.

Phone (202) 347-5028

ALEXANDER A. SOKHIN, M.D., PH.D.
Counselor in Medicine of the Soviet Embassy

URGENT!

I can't finish this small peek at *Sacrificing America's Women II* without acknowledging both Bob (RIP) and Pearl Estes. Without their help paving the way to the Soviets, the entire USSR adventure would never have taken place. It was a once in a lifetime experience that we were all privileged to be part of, thanks to them. G-D only knows how many women have been spared breast cancer because of my team and I bringing the Soviets Tamoxifen for prevention.

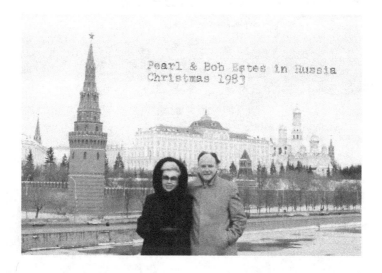

Me outside the Soviet Embassy in Washington

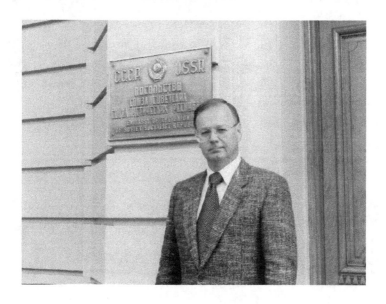

The Desert Sun

WEDNESDAY, June 27, 1990
Keith Carter, Managing Editor/N

VALLEY

Inside:
Across the valley/A4,5
On the record/A5
News from back home/A11 **A3**

Doctor touts breast cancer drug

Valley surgeon takes tamoxifen to FDA Friday

By KELLE RUSSELL
Staff writer

RANCHO MIRAGE — Dr. Phillip Bretz wants to put himself out of business.

Bretz, a breast cancer surgeon, believes women at risk for breast cancer should be given an experimental drug, tamoxifen, that may prevent the disease.

That would eliminate the need for radiation, chemotherapy and surgery.

"Breast cancer surgeons and mastectomies are on the way out," said Bretz, director of the Desert Breast Institute.

Breast cancer study at a glance

This is how the study would work:

■ Women thought to be most likely to develop breast cancer would be given tamoxifen and then closely monitored by breast cancer specialists to see whether the drug could be used in preventative treatment. The treatment involves two tablets a day.

■ The patients, about 10,000 each from the Soviet Union and

the United States, primarily would be daughters, sisters and mothers of women who have had breast cancer and thus are regarded as the most likely to develop cancer themselves.

■ Soviet women who were exposed to large amounts of radiation after the Chernobyl nuclear accident in 1986 would be included in the study, with the hope of preventing breast cancer among them.

Bretz will present his case for tamoxifen at a U.S. Food and Drug Administration hearing Friday in Rockville, Md.

FDA officials are expected to decide if Bretz can use the anti-estro-

gen drug in a landmark 10-year, $100 million study of 20,000 women in the Soviet Union and United States.

In March, Soviet and American

"Breast cancer surgeons and mastectomies are on the way out."

Phillip Bretz
Desert Breast Institute

cancer specialists signed an agreement for the study, the first undertaken on such a large scale between the two countries.

The project will be coordinated in the United States by Bretz and Dr. Phillip Strausberg of Eisenhower Medical Center.

Currently there is no drug that prevents breast cancer, which

strikes one out of 10 American women.

Tamoxifen, which is manufactured by the British firm Imperial Chemical Industries has been used with considerable success for 11 years in the post-surgical treatment of breast cancer patients to prevent a recurrence. Bretz said tamoxifen is a wonder drug because it also reduces heart disease, prevents osteoporosis — a disease that causes brittle bones — and has minimal negative side effects.

"In the study we want to find out if the drug prevents breast cancer and if it lowers deaths from heart disease," Bretz said.

The study's $100 million cost will be financed with grants from the United States and Soviet governments and by pharmaceutical companies.

Breast cancer surgeon

The Desert Sun
Staff writer 7-3-1990

RANCHO MIRAGE — Dr. Phillip Bretz remains optimistic about carrying out his ground-breaking U.S.-Soviet study of 14,000 women to determine whether a hormonal treatment can prevent breast cancer.

A federal advisory panel recommended last week that the Food and Drug Administration reject his proposal because of several flaws,

including how the study would be conducted and funded.

But the Rancho Mirage breast cancer surgeon said he plans to redesign and resubmit the study.

"Now I am going to talk to my Capitol Hill sources to get money and support," said Bretz, director of the Desert Breast Institute.

Bretz said his study was rejected because he did not have the academic ties of traditional researchers.

still pushing drug study

"I'm very proud of this. If I don't get to do this, fine. But we paved the way for others."

Bretz contends tamoxifen can prevent cancer in women, thus eliminating the need of radiation, chemotherapy and surgery.

In England, tamoxifen, an anti-estrogen drug, has been used with considerable success for 11 years in the post-surgical treatment of breast cancer patients to prevent a recurrence.

In March, Soviet and American cancer specialists signed an agreement for Bretz's study, the first undertaken on such a large scale between the two countries.

Participants for the study would be daughters, sisters and mothers of women who have had breast cancer and thus are regarded as the most likely to develop cancer themselves.

Currently, no drug prevents breast cancer.

As I said, we just touched the surface of the adventure that was dealing with the Soviets. It was cool, James Bond-style for sure. And you know what I found out? As I said, the real people of the Soviet Union and, for that matter, China really liked gringos. Maybe it's an important lesson for our senior diplomats. Don't start the conversation by saying you must relinquish your nuclear arms. Start it by engaging them on a subject you know to be important to them, like "breasts." Works every time.

Here is an article from *The Washington Post*. My prevention protocol would have solved the issue. My question is, who reads stuff like this and who does anything about it??

The Washington Pos

TUESDAY, JUNE 19, 1990

Study: NIH Slow to Include Women in Disease Research

By Susan Okie
Washington Post Staff Writer

The National Institutes of Health has made little progress in carrying out a four-year-old policy to include more women in government-funded studies of diseases and their treatments, according to a study by the General Accounting Office described at a congressional hearing yesterday.

Although an NIH memorandum acknowledged last year that underrepresentation of women in such research has caused "significant gaps" in medical knowledge, the agency has been slow and inconsistent in its efforts to get researchers to include more women in studies, said Mark V. Nadel, the GAO's associate director for national and public health issues.

"This is not a question of legal access or affirmative action. It is a question of health and well-being," said Rep. Henry A. Waxman (D-Calif.), chairman of the House Energy and Commerce subcommittee on health and the environment.

For example, a 1988 study of 22,000 male physicians, funded by the National Heart, Lung and Blood Institute (NHLBI), found that aspirin could prevent heart attacks in men. Doctors subsequently recommended that older men at increased risk for heart disease take an aspirin every other day but specifically said they could not offer women the same advice. Heart disease is the leading cause of death in both sexes.

"If heart disease studies use data solely on men, should women take an aspirin a day?" Waxman asked. The question cannot be answered authoritatively yet.

William F. Raub, acting director of the NIH, said in an interview the "vast majority" of NIH studies include adequate numbers of women and are in compliance with the policy. He said the GAO study had uncovered procedural problems within the agency, and that the NIH would follow the GAO's recommendations to correct those problems.

"I don't believe the NIH system is grossly out of focus," he said. "We do need to do some fine tuning."

The NIH, which pays for most U.S. medical research, first stated in October 1986 that it would encourage greater inclusion of women in studies, but it did not issue guidelines on the new policy for its officials until last July.

The GAO found variations among the NIH's various research institutes in how the policy is interpreted. A booklet sent to applicants makes no mention of the policy. The NIH has no central mechanism for counting the number of women or minority members included in its studies, and NIH officials have not encouraged researchers to analyze findings to reveal gender-related differences, according to the GAO study.

Raub said that in studies of diseases that occur more frequently in men, such as heart disease, researchers must often decide between doing an all-male study in order to get a quicker answer or doing a larger, slower study that includes both sexes in order to get results that can be applied to both.

Listen, I struggled a long time with the issue of detailing my experience with the NSABP, especially since Dr. Fisher is no longer with us (RIP) and, therefore, unable to respond. They might legitimately ask why I waited so long to publish what I did about the Tamoxifen trial. The answer is I was content to let it go since I had been to the White House and there was nowhere else to go. I was content with just letting the story lie, as it turns out, for decades.

However, with the advent of my demise in medicine and wanting to relay my story to my grandchildren, the Tamoxifen thing was a big deal and a significant part of my history. I think I am honest in presenting only the facts as they played out. I wish Bernie was alive to comment on whatever. Yeah, so it troubles me that I have to put to pen something said to me and the person has passed away. The quotes from Bernie came from yet unpublished Sacrificing America's Women II. That was written accurately as events occurred back in 1989 and 1990.

CHAPTER 13

THE CARNEGIE MEDAL STORY, BLIND LUCK OR DIVINE INTERVENTION?

CARNEGIE HERO FUND COMMISSION

2307 Oliver Building
535 Smithfield Street
Pittsburgh, Pennsylvania
15222-2394
(412) 281-1302

News Release

FOR RELEASE   Contact: Walter F. Rutkowski
JULY 1, 1993   1-800-447-8900

CARNEGIE HERO FUND COMMISSION
CITES 20 FOR EXTRAORDINARY HEROISM

PITTSBURGH, PA, JULY 1, 1993--In its third award announcement of 1993, the Carnegie Hero Fund Commission today named 20 individuals from throughout the United States and Canada as recipients of the Carnegie Medal. The medal is given to civilians who risk their lives to an extraordinary degree while saving or attempting to save the lives of others. Four of the awardees lost their lives in their heroic endeavors.

The heroes announced today bring to 49 the number of awards made to date in 1993, and to 7,744 the total number since the Pittsburgh-based Fund's inception in 1904.

Commission President Robert W. Off stated that each of the awardees or their survivors will receive also a grant of $2,500. Throughout the 89 years since the Fund was established by industrialist-philanthropist Andrew Carnegie, $20.3 million has been given in one-time grants, including scholarship aid and death benefits, and continuing assistance. The awardees:

Lisa Marie Griffith	West Liberty, Iowa
Theodore Griffith	West Liberty, Iowa
William H. Hopkins	Battle Creek, Mich.
Eric Jacob Ratke	Peoria, Ariz.
Joel F. Dubé	Methuen, Mass.
Larry DuBoise	Winslow, Ariz.
Paul Macsuga	Mississauga, Ont.
Salvatore J. Ciambrone	Pompano Beach, Fla.
James A. Whitley, deceased	Lilburn, Ga.
Heather Ann Stewart	Westlock, Alta.
Paul Edward Crawford	Antioch, Ill.
Joe Wayne Wheeldon	Lansing, Mich.
Phillip DeEvans Bretz	Bermuda Dunes, Calif.
Daniel Schneider	Kamloops, B.C.
Robert P. Cotter	Romulus, Mich.
Sue L. Brewer	Waterbury, Conn.
Jean-Yves Bernard	Lanesville, N.Y.
Chad L. Schneider, deceased	Streator, Ill.
Clinton Carl Quaka, deceased	Streator, Ill.
Kevin J. Shriel, deceased	Chestertown, N.Y.

Resumes of the acts follow.

To nominate someone for the Carnegie Medal, write the Carnegie Hero Fund Commission, 2307 Oliver Building, Pittsburgh, PA 15222, or call (toll free) 1-800-447-8900. The Commission's annual report is available to the public.

93-3

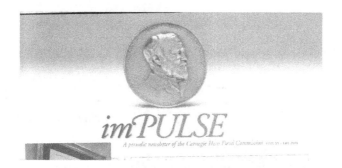

Carnegie Hero Fund Commission
Pittsburgh, Pennsylvania

This certifies that

PHILLIP DEEVANS BRETZ
has been awarded a Carnegie Medal
in recognition of an outstanding act of heroism:

Phillip DeEvans Bretz helped to rescue Frederick A. Garbutt from burning, Anza, California, August 14, 1992. Garbutt, 28, was trapped in the wreckage of his sport-utility vehicle, which had overturned and caught fire in a highway accident. Driving upon the scene within moments, Bretz, 46, surgeon, stopped and ran to Garbutt's vehicle, where he heard Garbutt scream that he was on fire. Bretz went to the rear of the vehicle, which lay on its passenger side, and entered through the broken-out window of its rear door. He attempted to remove Garbutt, but Garbutt was restrained by his safety belt. Bretz shouted to the others who had arrived that he needed a knife, and a police officer handed him one through the rear window. With flames growing inside the vehicle, Bretz returned to Garbutt, whose seat was aflame, and cut the safety belt, freeing Garbutt. Bretz dragged Garbutt to the rear window, where others helped to pull him out of the vehicle. Bretz and another man dragged Garbutt across the street shortly before the vehicle was engulfed in flame. Garbutt was hospitalized five weeks for third-degree burns and other severe injuries.

President   *Secretary*

COMMANDING GENERAL
MARINE CORPS AIR GROUND COMBAT CENTER
BOX 788100
TWENTYNINE PALMS, CALIFORNIA 92278-8100

July 19, 1993

Dear Doctor Bretz,

I was pleased to learn of your recent heroic actions when you risked your own life to save another from a burning vehicle. You are to be commended and congratulated for your bravery.

The Carnegie Medal is indeed a prestigious award. It is indicative of the example you have set for others to follow. Too often we hear of people in need of assistance who are passed by because no one came forward to help. Your actions are proof that even in today's society, there are people who care.

On behalf of the Marines, Sailors and civilians aboard the Combat Center, I salute you for your selfless action and concern for human life.

Sincerely,

R. H. SUTTON
Brigadier General, U.S. Marine Corps

Mr. Philip Bretz, M.D.
Naval Hospital

DEPARTMENT OF THE NAVY
NAVAL HOSPITAL
TWENTYNINE PALMS, CALIFORNIA 92278-5006

IN REPLY REFER TO:
1650
Code 060
30 Jul 93

From: Commanding Officer
To: Dr. Phillip D. Bretz, 318-26-0556

Subj: LETTER OF APPRECIATION

Encl: (1) CG MCAGCC ltr of 19 Jul 93

1. Enclosure (1) is delivered with my personal congratulations on being awarded the Carnegie Medal. You should be justly proud of your actions, and I am proud to say you are a member of my hospital team.

C. S. CHITWOOD

Copy to:

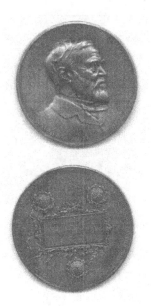

Qalifornia Ḥighwaȝ Patrol

CERTIFICATE OF COMMENDATION

IS PRESENTED

TO

DR. PHILLIP BRETZ

FOR

COMMUNITY SERVICE

This award is presented in recognition of your exemplary actions on August 14, 1992, when you stopped and rendered aid to Mr. Frederick Garbutt, who had been involved in a head-on collision. You acted quickly, entering a burning vehicle with complete disregard for your own safety in order to free Mr. Garbutt. Your high degree of concern and compassion for your fellow man undoubtedly helped save the victim's life.

done at Sacramento this 7th day of October this year

of our Lord one thousand nine hundred and ninety-two.

M. J. Ha~~ Commissioner, DEPARTMENT OF CALIFORNIA HIGHWAY PATROL

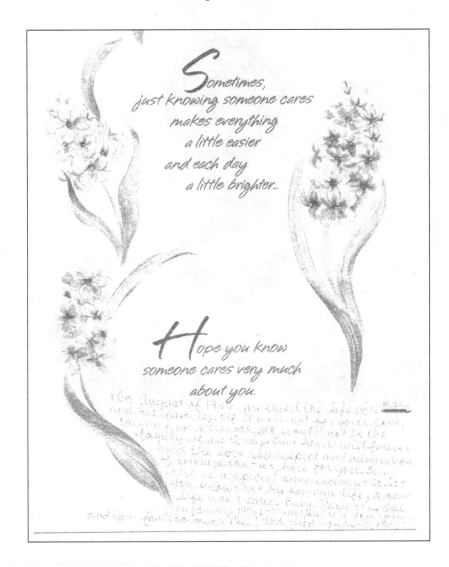

STRANGE LUCK OR DIVINE INTERVENTION?

It was January 1996 and I just watched a TV report hailing actor Mark Harman as a hero for rescuing two teenagers from a burning vehicle. They said he ran out of his house and before help arrived, he knocked the window of the burning vehicle in and pulled the two boys to safety. One of them while hanging upside down trapped by the seatbelt sustained third degree burns and was in critical condition but survived. During the broadcast by Dave Clark of Channel 9 (KCAL) in Los Angeles, he showed the tree the vehicle hit and it was charred black.

I paused for a moment and then as I had done a thousand times before, my thoughts went back to August 14th, 1992 when I myself was in the exact same position of rescuing a young man trapped inside an upside down burning Blazer S-10. He likewise was trapped by the seatbelt. Unknown to me at the time, as he lay there trapped and on fire, he was thinking, "Oh G-d, I'm going to die the same way my father did." Let's go back to the beginning of the story. While my story is not unique as shown by Mark Harman's story, there are only a relatively few, perhaps a few thousand in the world who have ever been confronted with the type of situation presented here.

At the time, my family and I lived in Rancho Mirage, Calif. My older daughter Ashley had been invited to visit a school girlfriend who had moved to La Jolla. The girl's family offered to meet us halfway in a town called Temecula. Going toward San Diego we would drive up Route 74 to 371 and head toward Temecula. Route 74 is otherwise famous since the film "It's a Mad Mad Mad Mad World," was shot there. It is a treacherous winding dangerous road climbing from sea level at the desert floor to about 5,500ft at the top of the San Jacinto mountain community of Idyllwild.

The family decided that after dropping Ashley off with her friends we would continue on to visit Wild Animal Park near San Diego. Before we started up the mountain, the answering service called and one of my patients, also a friend was having some urgent medical problem and needed to see me, I am a general surgeon. So everyone waited until I took care of my friend and then we were off up Route 74. This first episode delayed us about an hour. It was the first in a series of strange events that would ultimately bring me, CHP officer Durate and the accident together at the exact moment in history to intervene and save a life.

It's always great going up the mountain, as the air becomes noticeably cooler. The trip up was uneventful and we turned toward San Diego unto Route 371. At that particular intersection there is a rustic country restaurant now called the Paradise Cafe. Tamecula is another forty minutes winding along the countryside. We pulled into Carl's Jr. where we met Ashley's friend and her family. Since we hadn't seen them for some time, we decided to have lunch with them instead of just dropping Ashley off and then we would continue on to San Diego Wild Animal Park. This was the second event that was unplanned but figured critically into the plot of the day. By the time we finished lunch we had been delayed enough for us to say good-by to Ashley and the Corsinita's and head back down the mountain. It was approaching 2pm and we figured we could come back tomorrow to visit Wild Animal Park.

So back down we went. The third unscheduled event unfolded as we approached the Paradise Cafe, my youngest son Christian who was 11 years old at the time began persistently begging for some water. He had had a milkshake at Carl's Jr. and was decidedly thirsty. His insistence was convincing and so we pulled into the Paradise Cafe for him to get a drink of water and for the rest of us to have ice cream.

There were some scattered low clouds with a little rain slowly going by. We were watching those clouds cooling off the area and enjoying our ice cream when a CHP officer pulled a vehicle over for speeding. This occurred right in front of us and as we all do I thought, "better him than me." This was the fourth in the series of unplanned events. Without the CHP officer stopping that motorist for speeding, he would have probably been almost to Idyllwild and nowhere near the scene of the accident that was to come sooner than we all knew. As it turned out, we and the officer finished just at the same time and as I was preparing to pull out of the restaurant parking lot the CHP officer was preparing to go back down the mountain in the same direction as I needed to go. I thought the heck with this, I'm not going to have the CHP following me all the way down to Palm Desert, and so I let him go by. I waited a minute or so, giving him plenty of time to get away from me and then I pulled out. Well, wouldn't you know it, there he was about three-quarters of a mile down pulled off to the side of the road, like he was waiting for me to go by. I thought what the heck is this? He was pulled over just before the first sharp turn down from the restaurant. As it turns out he was probably trying to catch speeders coming around the turn from the other direction. As we approached, a car had just come around the turn and had stopped right by the officer and was apparently talking to him. I slowed down but went right through and around the corner and head long into the surrealistic scene of the accident. I put on the brakes the instant I realized what had occurred. Looking off to the left I saw a Chevy Blazer S-10 upside down on a little embankment and smoke was coming from the front of the vehicle. There was a man standing by it and I figured he must have been the driver. He had a little blood coming from his mouth but looked to be ok. Further down the road about twenty yards or so, there was another vehicle, a jeep pick-up kind of turned in the middle of the road.

There were a few people beginning to gather down the road a little. No one was behind me. I looked at my wife and said "Don't worry I'm not going any place and I'm sure (to use bad English), ain't going out to announce I'm a trauma surgeon." Everyone concerned seemed at first blush to be ok. I'm sure she was thinking if I got out and identified myself, that we'd be stuck there doing doctor stuff. We were about thirty feet or so from the Blazer. My daughter Alexandra (four at the time), came up in front with us. Christian couldn't believe his eyes as the story unfolded and was waiting for something to happen, he didn't have long to wait. The CHP officer came up right behind me and he was using his radio to call for help. As he walked by me he had a fire extinguisher with him. I thought he would just walk up and put out the fire, ascertain everyone was ok, re-route traffic and we would be on our way in short order. I had put down my window so I could hear, and as the CHP officer walked by and toward the man standing by the Blazer, the man started saying in a distressed tone, there was someone trapped in the Blazer that was on fire.

I turned to my wife and said, "Oh hell I have to go now." She nodded and with that I got out and walked toward the Blazer. As I approached some things were going through my mind. If I identified myself as a physician and trained trauma surgeon at that, I would be taking on a lot of liability. Would I get blamed if this guy was paralyzed? Since the Blazer was on fire and upside down, our natural inclination was to right it and get this guy out. I yelled into the Blazer, "Are you OK, can you move everything?" From inside came the words I didn't want to hear. "I can move, but I'm on fire!" Three of us were up by the Blazer on the passenger side. By now, you could see the fire was for real. I said let's get the thing right side up so we could get the trapped man out. We pushed it off the little embankment and it landed on its side with the driver's side up.

Immediately the CHP officer tried to put out the fire with his extinguisher. I looked at this effort and realized in a heartbeat it would be futile. I looked around and by this time there were a couple of other guys standing nearby, but I realized no one was going inside the burning vehicle to get this guy out. I thought to myself, "You have to go in there and just do it, that's why you're here." I walked around the back and just as I was about to go in, I had this thought, that Jesus wasn't going to let me die that day.

My dad was killed when I was twelve and if the guy in the Blazer died along with me then two families would be without dads. I knew I had been called to be there to do this thing and it was as if I had been programmed, it was effortless but maximally exhilarating. The smoke (in just a few seconds), was much darker. I was a swimmer in high school and college and I don't smoke. I took a deep breath and crawled through the back window which had popped out during the accident. I crawled in the space between the seats and the roof of the vehicle, remember the Blazer was on its side.

As I got up to the front, I could see the separated dashboard and the fire coming up on the left. I could see the victim's left leg was on fire and he was hanging off the seat toward the passenger seat with his right leg jammed into the passenger seat, it had sustained a compound fracture (where the bone sticks through the skin). While I'm not Arnold Scharzenegger, I'm not a weakling either. I grabbed him from the shoulders and pulled to get him out but he wouldn't budge. I thought what the heck? He said before lapsing into unconsciousness, "It's the f---ing seat belt." He was lying on the belt causing tension so the belt wouldn't relax and I couldn't push the release button. The smoke was getting worse and darker. I took a breath from the air that was least smoky. I looked down at Fred's (Fred Garbutt was his name) head and it was in smoky air and I wondered if he was about to suffocate.

I yelled out if anyone had a knife. The CHP officer (Officer Paul Duarte) yelled back that he had one so I made my way back to the rear of the vehicle. He handed me his knife and I took another deep breath and headed back in. As I did so, I could see the flames were getting large, the smoke getting blacker and I thought if I don't get him out this time we're both going to die.

Remember the movie Backdraft? For those who don't, it's about firefighters and in one scene a fireman was in a hallway and as the fire came out from under a door, it seemed to come up in front of the fireman and for a moment they both seemed to be communicating with each other. It seemed to be almost an understanding and like it was all taking place in slow motion. I had the same feeling, like I was moving in slow motion and that while my life was in obvious danger; it seemed I was being allowed to move alongside the flames to free Fred. I looked into those flames and it was like I was staring into eternity and both of us were a heartbeat away from knowing the ultimate truth.

As I got right next to him, by the grace of G-d I was able to see the seat belt coming over his shoulder and it cut like butter with officer Duarte's knife. I took a breath and started to cough as the air was so thick with smoke, and Fred was unconscious. I grabbed him under his arms and pulled him back. I had to dislodge his right leg with my right foot since his leg had the fracture and was still jammed under the passenger seat. I began to pull him back from the front seat along the space between the top of the seats and the roof, remember, the Blazer was on its side. I could see the flames go out on his leg and back as I pulled him out. I later found out Fred was about 6'2" and weighed about 210lbs. Officer Duarte and another man were there and helped me get him out and Duarte and I dragged Fred across Highway 74, the distance was only about thirty feet or so.

Just as we got Fred across the highway, the Blazer became engulfed in flames producing voluminous pitch black smoke. It looked like a jet plane crash. There was no explosion but that vehicle was immersed in an inferno of flames where Fred and I had been only seconds ago.

Having freed Fred, my attention then turned to his medical condition which looked to be precarious to say the least. Officer Duarte had brought oxygen and a cervical collar that we applied with care. I straightened his leg and wrapped it with a makeshift brace. In the fresh air Fred began to barely mumble. I looked him over and noticed blood coming from his left side. At first, I thought this is strange since third degree burns don't bleed and I knew that was what he had. The flames had burned right through the skin, they would require skin grafting. I cut off his shirt to see if I was right and sure enough there was a small hole in the lateral (side) of his left chest. I knew this was probably a pneumothorax (punctured lung). If they are not treated immediately sometimes the lung is pushed toward the heart because the air that you breathe in goes out through the hole and is trapped inside the chest. Depending on the size of the hole in the lung, the lung collapses and blood supply to the heart is cut off and the victim dies. The treatment is a chest tube that sucks the air out until the lung expands and heals. Obviously I didn't have a chest tube. At that instant the fire department showed up and I thought "good the paramedics will have equipment."

I asked the first fireman who came up if he had any gloves? If worse came to worse, I was going to put my gloved finger through the hole in Fred's chest and let the trapped air out. The fireman asked who I was and I said I was a trained trauma surgeon and he asked if I had any I.D.?

I didn't have anything that said I was a physician so I turned to officer Duarte and said, "If this guy has a pneumothorax and he doesn't get treatment, he won't make it to the hospital." Officer Duarte said, "Do what you have to do." The fireman didn't say anything and I went to work. I took the glove, put it on and gently stuck my index finger inside Fred's chest. You could hear the air come out in a SWOOOSH. I did this three times until the helicopter came. I tried to talk to Fred but he was in shock and not responding well. Right after the firemen arrived they put tons of water on the fire and it was out quickly.

Only a short time passed and the rescue helicopter arrived. The chopper was big and sounded awesome. It reminded me of the times back in my surgical residency at Loyola when I was on the burn team. If a call came in about a burn victim a long way off, I would call the Cook County Fire Department and they would land their big county helicopter at the hospital and we would fly to the victim many miles away. We would land in parking lots with many people surrounding the chopper. Sometimes I would do emergency surgery on the victims like a fasciaotomy (cutting the fibrous sheath around the muscle so it can get blood supply). I didn't have much time to think about that though. We transferred Fred to the waiting chopper and I said a few words to the crew about his condition. In a few seconds Fred was off to Desert Hospital trauma unit. Fred would be in the hospital a few weeks recovering from multiple skin grafts, having his spleen removed and lung fixed along with his broken leg.

As I watched the helicopter go off, I turned and walked toward my car. I thought to myself, "I really did something good here." It was a different good than just doing a surgery well.

I walked up to my wife and said just that. My wife as it turns out was not aware I had been in Fred's vehicle because of the smoke. I felt as though if you had cancer or something that if you would have touched me, you would have been cured on the spot. I mean I never had that type of feeling in twenty years as a surgeon. It was just a feeling of profound good. I took Christian up to the Blazer and looking in from the back, it was just a completely burned out hulk.

We listened to all the comments looked the scene over and quietly drove back home. The following morning a report of the accident was in the newspaper and TV interviews followed. Christian and I went to visit Fred in the hospital and his wife and kids were there. Fred is married to Kym, and they had two daughters at that time ages two and four.

We all kind of cried seeing him and reliving the story. He would be there many days recovering with multiple surgeries. He would eventually heal enough to go home and today he is almost back to normal. I learned from Fred much later, that as he was lying upside down and on fire, he was saying to himself that "Oh G-d, I'm going to die just like my father." I pondered more than a few hundred times what my intervention meant that day. Two fathers could have been lost that day but something more important needed to be done and that was two fathers needed to live. The preservation of life and helping someone who at that given moment in time could not help himself out of a death trap was the essence of that day.

Some months passed and I received a letter from the Carnegie Hero Commission that I had been nominated for the Carnegie Medal for and outstanding act of heroism. I must confess that I had never heard of the Carnegie Medal but it sounded intriguing. Interviews were conducted, information gathered and months passed. This next happening is what put the whole experience in the realm of a religious epiphany. I came home from work and there was a certified letter confirming that I would be awarded the Carnegie Medal. I looked at the letter a while and as I did, I reached into a box where I have a lot of VCR tapes many unmarked. Sometimes I like to look at them to see what I found interesting two or three years in the past. I reached into the pile and pulled an unmarked tape out and popped it into the VCR.

As the tape began not only was it Bill Moyers and Joseph Campbell on PBS, but it was them discussing why one man would lay down his life for another who he doesn't even know. I thought, "I've got to listen to this." For those of you who don't know, Joseph Campbell until his death a few years ago was the West's foremost authority of myths and religion. Bill Moyers interviews Mr. Campbell over several hours discussing almost all ancient myths and how they relate to our lives today.

Remember, I had just received the letter telling me I would be awarded the Carnegie Medal and I had just pulled an unmarked tape out of the about twenty and this story unfolds told by Joseph Campbell. So Mr. Moyers asks Professor Campbell, "Why does one man lay down his life for someone he doesn't even know?" I was riveted to the set. Joe started in with this story about two cops driving their beat in Hawaii (where Joe lived). There is a place going up to Diamond Head called the Pali.

There the wind blows hard and according to legend, the wind blew so mightily that it once saved the life of a princess as it blew her back to safety when she fell over the edge. This place is high up and unfortunately people also go there to jump off and commit suicide. Well, as the two cops rounded the corner they saw a man at the edge who was obviously preparing to jump.

They slam on the brakes and the cop on the right gets out followed by the cop who was driving. The cop in the right gets to the man first and grabs him as he is jumping over the edge. He begins wrestling with him to prevent him from going over the cliff. Well, the cop would have gone over with the man if it weren't for his partner coming and preventing the two from going over, and they saved the man's life. After the press picked up on the cop's heroic act, they asked the cop why didn't you just leave the guy jump? The cop's answer was, "If I would have let that man jump, I could not have live with myself another day." This is nearly the same feeling I had right after Fred's accident when people asked me why I went into the burning car not once but twice? If my dad knew his son was in the position I had arrived at, turned away from another human being in desperate need he would have turned over in his grave. Although a civilian I felt with my surgery training, that I had been prepared to act just the way I did without hesitation that day August 14, 1992. So that was a story of one man risking his life for another but Campbell was about to enlighten the viewers with the reason way people do those things.

Campbell talked of Author Schopenhauer (a German philosopher in the late 1700's) rational for all this. I really wanted to hear this because I had lived it. Well, Schopenhauer would have said that stories like the one above and mine were a realization of the metaphysical breakthrough that we are all one and the only thing that separates any of us is the temporal relationship of time and space. The cop and the man were actually one and in my case as well, I was actually saving myself from the burning vehicle.

This revelation together with the actual experience caused me to reflect profoundly on these events and how life is altered by them. I don't know if Schopenhauer was right but as far as I'm concerned, there is more to life on earth than meets the eye. Being in that fire was for me like being in and looking at eternity, putting it all on the line for that moment in time. I felt like I at last had a handle on life and what it meant to act in an unselfish manner. There is nothing like profound good to quench the soul. Like I always say to anyone who wants to hear the story, we looked evil in the eye that day and evil lost. In fact, many times I have wished I could experience that moment of profound good again because there is nothing like looking death in the eye and coming out on top. It was exhilarating to say the least.

Realizing that feeling, it was somewhat disappointingly enigmatic that my medal came by regular mail and the box was just stuck in the fence. What if I had died affecting that rescue? I think for what it is worth, the Carnegie Hero Fund should present these medals at an official awards ceremony. It would do the country good to see that in the hearts of many, honor has not left the stage. That year of Carnegie awards four died affecting their rescue and I thought maybe I should give the medal back. Receiving that medal in the fence like that well, I felt as though the purpose of the medal was dishonored.

The story doesn't end there. Fast forward to 2014. While I didn't know who I was rescuing back in 1992, the Garbutt's (Kym and Fred) have become very good friends. It turns out they actually live about two miles from us in La Quinta. We meet every so often and on that anniversary date every year we do dinner. They had a baby about a year and a half after the accident and we call that baby the miracle baby.

Over the years going to San Diego we have passed that turn many times and it evokes the adventure of that day. You have probably passed it as well. It's either the last turn before the long straightaway leading to the Paradise Café going toward San Diego or it's the first turn going down to Palm Desert from the café.

The lesson learned was be very very careful and drive slowly going up and down Hwy 74 unless you see me in your rear view mirror.

Take Care

Dr. Bretz

OBSERVATION POST

VOL. 38 NO.26   TWENTYNINE PALMS MARINE CORPS AIR-GROUND COMBAT CENTER   JULY 9, 1993

OBSERVATION POST   JULY 9, 1993   13

Hospital emergency room doctor receives Carnegie Medal

SSGT. SCOT JENKINS
Observation Post

A Naval Hospital civilian emergency room doctor received a Carnegie Medal for heroic actions he made last August. This medal, given by the Carnegie Hero Fund Commission recognizes individuals who have made an outstanding act of heroism.

Doctor Phillip Bretz risked his own life Aug. 14, 1992 on Highway 74 to rescue the life of Frederick Garbutt who was trapped inside a Chevrolet Blazer near Anza.

"I was kind of stunned," said Bretz. "I didn't correlate what I did with something like an award. It was a very strange set of circumstances. I hardly ever use this road."

I started grabbing him but he wouldn't come."

Bretz noticed Garbutt's leg was on fire and wanted to get him out of the vehicle.

"The guy told me the seatbelt was stuck and wouldn't budge," Bretz said. "I yelled out and said I needed a knife."

A cop yelled he had a knife. Bretz crawled back out to the rear window and took another deep breath and took the knife. He returned to the front seat and cut the belt.

"Flames were up in the front seat and black smoke billowed around," Bretz said. "The belt cut like butter so I started pulling him. Both of his legs were broken and his right leg looked like a Z. He couldn't help me."

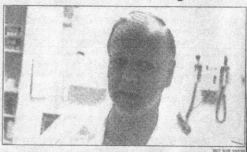

Doctor Phillip Bretz, a civilian doctor with the Emergency Room of the Naval Hospital, takes a break from his hectic schedule. The doctor recently received a Carnegie Medal for heroic actions he performed last August.

The doctor described the circumstances surrounding the accident and his actions as surrealistic. He lives in the Palm Springs area and his family had enjoyed a long leisurely lunch with some friends. On the Bretz' way back home they suddenly arrived on the scene.

"I stopped my car and got out," he said. "I saw this guy who had blood on his mouth who started yelling someone was trapped in the vehicle."

By this time, Bretz, said about 20 or 30 people had gathered around the accident. The first inclination was to push the vehicle to get it upright, but the doctor wanted to make sure the person was alright.

"I yelled in and asked the guy, 'are you all okay? Can you move everything?'," recalled Bretz. "He said, 'I'm okay but the vehicle is on fire.'"

The on-scene California Highway Patrol officer grabbed a fire extinguisher and started trying to put the fire out. Bretz said the fire just expanded too rapidly and the patrolman had no way of putting out the fire.

"I knew in a heartbeat that the situation was deteriorating quickly," Bretz said. "The extinguisher just wasn't doing the job."

The doctor waited a couple seconds to see if anyone else was going to do something. He said they just sort of stood around and then he noticed the vehicle's back window had popped open. He decided to crawl into the smoke-filled vehicle and rescue Garbutt.

Bretz climbed through the back window of Garbutt's overturned vehicle, cut the safety belt and pulled him free. Seconds later, the vehicle turned into what Bretz said was a big puff of smoke.

"There was a lot of smoke, so I took a deep breath before going in. I had been a swimmer in college," Bretz said. "I crawled over the top of the seats until I got to the driver.

Bretz used his strength and pulled Garbutt out of the vehicle and took him across the road.

"By the time I got him out of the vehicle and across the street, the vehicle was engulfed in smoke. It looked like an airplane accident," said the Desert Breast Institute doctor.

Another person grabbed some water and put the fire out on Garbutt's leg. The firemen had arrived on scene, and Bretz felt a sigh of relief.

"I saw the firemen and thought to myself, 'good, the paramedics are there,'" Bretz said.

Unfortunatley, only firemen arrived at the accident's scene. Bretz used his medical skills and put a splint on Garbutt's legs as well as a cervical collar around his neck.

"I noticed he had blood coming out of his chest," said Bretz. "I wondered how this could be because third degree burns don't create bleeding."

Bretz quickly pulled up Garbutt's shirt and saw blood coming out of the driver's left side of his chest.

"I put a glove on and put my finger in his chest," he said.

He did this because when someone has this type of chest injury whenever they breathe, their lungs shifts. Bretz said it would not have taken long for the lungs to shift and crush the heart.

"This would have killed him," Bretz said.

The doctor was able to keep Garbutt alive and get him ready for a helicopter ride to medical facilities.

Once Bretz returned to his car and his family, he said, "oh my God, I did something good. As a surgeon of 20 years, I have never experienced anything like that. It was split-second timing and it was like a Hollywood script."

The doctor said the action created a rush of adrenaline.

The doctor received a Carnegie Medal, $2,500 and eligibility for scholarship assistance.

This article is from imPULSE, a periodical from the Carnegie Hero Fund Foundation. I submitted this piece.

CARNEGIE HERO MUSES 'BLIND LUCK OR DIVINE INTERVENTION'?

*Editor's Note: Carnegie Hero **Phillip DeEvans Bretz** was awarded the Carnegie Medal in 1993 for the rescue of Frederick A. Garbutt, 28, whom he pulled from a burning vehicle Aug. 14, 1992, in Anza, Calif. He submitted this essay to imPULSE anonymously, but as it is against policy to publish anonymous works, he reluctantly agreed to identify himself. His essay has been edited for grammar, style, length, and clarification.*

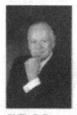

Phillip DeEvans Bretz

In my almost 72 years on this planet, I have come to realize certain things about the human experience. One of these is that whenever a person is awarded the Carnegie Medal, it becomes a personal, life-changing event. When I was awarded the medal in 1993, four people out of the 20 were awarded it posthumously. I felt like I should have given the medal back as I hadn't done enough.

In my caring for people throughout my medical career, I was fortunate enough to meet and care for Medal of Honor awardee Mitchell Paige and his family. Meeting Col. Paige was something very special. You just sensed the importance of this man, that somehow this encounter was very different. That is, this man was ready to lay down his life acting to protect his fellow soldiers. We've all heard the quote, "no greater love has a man than to lay down his life for another." But when time comes to actually live up to that, how many people are actually prepared and understand the potential consequences (meaning death to yourself)? How many would actually do it? It's the whole ballgame, everything is over for you if you don't make it. It's over for you, your family, your friends, your work, aspirations, and hopes are all gone in a heartbeat.

By the time you've reached my age, you have buried a lot of people, and you know the finality of death. Everything the deceased was working on comes to a halt and remains forever incomplete. I wonder at times how rare Carnegie awardees are in a world where many people can't commit to a full day's work let alone their lives ending just to help another who you might not even know. The character showed by Carnegie awardees is the very definition of character, courage, and commitment.

In my career as a surgeon, I had reached a level where I thought I had tasted rarefied air, but I had no idea what rarefied air was until that fateful day when we looked evil in the eye, and evil lost, Aug. 14, 1992. That was the day I did not allow Fred to die in a fiery crash. Throughout the years I have often wished I could go back to those precious moments where ▶ p.16

▶ from p.15

BLIND LUCK OR DIVINE INTERVENTION

I was caught up in saving Fred. While he sustained third-degree burns, I, right next to him, was allowed to move, in slow motion it seemed, around that fire. It was just like the movie Backdraft (1991) when the fireman had the fire come up and seemingly talk to him. Without a doubt it was the most exhilarating moment in my life, looking eternity in the face.

My father was killed in a work-related accident when I was 12, and Fred's father had died in the same kind of crash. With my family watching a few feet away, if both Fred and I hadn't made it out, it wouldn't have been good. We were "all in," as the saying goes. When they hear the story, many people have said that I acted without knowing what I was doing. No, not at all, as a surgeon I knew exactly what I was doing. If I hadn't have acted in the manner I did, my dad would have turned over in his grave.

Just before I entered the burning vehicle from the rear window, as I took a deep breath (I was a swimmer in high school and college), I had the sense that not only was Jesus not going to let me die that day, but, perhaps, I was the chosen one to be there at that very spot at that moment in time. While not a trained rescue member, such as a firefighter, a surgeon is confronted daily for decades with life and death scenarios in the operating room, which involve split-second decisions that no one else can make. So maybe I had the edge on the fire.

My wife said that this piece must have been difficult to write since I call these awardees such special people, and I apparently am one. It's like being between a rock and a hard place. The word needs to get out (since we are inundated daily with horrific events), but no one can adequately express what occurred except for the actual heroes themselves. Like all these awardees we don't walk around with our chests stuck out. The experience is carried inside. If someone wants to know about it, fine, otherwise boasting in any respect just isn't on the agenda. It's hallowed ground. But I have often thought there should be an annual meeting where we can just share our feelings among ourselves. I want to know their personal thoughts. Perhaps in the future we can.

If you are ever fortunate enough to meet a Medal of Honor or Carnegie (Medal) awardee, you know all there is to know. That is, when the chips are down their true character came through in an instant overshadowing everything so evil loses. It reminds me of my favorite movie, *The Magnificent Seven* (1960). There is a scene I have run over in my mind countless times that I wish I had the guts to pull off. That scene is where the star, Yul Brynner, (who plays Chris Larabee Adams) is listening to a discussion between the town's mortician and the town's people about how he can't bury Indian Joe because no one will drive the horse-drawn hearse. Their town was reluctant to let Joe be buried on Boot Hill since he was a Native American. Brynner, listening to this, says, "Oh hell, if that's ▶ p.17

▶ from p.16

BLIND LUCK OR DIVINE INTERVENTION

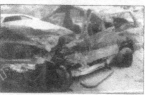

The wreckage of the burned sport utility vehicle from which **Phillip DeEvans Bretz** *freed its driver, who was trapped in the driver's seat after an accident in which the car overturned and flames breeched the passenger compartment. With the driver's seat aflame, Bretz entered the vehicle, used a knife to cut the driver's seat belt, and then dragged him to a rear window where others helped remove him from the car.*

all that's stopping it, I'll drive the rig." Brynner saw the problem and acted with utter confidence against unknown odds. It took guts, but he had it in him and did what was right. I don't know where supreme confidence comes from but it resides in these medal awardees' souls, and it permeates every aspect of their lives. That's the difference between those who act while everyone else stands by or turns their back. It's doing what's right at that moment in time because you know in your heart there is something overridingly profound to which we, as humans, aspire that's bigger than any individual.

They don't have to read in the paper about a heroic act and ask, "Could I pull that off?" It brings you into true rarified air that few have had the privilege to breathe.

In the movie *Ladder 49* (2004) there is a scene where John Travolta (who plays station Capt. Mike Kennedy) is giving a eulogy for a fallen firefighter and he asks, "Why is it that firemen run into a burning building when others run from it?" He answers, "It was your courage, Jack." And to each awardee, it's your courage. If all of mankind behaved in like terms the world would be a better place.

Of all the awards and certificates on the wall of my accomplishments though, I've missed the one for which I would give them all up: my dad having his arm around me saying, "You did ok!" I'll never have a chance to meet all the Carnegie awardees but I say to all of you, "You did ok!" and as they said of Richard Burton in the movie *Where Eagles Dare* (1968), "All sins forgiven."

God speed Carnegie Medal awardees.

— Phillip DeEvans Bretz, 1993 Carnegie Medal awardee ✖

Carnegie heroes interested in interacting with other Carnegie Medal awardees are welcome to join the Commission's private Facebook group for Carnegie Heroes at facebook.com/groups/781943251163346?/

OFFICE OF THE GOVERNOR
State of California

August 24, 1993

TO: DR. PHILLIP BRETZ

    I recently learned of your heroism that earned you the
Carnegie Medal, and I'd like to offer my sincere
congratulations.

    Your courage and presence of mind to cut Fred Barbult
free from his burning Blazer with your handy knife was
remarkable. The vehicle, I understand, exploded just after
you rescued Mr. Barbult.

    Few things give me greater pleasure than thanking
Californians who have performed heroically to save lives.
You are such a man, Dr. Bretz, and you have my best wishes
for every future success and happiness.

Sincerely,

Pete Wilson

PETE WILSON

Doctor climbs in fiery car, frees crash victim

The Press-Enterprise 8-19-92

Dr. Phillip Bretz, who is standing by a reflective window, used a buck knife last week to cut a man free from a burning car.

Steve Medd / The Press-Enterprise

By Mike Kataoka
The Press-Enterprise

RANCHO MIRAGE

Dr. Phillip Bretz saved a life, literally under fire, in the Santa Rosa Mountains Friday afternoon by relying on a buck knife and raw courage instead of a scalpel and surgical skill.

Bretz, California Highway Patrol Officer Paul Duarte and another passerby teamed up to rescue a Palm Desert man who was trapped in a 1989 Chevrolet Blazer that overturned and caught fire on Highway 74 near Highway 371. The Blazer had collided head-on with a Jeep pickup that had swerved out of control.

"If we had a video camera, that would have been on 'Rescue 911,' no question," Bretz said yesterday. "It was like a Hollywood script."

Bretz, a 46-year-old Rancho Mirage surgeon who directs the Desert Breast Institute, was heading back to the desert from an outing in San Diego with his family when the relaxed drive took a dramatic detour.

Bretz climbed in the fiery Blazer through an open back window and used a buck knife to cut the seat belts and free the injured driver, Fred Garbutt, according to CHP reports and Bretz' own account.

The three rescuers pulled Garbutt to safety moments before the vehicle was engulfed in flames. The other man who assisted was Raymond Schwinn of Los Gatos, according to the CHP.

"Without those three working together, the outcome could have been pretty grim. This guy could have died," said CHP Officer Craig Rentie, spokesman for the Indio office.

Garbutt, 28, remained in critical condition yesterday at Desert Hospital in Palm Springs. He suffered internal injuries and third-degree burns on his left leg and left arm.

The driver of the Jeep, John B. Baker, 50, of Buena Park, was released yesterday from Desert Hospital. His passenger, Ventilon Mayer, 52, of Palm Desert, suffered minor injuries and was not admitted to the hospital.

Larry Brett, Garbutt's father-in-law, said yesterday Garbutt is unable to speak but can communicate by writing. The first thing he wrote was "Why me?"

"He is coherent and knows what's going

Please see CRASH, B-10

CRASH

Continued from B-1

on," Brett said. "Every day he gets better but he is in tremendous pain." The prognosis "looks very good," he said.

Brett said Garbutt, the father of two young children, owns a liquor store in Anza and was on his way to work when the accident occurred.

Brett said the family is appreciative of the heroism that saved Garbutt from sharing the fate of his father, who died in a car accident when Garbutt was 8 years old.

Bretz yesterday emphasized the teamwork rather than his individual courage in recounting the dramatic rescue.

He also noted the "unbelievable set of circumstances" that put him and the others in the right place at the right time.

Bretz said his son, Chris, had been thirsty, so they stopped at the Backwoods Inn near the junction of Highways 74 and 371. It was there that Bretz first saw Officer Duarte, who was citing a motorist.

Without those delays they would not have met again a couple of minutes later at the accident scene, where the Blazer was on fire

and the driver was trapped inside, yelling.

"We just had a couple of seconds to decide what to do, otherwise this guy was going to burn in front of us and I was not going to allow that to happen," Bretz said.

Officer Duarte used a fire extinguisher to contain the flames and enable Bretz to enter the vehicle. Schwinn helped Bretz and Duarte push the Blazer, which had landed upside down, on its side to ease Bretz' access to the driver.

Bretz said he reacted to the emergency without pausing to weigh the risk to his own life.

"That really didn't cross my mind," he said. "I felt I had enough time, which was naive, to get in there and get out of there. How tough could that be?"

It turned out to be extremely tough because flames were shooting out of the dash and the cab was filled with black smoke plus eye-

stinging fire retardant. Worst of all, Garbutt was restrained with the lap and shoulder belts.

"I just took a deep breath and went in," Bretz said. "I grabbed Fred and he wouldn't come out."

Realizing he would need something to cut the belts, Bretz backed out of the Blazer and got Duarte's buck knife.

He crawled back inside and cut the shoulder strap but Garbutt still would not budge. "Everything was black, but by the grace of God, I looked up and saw the (lap) belt and cut through the belt like butter as the flames were right in the front seat," Bretz said.

They pulled Garbutt across the street and "by the time we got there, flames were shooting out and there was billowing smoke. It was unbelievable. We had 20 seconds to spare."

Firefighters arrived to extinguish the fire and avert an explo-

sion and Garbutt was transported by helicopter to Desert Hospital.

"I was extremely elated when we got out of there," Bretz said. "The whole thing took place in probably 20 minutes. It's very compelling when someone is burning to death," he said.

Bretz said he has training as a trauma surgeon and is used to dealing with emergency situations.

"Maybe there is an edge there. Either you act and it works or don't act and it's really tragic," he said.

But Bretz said he hopes he never again has to face a life and death situation outside of a hospital.

Bretz and Schwinn are each likely to be awarded a Certificate of Community Service, among other possible awards for heroism, said Rentie, the CHP spokesman.

Duarte, who is in a training session this week at the CHP Academy, is being considered for special recognition.

CHAPTER 14

SHORT STORIES OF
A SURGEON

THE FOLLOWING ARE stories I hope you will find interesting. They mean a lot to me because they are all true but they are separate from the rest of the book so as not to take away from the main theme.

PROLOGUE

Having just witnessed the funeral of our thirty-eighth President, Gerald R. Ford, I felt compelled to put to pen (before it's too late) some true stories of life experiences that happened to me in my quest to become a surgeon. The Ford family and another president figure into two of the stories, so I thought it would be of interest to start with the funeral.

Some might call this little story strictly a coincidence, but it was one in a long line then and makes one wonder. I thought that we would simply drive up to Palm Desert (avoiding the buses at the tennis garden that carried people to the church) and park at our friend Jay's house and walk to St. Margaret's where President Ford's body was lying in state.

We parked at Jay's and began to walk towards the church; there was heavy traffic coming down Mesa View as Highway 74 was closed. We were walking, and suddenly we saw a little rabbit pulling itself out from under the tire of an SUV driven by a woman talking on her cell phone. The little guy who had been hit was bleeding but dragging himself by his front legs and was going back under the car. Joan and Alexandra screamed and held each other. I just walked out into traffic, stopped the cars, and grabbed the rabbit.

I put my other hand down to hold him at the same time so he would not bite me. I told him he was okay and that I was sorry. I picked him up with my hand around his neck and looked at him. It was obvious he was mortally wounded.

I made the split-second decision to put him down with my hands, all the while saying I was sorry. It only took a few seconds, and he was out of his misery. I put him down and went across the street and told Joan I wished this cross were not on me anymore.

We walked further up the road, and some people were coming down and said it was all blocked off. That meant if we wanted to see the President, we had to go to the tennis garden like everyone else. I stopped to pick up the rabbit. I felt responsible since it was I who put an end to its life. I buried him later. I thought, why was I there at that split second in time to see him? I was not only there but acted in a split second to deal with the situation. I realized it was all these things you are about to read that put me in a position to act; some would say in a small way then but at other times much more significant. For some of you who read "Blind Luck or Divine Intervention," and my story of saving Fred Garbutt from a burning vehicle, I thought the same thing.

While this story ended with the death of the rabbit, without my being there, that little guy would have suffered untold misery for hours, perhaps days, before dying. Instead, my action was swift and sure. I wondered, like Fred's case, if I was there by luck or not. How can there be all these coincidences? It is my thought that these are not just coincidental happenings. In the life of any physician, they sometimes bring untold suffering on people, and one has to be prepared to take that and move on every day. You've got to be tough. Here is the rest of the Ford funeral story.

THE GERALD FORD STORY

For those who missed the funeral, it was like saying goodbye to "our" President. Sometime after the funeral, someone sponsored a big billboard that said, Gerald "our" Ford. It wasn't until I reflected on his career that I realized Mr. Ford was perhaps the only President who served in the House (for twenty-five years), then Vice President, and finally President without so much as a single vote being cast. Seeing the flag-draped coffin with the four men from each branch of the service guarding him felt a little like the feeling one gets setting foot into Arlington cemetery. I wanted our youngest daughter Alexandra to see this and remember this. The funeral procession traveled the same streets we locals used every day to bring him to St. Margaret's Church in Palm Desert and then on to Palm Springs International airport for the final trip back to Washington on Air Force One and finally to Grand Rapids, Michigan.

Our family, like thousands of others, traveled to Indian Wells Tennis Garden to be bused to St. Margaret's to view the casket draped in an American flag and an honor guard standing at attention for hours on end. As Dr. Blakeley always said, it was a fundamental day. Mr. Ford represented the last of the real famous people who called the Coachella Valley home that I had met. There was Frank Sinatra, Red Skelton, David Jansen, Bob Hope, and Ford was the last.

While the rest of the country was enduring brutal winter weather, Air Force One stood on the PSP tarmac bright and glistening in the warm California sun with a backdrop of the 8,000-foot Mount San Jacinto. The deep blue of the cool, cloudless desert sky against the mountains with a dusting of snow and the most magnificent plane known to man was almost surreal. I'm sure the rest of the country was eating its heart out, seeing that sight. We saw Air Force One go wheels up at 10:15 a.m. (then called SAM 29000) on Fox News, and as it lifted from the runway, we went outside and looked up, and there she was headed east and climbing into the sun.

It was a perfect send-off from the desert. Later that day, I watched the plane arrive at Andrews Air Force Base in Maryland. Just hours ago, I was not ten feet from his casket, and now it was surrounded by thousands of people in Washington. I had lost a friend. I felt as though he should be brought back here to the quiet, peaceful, beautiful desert he loved so much. My connection to President Ford is through Betty and her heart surgery. The true story will follow with the rest.

I suppose whenever anyone reaches a point in his or her career where a series of significant things have happened, they seem to have all come together to make that person who they are. To put it another way, what has happened that a person has significant things happen to them? When does this all start? I suppose with me, it started in college where I met Bernard Lerner, whose father was a surgeon and whose brother was in medical school. Bernie and I were in pre-med at North Park University (then College). You have read the story of my transition from going into construction to events that turned me into a surgeon. A lot of things had to fall in place.

Next is an article in *The North Parker* and it appeared in the Winter 1998 issue. They actually flew out to do the interview at my office on Bob Hope Drive. Back then I thought I was doing the best there was performing my cosmetic lumpectomy technique. My complaint with the system though is pretty much the same now as it was back then. It was just a few years later that accelerated partial breast radiation (APBR) came out, which changed the ballgame to five days of targeted radiation instead of six weeks. That was followed a few years later by intraoperative radiation therapy (IORT). That pushed the envelope further by applying only twenty minutes of radiation during the lumpectomy instead of the five days or six weeks. Next came my epiphany of a targeted kill of breast cancer with liquid nitrogen. The trick was being able to find nascent tumors before they had the capability to metastasis (spread). As you're aware now that's the Lavender Way which portends the Lavender Procedure.

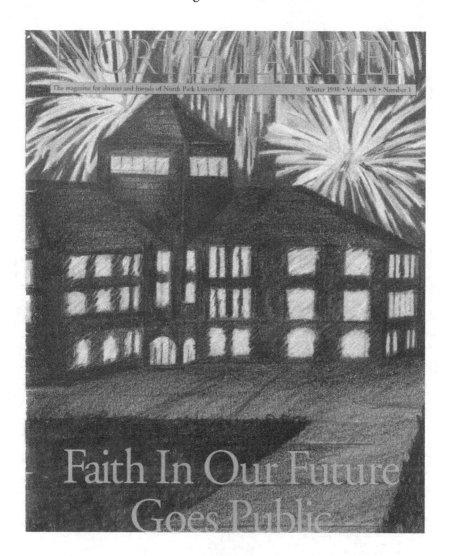

QUIET LIVES OF INFLUENCE

"Preserving mind, body, and spirit"

by John Baworowsky

Phillip Bretz, M.D., is angry. Women are dying needlessly. They are having breast surgeries that are unnecessary. Many are waiting too long between breast examinations or are being examined by physicians who are not trained to detect cancer in its earliest stages.

Dr. Phillip Bretz is also tenacious. In response to his belief that the United States has a lack of long-range healthcare and treatment for breast cancer, this 1967 North Park College graduate decided to challenge the accepted care and treatment of women's health. He founded the Desert Breast Institute in Rancho Mirage, Calif.

Dr. Bretz' anger and tenacity comes from a sincere desire to improve women's health and from a frustration with the country's current system for providing women with check-ups, test, diagnoses, and treatment.

Bretz credits his father's death as one important source of the tenacity and passion that fuels his drive. After Bretz graduated from North Park Academy, the admission director told the young Bretz that he didn't have the requisite skills to make it academically at North Park. Bretz enrolled in summer school to prove him wrong. The Bs he received earned Bretz a place in the freshmen class.

Although not a standout athlete, he competed at football, tennis, and swimming as an undergraduate, earning letters. Bretz first met his wife Joan Pedersen at North Park Academy, even though they grew up only a mile from each other. Even in college, Bretz' tenacity was apparent to his classmates. When Joan was elected homecoming queen, the king asked Bretz' permission to kiss her. He was afraid he was going to get punched.

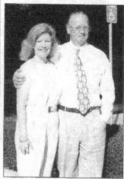

Joan and Phillip Bretz at the Desert Breast Institute in Rancho Mirage, Calif.

Phillip and Joan were married by Rev. Ronald Magnuson. They have four children: Jason, 23; Ashley, 21; Christian, 15; and Alexandra, 8.

Bretz wanted to be either a minister or a contractor until a classmate introduced him to his father, a local surgeon. After making the rounds at the hospital with the doctor, Bretz knew this was what he wanted to do.

I don't like it when I have to refer a patient to an oncologist for chemotherapy because that means that either the system failed or the patient somehow failed.

After graduating from North Park College with average grades, Bretz was determined to attend medical school. He and Joan decided to go to Mexico, where Guadalajara Medical School offered him admission. Not speaking Spanish, the by now famous Bretz tenacity and perseverance motivated him to learn the language the summer prior to enrolling. Although the Spanish-taught medical school heavily stacked the odds against Americans, Bretz thrived in the environment.

Upon graduation, he returned to Chicago, participating in a surgery residency at Loyola University Medical Center. There he learned an important lesson that would shape his future: as a resident, you can call upon more experienced doctors to assist you with a problem. When you have your own practice, you are on your own.

After completing his five year residency, the Bretzes moved to Rancho Mirage where he joined a general surgery practice specializing in heart surgery. According to a 1984-85 Medicare study, the open heart team earned the lowest mortality rate in the country. Among his patients was Betty Ford, wife of former President Gerald Ford.

In his spare time, Bretz tried his hand at politics, unsuccessfully challenging Sonny Bono for a congressional seat.

Success came at a price – working 14 hour days seven days a week, he became concerned about the quality of his life and the lives of his family members. He also noticed that care for and treatment of women's breasts was being done primarily by male doctors who operated in the old tradition of radical surgeries.

He thought he could do it better.

Bretz created what he calls a "compre-

As soon as you tell me I can't do something, I have to prove to you that I can do it. Not only do it, but make things happen.

hensive breast center." His approach is to provide very regular check-ups from a physician specially trained at detecting breast tumors who is supported by similarly trained radiologists and oncologists. Because of how rampant breast cancer is in our society, he feels that women should receive regular, specialized examinations in addition to their regular visits to gynecologists.

"You make the diagnosis," he explained. "You help formulate the treatment. You execute the treatment so it's on your head. And then you follow that patient."

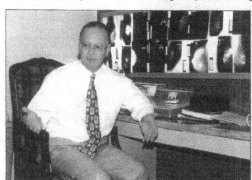

Dr. Bretz believes, *"a mammogram is a small price to pay because you only have one chance to treat this disease."*

Patients become partners with Bretz. He interprets their x-ray films with them so that they stay involved in the process. If a further test is called for, he can do it right in the office and give the patient immediate results. If a tumor is detected, he combines lumpectomy with radiation and sometimes chemotherapy as an alternative treatment to the more common mastectomy.

Continued on page 30

Bretz awarded Carnegie Medal for Heroism

In January 1996, Dr. Phillip Bretz and his family happened upon a serious car accident near Temecula, Calif. They were driving along Highway 74, a winding road made famous in the movie *It's a Mad, Mad, Mad, Mad World*.

The Bretzes saw smoke coming from an overturned Chevy Blazer. As a California Highway Patrol officer came by their car, the driver of the Blazer said in a distressed tone that there was someone else trapped in the burning car.

"I turned to my wife and said, 'I have to go now,'" Bretz remembered. "I yelled into the Blazer, 'Are you OK, can you move everything?' From inside came the words I didn't want to hear. 'I'm OK, but I'm on fire!'"

Bretz, the driver, and the officer pushed the car over so that it lay on its side with the driver's door up. Immediately the officer tried to put out the fire with his extinguisher.

"I looked at this effort and realized in a heartbeat it would be futile," he continued. "I thought to myself, 'You have to go in there and just do it, that's why you're here.' I walked around and just as I was about to go in, I had this thought that Jesus wasn't going to let me die that day.

"The smoke was much darker. I took a deep breath and crawled through the back window which had popped out during the accident. I crawled in the space between the seats and the roof of the vehicle, remember the vehicle was on its side.

"As I got up to the front, I could see the victim's left leg was on fire and he was hanging off the seat toward the passenger side with his right leg jammed into the passenger seat. It was fractured. I grabbed him from the shoulders and pulled to get him out, but he wouldn't budge. He was lying on the seat belt causing tension.

"I yelled out if anyone had a knife and I crawled through the back. The officer handed me his knife and I took another deep breath and headed back in. As I did so, I could see the flames were getting larger, the smoke blacker, and I thought if I don't get him out this time he's gonna die, maybe me too.

"As I got right next to him, by the grace of God I was able to see the seat belt coming over his shoulder and it cut like butter with the officer's knife. I took a breath and started to cough the air was so thick with smoke and Fred (the victim) was all but unconscious. I grabbed him under his arms and pulled him back. I had to dislodge his right leg with my right foot since his leg had sustained a compound fracture and was stuck under the passenger's seat. It took all I had to get both of us away from the flames. The vehicle became engulfed in flames some 30 seconds after we got out."

Immediately after pulling the victim from the car, Bretz administered emergency medical treatment. Besides the broken leg, the victim had a punctured lung, and without Bretz' quick thinking, would have died from that before reaching the hospital.

Media stories about the rescue led to a nomination by the Carnegie Hero Fund. Dr. Phillip Bretz was awarded the Carnegie Medal for Heroism.

"Preserving mind, body, and spirit."
Continued from page 19

"Women were dying before our eyes and we didn't even know it," he explained. His hand shakes as he waives a folder filled with the files of women who came to see him too late. "I don't like it when one of my patients dies. I really don't like it. I have to die with them. I have to talk to the husband. I have to see her deteriorate. So you can bet I learned early on to take steps to maximize their chance of surviving so that we preserve mind, body, and spirit. So when I am done with them, they can look in the mirror and say, 'I'm still intact.'" Soon to be published data he has gathered from his 10,000 patients will show significantly better results than standard treatments.

"I enjoy dealing with women," he said. "After 10,000 patients and 100,000 mammograms over nine years I know this little (he holds to fingers an inch apart) about women. I know there is so far to go.

"We (the medical community) haven't learned our lesson after 15 years of clinical trials," he confidently explained. "For Medicare patients, surgeons are still relying on mastectomy 75 or 80 percent of the time in this country. We proved 20 years ago that we shouldn't be doing that kind of surgery. Until we get comprehensive breast centers and take it out of the hands of the old referral patterns women will be butchered and die needlessly."

"We need to form a partnership with women in this country," he explained. "We need to preserve mind, body, and spirit, and not just mutilate them. We call this partnership the compass treatment, because it is 180 degrees from how our predecessors taught us to treat breast cancer. We as surgeons need to be cognizant of the fact that we leave lasting impressions on people."

Bretz believes that the devastating effect of mastectomy scares women from having regular mammograms. If you have less invasive forms of treatment, women are more likely to come in for regular check ups which can detect illness at an earlier, more treatable stage.

We proved that lumpectomy is superior and yet women are losing their breasts for no good reason.

"If they think you are caring for them," he said. "If they trust you. If they think they won't die because they come here. They'll do whatever you tell them."

Bretz believes all women without a history of breast cancer should have mammograms beginning at age 35. Ideally, every woman should have individualized guidelines. "A mammogram is a small price to pay because you only have one chance to treat this disease," he said. "If you don't do it right the first time, that patient is going to die."

Bretz was the author of the first large scale breast cancer prevention trial of the drug Tamoxifen in 1990. At their invitation, he worked to involve the Soviet Union in the project. Sixteen thousand patients enrolled with the last enrolling in 1997. Next year, the National Cancer Center will publish the data.

Bretz believes that if tumors can be detected when they are five millimeters or less, the patient can be treated without aggressive surgery and possibly without radiation. He analyzes tumors, regardless of their size, to chart an appropriate course of treatment.

"I am convinced that there are patients who are dying but we can't diagnose it. But we know now that with tumor analysis, we can identify those tumors that have metastic disease, whether or not they are large or small tumors. On the basis of that, we can counsel that patient that it is an aggressive tumor, we think you need primary chemotherapy."

Bretz uses an analogy of common bacteria mutating into organisms resistant to antibiotics to explain how early cancer cells mutate into more aggressive cells which are resistant to chemotherapy. "The (cancer cells in the) tumor that kills the patient are not the same ones that were there when the cancer was born," he explained. "They mutated into an aggressive form. We can identify those tumors and take action appropriately."

"When we told somebody that we had gotten it all and then three years later the cancer is back in the bone or somewhere, we say 'gee Mrs. Smith, the cancer is back!' For decades, we haven't answered the real question: We told Mrs. Smith three years ago that we got it all. 'How did it come back?' The answer is that it didn't really come back. It never left. It was out there all along and was there long before the person ever walked into our office in the form of micromastastices, cancer so small we can't identify it in a scan."

"Increasingly, we give chemotherapy first if we can detect the tumor is aggressive, even without demonstrable mastastices and in 80 percent of such cases, there is at least a 50 percent reduction in the size of the tumor. We can then down stage the patient from mastectomy to lumpectomy and in some cases, the tumor disappears altogether and we haven't operated on the patient." (Published in the Scientific proceeding of the American Society of Clinical Oncology.) Dr. Bretz was invited and traveled to Vienna and Canada at the World Conference on Breast Cancer this past summer to present the data.

Even though the compass treatment is based on chemotherapy, that is not the message that Doctor Bretz wants in the community.

"The real message is that I cannot prevent breast cancer," he said. "But if you come to a comprehensive center early on, the chance of you dying or losing a breast, or even having to have aggressive therapy is remote. Because the present system doesn't work, we haven't seen the mortality rate decline in 60 years."

SOME LOYOLA STORIES

This is what happened to my first surgery at Loyola, attempting to repair an inguinal hernia. The Chief Resident Phil Rice and the junior resident (Charlie Voss) did the one side, and I had the attending (great). I studied where to make the incision, etc., and looked at it ten ways from Sunday. Knowing what I know now, I could have made that incision anywhere and repaired the hernia but not back then, my first time. I remember the attending saying, "we're slow but poor." I have learned throughout the years, doing thousands of "big cases," that even the biggest baddest surgeon can get up to his/her ass in alligators, and that attitude really wasn't necessary.

Throughout my time at Loyola, I remember many things. I remember a sign posted in the locker room that said there was a shortage of blood and that we couldn't operate on elective cases. Someone crossed out the words and inserted, "we can, and we will." That was the attitude around that place. Dr. Freeark (our commander in chief) had come right from Cook County as Chief Resident to taking charge at Loyola. He was, in large part, responsible for the first blood bank and trauma center in the country at Cooks. He had a favorite saying when someone would say, "This tumor is unresectable," meaning the surgeon couldn't get it out, he would say, "It's unresectable for you." I remember doing a trauma case with him when I was Chief Resident, and the guy had a liver injury. We probably could have sewn that liver up, but he said to resect it because he wanted me to know how to do it with him guiding me.

I remember being on the burn unit rotation, and when a call came in of a bad burn downstate, I would call the fire department helicopter, and Chicago's big red chopper would land on the pad outside and I would ride with. Sometimes when we landed, it would be in a small hospital parking lot with a hundred people watching. It was good for my ego. Sometimes I would have to operate right there on a third-degree burn cutting the fascia so the person wouldn't get a compartment syndrome. Tissue swells a lot when it's burned, so much so that it cuts off the blood supply if the fibrous tissue encasing the large muscles isn't cut. Then there was the time when as Chief Resident, I was at my Hines VA rotation, and I wasn't getting lab results for this critically ill patient because of some lazy guy in the lab, I actually ripped the phone out of the wall because I wanted that guy taken care of right now, because his sacrifice in World War II made it possible for us to be there. I think the hole in the wall is still there. As a surgeon, some things need to get done right now or never. I also remember being near the top floor at Hines when a DC-10 went down at O'Hare Field. You could see the big billowing black clouds of smoke.

On a happier note, during my fourth year, I had a rotation at Chicago Children's Hospital. I really learned a lot there. Bernie Lerner (my best man) and I were there at the same time. He was doing his neurosurgery rotation and, at the time, had a Mario Andretti commemorative edition Lotus Esprit. I convinced him he shouldn't leave the car unattended at night and that I should take it home for safekeeping.

Also, while at Children's, a prominent politician's little son came in with an intussusception; that is when the small bowel telescopes into itself. I also remember while at Children's that Dr. D. (initial changed) had just completed her thoracic surgical residency at Loyola and started her pediatric surgery residency.

She and I were repairing a hernia on a little baby. It was her first case as a big shot. She/we hunted for some time for the hernia sac, and she finally had to call the boss Dr. John Raffensberger, which was the last thing she wanted to do on her first case. He came in and, without much ado, found the sac and repaired it. A little ego-bruising, but such is the life of a surgeon.

What else. Oh yes, there was the GW story. AC (initials changed), and I were on the transplant service as Chief Residents. That rotation was really a trip, sometimes literally. We were one of the only facilities doing transplants, and Dr. Peter Geis was our mentor. We would get a call that there were organs available at such and such hospital, and the team would go into action. The first time was a bit of a shock. The patient was brain dead but on the respirator. We wheeled him into the operating room and started taking his organs out one by one, kidneys, liver, and heart. When Dr. Geis clamped the ascending aorta, he told the anesthesiologist to turn off the respirator, and the guy looked at him like, "If I do that, I'll kill this guy." As I said, it was a little unnerving. Anyway, AC and I took turns staying at night looking out for the patients. Well, blood had been ordered and was given to GW (our patient), and there turned out to be two GWs, and ours got the wrong blood and had a major reaction and died. It could have been my night, but just another thing you have to carry forever being a surgeon.

The AB story (initials changed): AB was the fellow on the cardiac service, of which I did two rotations. Dr. Roque Pifarre (Chairman of the Department, RIP) invited me to stay on as a cardiac fellow after my five years of general surgery, but I don't think Joan could have taken it. Anyway, one day we are doing a routine bypass, and I'm taking out the saphenous vein in the leg to be used as the bypass, and AB and Roque (Rock) were opening the chest and going to cannulate the right atrium to prepare for the heart-lung machine. A big cannula (tube) goes into the right atrium of the heart to take blood away to the heart-lung machine, and the aortic cannula gets it back once oxygenated by the heart-lung machine into the body. The venous cannula is larger than your thumb is around. It has to carry a lot of blood, and usually, one puts a simple purse-string suture around the atrium, clamps it just beyond the suture line, makes an incision, and simultaneously releases the clamp and pushes the cannula into the atrium and superior vena cave (SVC) and simply ties the purse-string suture. The above is why we are all not cardiac surgeons. As fate would have it, as AB released the clamp, pushed the cannula in and tried to tie the suture, the purse-string suture broke, and blood started welling up and damn fast. Soon the heart was almost out of view. AB just stood there without acting for about three seconds (an eternity in such instances), and Pif said calmly, "AB, stop the bleeding." AB said, "I don't know if I can."

Now the heart is out of sight, and the anesthesiologist is panicking, and I am riveted to the chest filling up with blood. At the same time, I am learning an invaluable lesson on what separates the men from the boys. Pif drops his DeBakey forceps and leans over the table toward AB, and says calmly, "AB, you have to stop it."

Meaning that Pif wasn't going to be there forever. If AB was going to be a "real" cardiac surgeon out in the community, he would have to handle situations like this with relative ease. You see, a good surgeon makes everything, even the most difficult maneuvers, look easy. With that, Pif puts his hand into the pool of blood, grabs the atrial appendage and re-clamps it, while sucking the blood out to the heart-lung machine, and all is well. You're either a surgeon in command or you're not; it's that simple. Stuff like that was why I was trained well.

Every week at Loyola, we had mortality and morbidity (M&M), and each Chief Resident would have to get up on stage before about a hundred people and say, I did this, I did that. Usually, it was his underclassman that had done something, but it was always your fault. You had to take all the questions from the audience. One time, my junior resident and I were taking care of an Illinois senator who had come to Loyola to get the best of the best care. He had a pneumothorax (a hole in the lung). With each breath, air in the lung comes out through the hole, filling the potential space between the lung and the interior lining of the thoracic cavity. That cavity fills with more air every time you breathe, and eventually, the pressure builds up and shifts the mediastinum and heart, and blood is cut off to the heart, and you die. The treatment is inserting a chest tube. What my junior forgot was that when you look at a chest X-ray, what is on your right is actually the patient's left and vice versa. I let him on his own to put the tube in (so he could learn). We went down to look at the portable chest X-ray, and the tube was on the wrong side.

We had a resident from China on one night, and when I came in the next morning, he was very excited. He had just done a colostomy (colloquially known as a bag where the colon is brought out to the skin, so you crap into the bag). The reason was this patient had had several large rubber balls shoved up his rectum, and his partner, in an attempt to retrieve the balls, put his hand up his rectum and put his hand right through his colon. Such was life at Henrotin.

VISITING PROFESSORS AT LOYOLA AND EISENHOWER STORIES

Intermittently, Loyola would have visiting dignitaries in the form of iconic surgical pioneers. It fell to the Chief Resident on the boss's service (Dr. Freeark) to conduct rounds with the visiting chief. I won't tell you the name of this individual but every general surgeon knows him and probably had his book, which was big and blue and green in color. I had mine with me and asked him to autograph it, which he did. In addition, he was from Ohio State and had a very well-known syndrome named after him. Aside from dinner and the professor giving an oral presentation to the staff, I took him on rounds with us and discussed the patient's symptoms, differential diagnosis, diagnostic work undertaken and the treatment and outcome. If we didn't perform, he would go back to Ohio State and say those jackasses at Loyola don't know anything. This was exceptionally stressful as not only was our reputation on the line with this guy, but the boss and several of the senior attendings, along with the medical students, interns, and junior residents, were closely bunched to hear how I presented the case and what the professor had to say.

Fortunately, the rounding turned out well with him asking questions and people responding, and as we neared the end, he stopped the entourage to look out a bay window that in the distance was the skyline of Chicago. He held up his hand and everyone stopped. Mind you, the boss and everyone else were still there hanging on his every word. We gathered close and he said in effect, "Look at that city, do you know what caused all this?" We gathered closer hoping to hear the next pontification that would enlighten us from this exalted surgeon that we could tell our grandchildren. He repeated, "Look at that city, do you know what caused all this?" We listened harder, until he finally said,"F——-g." The boss said something like, "That wraps up a good visit."

At Eisenhower, as I related before, I suggested the cardiac surgeon invite Viking Bjork (co-inventor of the Bjork-Shiley heart valve) out to possibly join us. While it looks like his first name is pronounced Viking like the NFL Minnesota Vikings, he is from Sweden and it's pronounced Vicking. In fact, he and his wife traveled from Sweden. Viking watched us operate, stayed and eventually joined us and bought a home at the Springs Country Club directly across from the Heart Hospital. He turned out to be a very personable guy and played golf. It was my privilege to play several rounds with him at Morningside Country Club in Rancho Mirage.

One anecdote about Morningside is that before Jack Nicklaus was brought in to design Morningside, there was a dirt road with a long wooden fence that would ultimately be the back end of Morningside. We would drive the kids at night along that road. The cool thing was, almost every time we would see one or two great horned owls sitting on the fence. They were really big and almost white. They would swivel their head like owls do and stare you down. You could get close to them and just watch for a minute or two. While it's great to have a beautiful country club put in, we lost the opportunity to enjoy mother nature.

BLOOD DONATION DURING OPEN HEART SURGERY STORY

Back then (late 1970s), open-heart surgeries lasted several hours, and all during that time, the patient was on cardo-pulmonary bypass via the heart-lung machine. That kept the patient alive but prolonged surgical times meant big-time clotting problems even when we reversed the effect of heparin.

One time at Loyola, I was assisting Dr. Moran on an open-heart case, which took several hours. At the end, we couldn't get the patient to clot. What to do? I asked what the patient's blood type was and it turned out to be "A", my type. I told Dr. Moran, nothing clots like fresh whole blood. Let me go give blood and I'll bring it back. He agreed and off I went.

They called ahead from the OR so the blood bank people were aware of the time factor. I gave the blood and ran back with my blood in the bag. While I scrubbed in, the anesthesiologist gave the blood, and what do you know? As luck would have it, the bleeding stopped and the patient lived, where he might not have. See letter from Dr. Moran below. I could have just let that patient possibly die on the table and no one would have been the wiser. But they trained me to care for people no matter what.

LOYOLA UNIVERSITY MEDICAL CENTER
2160 South First Avenue, Maywood, Illinois 60153   312   531-3000

February 14, 1975

Phillip Bretz, M.D.
1202 Woodbind
Oak Park, Illinois

Dear Doctor Bretz:

    I want to thank you personally for your response to our request
for fresh whole blood for the case of ▮▮▮▮▮▮ on Tuesday, February
4, 1975. Your response and that of others was truly lifesaving in his
particular case, and his family and I would like to express our appreciation for your timely blood donation.

    Mr. ▮▮▮ is doing reasonably well in his convalescence following
his extensive heart surgery, and I believe he should be able to look
forward to a reasonably bright future. Again, thank you for your donation which has helped to make this possible.

Sincerely yours,

JOHN M. MORAN, M.D.
Associate Professor of Surgery

JMM/kjc

I remember my final act as Chief Resident. It was to hand off my
"beeper" to the next poor guy in line who would have ever-increasing
amounts of responsibility on his shoulders. And worse, to have
whatever he did on his soul for all time instead of just selling balloons
at Disneyland. The worst thing that can happen there, is the balloons
escape into the air and everyone claps. This as opposed to the everyday
life of a surgeon that a mistake might cost someone their life.

I walked out of Loyola, I suppose, with a deep sense of accomplishment, having been through medical school in Mexico and finishing a prestigious fledgling surgical career at Loyola. They gave us a party and presented each Chief Resident with their certificates. Those certificates said we had faithfully and successfully completed our residency in general surgery. In the future, I would wonder if those words meant anything? On to Eisenhower.

THE EISENHOWER STORIES

Joan and I flew out with Jason and Ashley the day after my residency ended. I started work at Eisenhower Medical Center (EMC) in Rancho Mirage, California, with Dr. Lesser (the surgeon who took me in, so to speak). I worked in the ER for extra money and also took surgery call for Dr. Lesser and Dr. Garrett since I was the new kid on the block. One story from Loyola that I utilized at EMC was my "Palm Springs" hernia incision. I guess I was about twenty years ahead of my time with small incisions or minimally invasive surgery.

At EMC, my reputation grew as I would have around ten to fifteen patients in the house all the time. One of my first introductions into "private" practice was a small bowel obstruction that came into the ER around 9 p.m. I was manning the ER all night so I took personal care (as I was taught), putting down an NG tube, irrigating it, etc. In the morning, she was transferred up to the floor. After my shift ended, I went up to see her, and she was better. Her belly wasn't as tense, and no pain. I sat down to write a note in the chart when the attending came up to me and said (didn't introduce himself), "Are you going to operate on her?" I said I didn't think so as she was getting better, but if it came to that and she wanted me to, I would. He said, "Like hell, you will," and grabbed the chart right out of my hand. I failed to realize the pecking order, and my trying to provide good care didn't mean anything. I suppose it was partially my fault, but that remains in my mind thirty years later that he could have handled it differently. Later, he was thrown out for drinking.

I remember I gave a Grand Rounds on breast-conserving surgery, i.e., lumpectomy. Dr. Umberto Veronesi (RIP), from Italy had just published his seminal paper (in 1979) about lumpectomy and radiation having the same results as mastectomy. I thought I was going to be thrown off the staff. I was cornered in the locker room by the old guard surgeons and told they realized I just completed my residency but if I didn't do mastectomies, all my patients would die. I had just started doing lumpectomies at Loyola and vividly remember doing mastectomies with Dr. F. and having about ten clamps in the field with some falling on the floor, those horrendous incisions destroying women's bodies for all time. I vowed I would do it differently. To be fair, though, mastectomy at that time was realistically a patient's only hope. I remember a doctor went on vacation, and I saw his patients. It was a woman he had done a lumpectomy on and sent for radiation. She was about halfway through and called the office as she thought something was wrong. Luckily, that was the first and last time I saw a charcoal black dead breast from radiation. I can't remember what happened to her, but I'm sure that breast came off at another institution.

THE NATIONAL INQUIRER STORY

One morning of my three weeks on ER call out of the month, I got a call at about 5 a.m. that there is a woman in the ER that had been hit by a car. So I rushed in and tuned her up, did tests, and took her to surgery. At surgery, she had her colon ripped off its attachments, ruptured spleen and pancreas, two fractured legs and pelvis.

She got through the surgery and then started about a three-month ordeal of ICU care and several other surgeries, including a tracheostomy, bilateral chest tubes (put in because we had to go so high on the respirator to oxygenate her, it would blow her lungs out, a pneumothorax). She developed multiple organ failure because of the trauma and infection, etc. Over the months, she had about six "code blues." I remember one I handled right from my shower at home. One night (the day her son was graduating from high school) she was going down the shoot. There was nothing more I could do. She was on multiple IV drips to maintain her blood pressure, but it wasn't holding her. Then while in bed at about 2 a.m., I remembered at Loyola we used to use the balloon pump (a machine that had a long balloon that was inserted into the patient's femoral artery, and the balloon, when blown up and down, acted like a second heart). It was used for patients who had a heart failure awaiting surgery and after for support. Anyway, I called the cardiac surgeon and convinced him to come in, and we put a pump into her. That turned the tide. She ultimately recovered and was released from EMC after about three months. There was all kinds of press coverage because of the severity of her case and surviving. At the time EMC was trying to get the designation as "the trauma" center in the valley, and it was played up in the TV, papers, etc. There was a nice piece in EMC's newsletter with my story on how "the team" saved this woman alongside pictures of the Bob Hope Classic Ball with (Bob Hope, Jack Nicklaus, Arnold Palmer, etc.). Then the interview came from what I was told was a women's magazine.

Initially and throughout her stay, she was called the "Bird Lady" because when she was hit by the car, it knocked her into the side of the road in a little gully so no one saw her. After a while the ravens started picking on her. We never really resolved the issue of why she was jogging at 2 a.m. up in Anza. Months went by and I was in the hospital making rounds, and a nurse came up to me and said, congratulations, you made the *National Inquirer*. It was billed as "The Miracle Woman." It was my first paper to be published nationally, ha. Years later, I took care of her breast cancer, then they moved away, and I lost track of her. But that was a real defining point in my opinion of myself as a "can do surgeon." I earned my bones on that woman, as they say.

THE BETTY FORD STORY

I had been on the heart team at EMC for about three years. The heart surgeon had asked me to join the team presumably for my reputation of being a damn good surgeon. And having had rotations on the cardiac service at Loyola and with he and I saving the "Bird Lady" at 3 a.m., he made the call. Betty had been having chest pain, and one thing led to another, which was the angiogram. She needed bypass surgery and her carotid artery done because of obstructions in that artery. As soon as the press found out, it was a media frenzy. I had never seen anything like it. There were mobile stations with big dishes and antennas, all ready to record her death at EMC while undergoing heart surgery. Jack and I couldn't walk out of the hospital without microphones put in our faces about her condition. We practiced what to say.

The night before the surgery, we went up to see President Ford, the First Lady, and the family a final time before surgery. My father-in-law, Roy, joked with me (as we were having dinner at his house) as I said I'd like to stay, but I have an appointment with the President. We assured the President that we were up to the task. This was a very risky surgery, though. Usually, one does the carotid artery first (as a separate procedure) and makes sure the patient doesn't stroke from the carotid surgery, then schedule the heart. We did them simultaneously. We told the press we were starting at 10 a.m., but actually, we started at 6 a.m. We did the carotid first, woke her up from anesthesia, and made sure she moved all four extremities, and then put her to sleep again and did her heart. We used both internal mammary arteries, and I took one vein from her leg.

You always look like a hero if you come out of surgery sooner rather than much later. She had come through the surgery and was moving along but slowly. Remember, she was an alcoholic and had had a modified radical mastectomy earlier. Those things add up to a very high risk for any surgery, let alone simultaneous carotid and a triple bypass. There was a push by the media, "When can she go home?" Of course, the sooner she went home, the better we looked as in "wow" she had open heart surgery and is home the next day, really? That didn't happen and it was relatively slow going for a few days.

On the day she was to go home I said to myself, she really doesn't look like she should go home. Anyway, she went as they only lived a few blocks from EMC. A couple of days passed, and I was at home (at Thunderbird, the Fords only lived the next hole down). I had turned off my beeper and unplugged the phone as Betty had been home for some time apparently doing fine. It was Joan, the kids, and me having dinner when there was a pounding on the front door. It reverberated throughout the house like a shot, bam, bam, bam. I got up wondering what the hell as we were in a very secluded part of the city where I paid for privacy. I opened the door, and everyone was shocked to see a very tall state trooper in full dress (hat with braids and all). He asked if I was Dr. Bretz. He said I was needed for the First Lady at the hospital. I thought, "Oh shit," the phone was off, and they couldn't get to me. As I left, I told the trooper that I had to get there fast.

At the time I had a Porsche 928. He said, follow me. I looked at the speedometer and we were doing in excess of 120 mph down Country Club Drive with the trooper's lights and siren going like mad. He was ahead of me and actually spun his car out at the intersection of Country Club and Bob Hope, got out and stopped traffic, holding his arms out and let me through.

It turned out that Betty and the President were at Leonard Firestone's (Firestone tires) for dinner. They had Jello for dessert. The President looked at Betty and said in effect, "You dropped some Jello on your blouse." It was actually blood. She was rushed to EMC, and we ended up in the OR right away. In heart surgery, you don't know if bleeding is from the sternum or the bleeding is from an anastomotic leak which could be fatal.

So off to the OR we go. It turned out to be just from the sternum, probably because of lack of healing power from the mastectomy and both internal mammary arteries being used for the bypass. Incidentally, we use the internal mammary arteries because theoretically 90% remain patent ten years after surgery.

It wouldn't have looked too good if we had knocked off the first lady a few days after surgery. Anyway, with the bleeding controlled, we waited an extra hour just to make sure. Because now we had to take her back to surgery, "What went wrong?", etc. from the media. We didn't want to take her back a third time; as then she might not leave the hospital.

I remember I came out of surgery around midnight. Although no media were there, I turned on the radio and they were announcing in a bulletin that Betty Ford had been taken back to surgery. The nation's eyes were on us again. Luckily, she did well and, indeed, had done well ever since and outlived the President. We became good friends and every time she saw me, she said that every time she takes a shower, she sees the scar I put there, ha. The incision I think was only about an inch long. As time passed and I opened my breast center institute, she would intermittently drop in (unannounced) to bring me a new patient. Her Secret Service detail would come in and visit every room to make sure she would be okay, then bring her in. I felt proud that she would be my friend and trust me to care for her friends.

WILLIAM P. LONGMIRE LIVER SURGEON AT UCLA AT A DISTANCE

One of the first cases when I started at Eisenhower was a patient brought in that was near death and in shock from a botched surgery done outside the valley. I resuscitated the patient with fluids and antibiotics, then it was off to the OR for what is termed an exploratory laparotomy. He presented with an acute abdomen following a gallbladder operation in which the surgeon injured the common bile duct (where the gallbladder empties into). The gallbladder stores, concentrates, and secretes bile which aids in digestion of fats. In any case, on opening the abdomen, I was met with a lot of free bile indicating some major injury to the biliary tree. After some time, I was able to identify the problem—a big rent in the common bile duct. Sometimes after the gallbladder is removed, a surgeon will do a cholangiogram, which is a dye test that outlines the common bile duct.

If there is a gallstone in there, the surgeon opens the duct, removes the stone and closes with a T-tube that serves as a drain and later removed. A hole like that in the common bile duct is well controlled. A false move at surgery resulting in extensive destruction of the common bile duct requires some major reconstruction.

For a moment I thought of trying to repair it with either a vein patch or bringing a loop of small bowel to hook up to the duct. Then in a flash I thought of Dr. Longmire at UCLA, one of the world's leading liver surgeons. I decided to not try and repair this as I knew Dr. Longmire could probably do it better than anyone. This case shows my ability to delegate surgery to a higher authority than myself (at that time).

I just drained the common bile duct, and with adequate drainage, the patient was stable. I called UCLA and was able to get to Dr. Longmire's resident and told him the story. He accepted the case and the patient was transferred as soon as that was arranged. Some days later I got a call from that resident who told me that the patient arrived "as advertised" and initially he thought about taking the case on by himself but then had second thoughts. Upon reflection, he said there was only one man who should do it, and that was Dr. Longmire. As I remember, I think they did a (Longmire I) procedure where the small bowel is hooked up to the liver so the bile flows into it directly instead of trying to repair something that is not repairable.

Dr. Longmire was a legend in general surgery. He studied under Alfred Blalock, the surgeon who developed the operation to save "blue babies," the term used to describe a congenital condition known as the Tetralogy of Fallot. There is an article on Dr. Longmire by one of his residents who remembers that the thing about Dr. Longmire was that he'd never be content with just doing an operation. He was always trying to make the procedure better. Sound familiar?

THE APPENDIX STORY

This was definitely one of those times in a surgeon's life where he earns his bones and thereafter can feel confident standing toe to toe with anyone. As Dr. Blakely would have said, "It was a fundamental day." This story involves KS and his family. K was my medical student when I was Chief Resident at Loyola. He wanted to become a surgeon, so I kept track of his progress. I had him come out to Palm Springs after his residency. He was supposed to learn enough in the heart room to relieve me so I could go on vacation (which I hadn't been on for six years). While that didn't work out, this episode did.

One day K's wife called that their two-year-old child (a girl) was not looking good. She had a fever. She was listless and getting to be unresponsive. We told her to bring her into the ER, and as soon as we finished the case we were on, we would come down. Now with my rotation at Chicago Children's Hospital, I learned that these small kids could go down the shoot very rapidly. One minute they are looking at you, and the next, they are near death. This kid was obviously very sick, and something rapidly had taken over her body. We put her in ICU and reviewed her labs. She had a temp of about 103 (kids can run high temps), and her white count was elevated (it gets elevated in infections), and she was moribund.

In examining her, I noted that she winced when I pushed her abdomen in the right lower quadrant (where your appendix is). The odds of a two-year-old having appendicitis were small, but it sure looked like a surgical disease to me and not viral which is so often the case. With the kid going downhill fast, we had to decide whether to treat her at EMC or have her helicoptered to Loma Linda where they had a children's ward. I asked K if we thought she had appendicitis, and if so, could they do a better job than us? The answer was no. The problem was if we (meaning me because I made the diagnosis) were wrong, his child might die from something treatable non-surgically like a viral infection.

We decided to take her to surgery, a bold move. While we were scrubbing, I looked at K and asked him, "Who's the best surgeon you ever saw?" before he could reply, I continued with, "You're looking at him." It is a line out of the movie *The Right Stuff*, only it was an astronaut asking his wife, "Who's the best pilot you ever saw?"

Well, talk about pressure, everyone in that operating room wondering if this kid was going to die, and we had overstepped our bounds. You could cut the tension with a knife. With the child teetering on death and her father assisting me, I made the tiny incision. I got through the abdominal wall, and the moment of truth was at hand. Did this two-year-old have appendicitis? It is the moment of truth with any surgeon who takes a person to surgery for appendicitis, and maybe you take out a normal appendix. I stuck in my finger and fished around a little, and there it was. You can feel the inflamed appendix before you see it. I think I said something like, "Thank God." Yes, I delivered an infected appendix that was about as big as your thumb through the small incision, much to everyone's amazement. The heat was off; we had done it. Perhaps others could have done it, but others were not there to make that life and death decision. Needless to say, your stature increases several fold after something like that where you're playing for all the marbles. All these cases add up in their ability to make a real surgeon out of you.

THE PHIL STORY

No, it's not about me. It's about another Phil who again had sustained what would ultimately turn out to be a mortal complication done by another surgeon in town. Remember, I wrote before that a surgeon who says he/she hasn't been up to their ass in alligators is a liar? Well, this was my case. A surgeon has to take cases like this one and after, get up and face a new day. Sometimes it's hard to do. As a result of this, I remember Phil in my prayers every night though I did the best I could.

I felt I had been trained at Loyola to take on most anything, that is from start to finish, where you're the one responsible for keeping everyone else out of trouble. Taking on another surgeon's life-threatening complication is another matter. This case occurred during my first year at Eisenhower and resulted in a wrongful death suit. It was my only lawsuit in the thirty years at Eisenhower where I performed thousands of surgeries. This covers the thirty-three years since I became a dedicated breast surgeon. That takes into account that breast cancer surgeons are the most frequently sued surgeons, aside from obstetrics. The reason is, as the lawyers say, it's the failure to diagnose cancer in a timely fashion.

That's over 13,000 patients in those thirty-three years since 1988, so I must have been doing something right all the time. Phil came by ambulance to Eisenhower ER, where he was another patient near death around 3 a.m., in shock and had obviously had sustained a severe complication from another surgeon in town. It turned out Phil had had a subtotal gastrectomy (removal of most of his stomach) from bleeding. The surgeon used a family practitioner as the assistant. Well, upon entering the abdomen I was met with a "sea of pus" as I remember I said in response to questions. His surgery was over ten days before and the bowel was matted together and very fragile where it could tear apart and make things dramatically worse in an instant.

It turned out almost the entire anastomosis (where the surgeon had sutured small bowel to the remnant of the stomach), had fallen apart. I repaired this the best I could. He stabilized and I waited about ten days until I tested the new repair with methylene blue down the nasogastric tube (a tube into the stomach to suck fluid up when the bowel isn't working). Sure enough, while there wasn't an outpouring of methylene blue, there was some staining on the drain when I removed it. This meant another surgery before he again became septic. Probably about two to three other surgeries followed, it's hard to remember now. He spent weeks and weeks in the ICU and Dr. Curry was instrumental in helping with his endoscopy evaluations. But I got him through all that. Phil had been on total parenteral nutrition (TPN) for all that time. In spite of that, he had lost a lot of weight.

Upon discharge he was eating a soft diet and I visited him at home a couple of times. The problem was his dentures didn't fit anymore, resulting in his inability to eat solid foods leading to further weight loss. Eventually this led to his re-admission to a VA hospital. Their insurance had been maxed out.

Upon entering the VA some intern or resident started a central line (a large IV) going into the subclavian vein under the collar bone which was well within standard of care. The problem was he developed a yeast infection which ultimately did him in. When a lawyer sues a doctor, it always says and "50 John Does." Why fifty? Because they can. In any case, because while I was not responsible for the fatal yeast infection, I did perform multiple surgeries on Phil. So, I was included in the suit along with the VA people and the original surgeon. Lesson learned on that case was that probably a major surgery should be performed with another surgeon, not a family practitioner. That's one of the reasons Dr. Kopp and I assisted each other. Of course, functionaries have outlawed two surgeons assisting each other probably just to save money. As I said, I remember Phil in my prayers every night and carry his memory every day of my life.

THE BOMB BOY STORY

I was on ER call (of course) and I heard the ambulance siren and I just waited for the call to come. It was a young boy brought in from the high desert having been the recipient of his homemade bomb going off. I came right in and we got IVs going, limited X-rays, blood work and type and cross. He had sustained, that I could see, multiple lacerations on abdomen, chest, arms and face. But the kicker was the open wound in his abdomen and on portable chest X-ray, his liver was in his chest indicating at minimum a major diaphragmatic injury. He was going downhill and there was no time for further studies or consent from his parents. It was just him and me. Dr. Kopp assisted me. As soon as the OR crew was ready, we rushed him to the OR. He was not able to understand anything or sign anything, thus no informed consent.

We prepped both his abdomen and chest just in case we needed to extend our abdominal incision into a thoracotomy. I did a midline incision from the xiphoid to past the umbilicus giving us plenty of room. With cases like this one, there was no minimal incisions. On entering the abdomen, I suctioned out the blood and noted his liver had disappeared into his right chest as advertised. A cursory inspection of the stomach, and large and small bowel did not disclose any damage. I then slowly insinuated my left hand up into the chest just above the liver. Once reaching the dome of the liver, I gently (and gingerly) inched the liver back into its proper resting place. I patched up the liver lacerations (thanks to Dr. Freeark insisting I resect that one trauma patient's liver). Once that was done without further injury, I repaired the diaphragm and inserted a chest tube. In short order, he was stable and the anesthesiologist was relieved. We checked his abdomen again and closed. I turned my attention to his multiple skin laceration and cleaned them and sutured with a subcuticular stitch so he wouldn't have any railroad marks from sutures on the face. He had an uneventful recovery. I think we nicknamed him "Fast Eddy."

THE JEFF LEVINE STORY (SENIOR MEDICAL CORRESPONDENT CNN 1990)

Our open hearing with the FDA of their Oncology Drugs Advisory Committee for my prevention trial was on June 29, 1990, at the Crown Plaza Holiday Inn in Rockville Pike, Maryland. As I said before, by that time I was calling the team, "Showtime." Back then, cell phones weren't ubiquitous, talking heads weren't on every TV station 24/7, and CNN was the only TV corporation to show up. It turned out covering the hearing was Jeff Levine, at the time their senior medical correspondent.

While we didn't achieve our goals that day, Jeff did interview me afterwards, stating that he wanted to do a story on me and the prevention effort. He and the crew came out to the Desert Breast Institute in Rancho Mirage. My friend and colleague, Brigadier General Lynch, was in Bulgaria listening to CNN getting ready to go to dinner and he was shocked to see me being interviewed. Following that interview, I received a letter from people in Sophia, Bulgaria, saying they wanted to be part of the trial and if it could be done involving the Soviets, it would be a Nobel Peace Prize.

Jeff soon came out and did a three-part series on my prevention efforts. Off camera he told me, it's like you're "the champion of women's rights." He said it, I didn't. He would invite me to the National Press Club for lunch on one of my trips back to DC. I think while CNN wasn't afforded any official capacity, their involvement helped to get the message out that it was time for Big Pharma and the NCI to look at prevention. Remember, this was 1990. Jeff and I have remained friends over the years. He is a good guy.

In the movie *The Hospital* starring George C. Scott, he says after losing his desire to work, "We have established the most enormous medical entity ever conceived and people are sicker than ever. We heal nothing, we cure nothing," he yells out the window. The question is, how do we change all of this?

A BAND OF BROTHERS

I feel sorry for the doctors (or should I say providers) of today that perhaps don't have this relationship with their fellow comrades in arms that I did. I can't think of a time in all my thirty years at Eisenhower where I ever felt alone in my daily work as a surgeon. It was all unspoken, of course, but I knew that if I needed anyone (like the men I mentioned before), all I had to do was ask and they would drop everything and anything they were doing to render assistance. There was no getting requisitions from any gatekeeper, you just went. We worked hard to care for the patients like we would want to be cared for. In the process, Eisenhower enjoyed a very good reputation in the community as the go-to hospital. If one of the guys got a new car, there was a tradition that he would put a card in the window that said, "Don't touch this car unless you are completely nude." There was even a time when a group of us contemplated buying a jet. When we came back to Earth, often there would be parties, especially on Halloween. Desert Orthopedics would always throw a big one and everyone looked forward to it. Below are a couple of photos from one party. I thought the reader would get a kick out of seeing how the docs at EMC partied. Joan went as a brick and I was the bricklayer. We won first place!

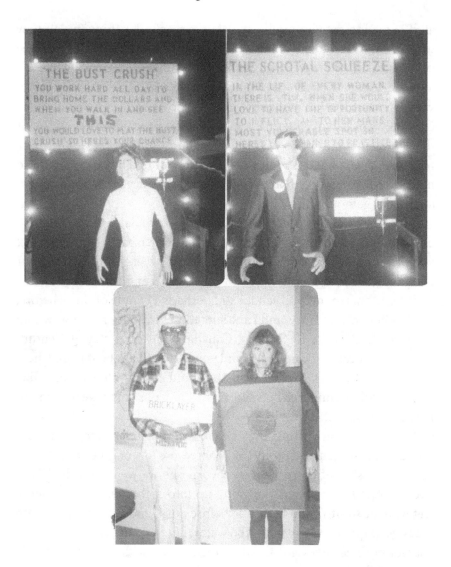

FISHING STORIES

I think being able to outwit the fish is the essence of fishing (aside from eating the fish). To come into a bay and determine where that big fish might be is the real hunt. Nowadays, there are all sorts of fishing aids from depth and fish finders to scents you put on the lure, etc. They are all designed to get you more fish. We have a similar thing in golf now with distance finders. Fishing should be just you and the fish. To see if you can outsmart that fish without all the equipment is where it's at for me. Any idiot can get fish if you have a fish finder and scent on your bait. But it takes real know-how to decide where in that cove (in Canada) your fish of a lifetime awaits. To make the odds even more for the fish, you could make your own lure and use light tackle so you're really at a disadvantage. I once made a lure out of a bypass graft. I also made a lure out of one of my patient's earrings she gave me and caught a ton of largemouth bass on it.

Then the catch is all the more satisfying, especially if it's a big fish because that fish has seen a lot of lures and other bait and is wise, but you fooled him. That's real fishing, just like it's real golf to rely on your gut instinct as to what the yardage to the hole is and what club to use.

When I was in medical school and perhaps a couple of times before, my brother-in-law, Gary, and I and sometimes my father-in-law, would go up to Eagle Lake in Ontario, Canada. We would stay at Century Lodge. It is located on an island, and you had to take a boat from where you parked the car. We were in the "land of sky-blue waters" like Hamm's beer commercials (sponsor of the Cubs thirty years ago) or now called "sunset country."

You knew that during that twenty-minute boat ride, you were probably passing many trophy fish. There were lots of little coves where you could fish, but there was one special one we went to (called "The Creek") that had a channel opening up into it that was about twenty feet wide or so. It would be a little before dusk, and we would slip into the cove as quietly as possible. The water there was like a mirror. It was a larger cove as coves go, about a block across with thousands of lily pads, and then there was the clear area leading into the channel where it was about a boat wide. The water was relatively clear, and you could see about thirty yards or so on a good day. You could see the fish many times. For some reason (probably feeding), there was usually a big fish in there. It was really neat to cast the lure down the narrow channel and see it splash in mirror water and slowly retrieve it anticipating that big swirl in the water just before you felt the strike. Doing that kind of fishing during a Canadian sunset recalls for me one of the most cherished times in my life.

When Jason was smaller, around twelve, we went to Northern Manitoba to an outpost camp, living in tents for a week, taking swims in icy cold water for bathing, eating shore lunches, the kind of experience that creates real lifelong memories. It was so cold the mosquitoes were flying in slow motion. Our proprietor said they were much more than a tent. Upon arrival, Jason was the first in the tent and came back to me and said, "Don't get your hopes up."

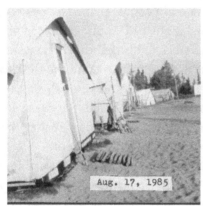
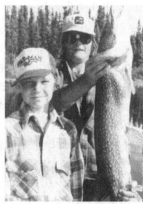

Aug. 17, 1985

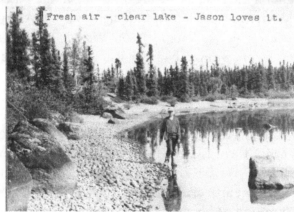

Fresh air - clear lake - Jason loves it.

I always listen for the distinct sound of the Otter seaplane as the props change pitch, and I watched it take off, and there was nothing but silence and the beautiful Canadian north. The tent had two cots, one bowl, one roll of toilet paper, and a little stove with scant wood and one candle.

The mornings were frigid, and since Jason wasn't moving from his bed, I went down to the lake for water to wash at least. We laughed as he said, "We'll have to go to the guide and ask them to start our fire." But little did Jason know he was with "Nanuk of the North."

Our fire was always going in the morning. We would be up early and walk over to the breakfast tent for a hearty bowl of Red River, eggs and pancakes, all the while thinking about the lucky guys who had coffee brought to their log cabins at the main camp. That first day we caught well over 200 fish. The largest was about a 15-pound northern pike that Jason caught. Our shore lunches were nothing short of magical with a lot of lard for the potatoes (just what a guy likes), and the fresh-caught northern were crispy and sweet. As the days wore on, going without a shower proved to be more than I could handle. So, every so often during shore lunch, I would strip down and wade out into the lake, which was very cold. Luckily, I didn't get anything bit off.

Then one day Jason, who had become quite adept at casting, threw his lure out a good distance, and he must have hit this 20-pound northern right on the head as the big thrashing in the water occurred just a second after his lure hit, and the fight was on. As it turns out, the fish was just about as long as Jason was tall, and the fight took some minutes before we even had a look at the big guy. It is those few precious minutes when you know there is a big one on, and he's down under for five minutes, that you don't know how big it is.

Then he surfaces and trashes around, and it's something I hope Jason never forgets. Another time we were back at Century Lodge in Ontario, Canada. There is a creek there that is probably my favorite spot on Earth. This year, 2017, Jason and I were fishing the creek. I had thrown almost all my artificial baits and nothing. Then I reached for my homemade lure, and no sooner did it hit the water than I felt the tug of a big fish. We don't use heavy lines, so it creates a level playing field for the fish. That is to say, you can't just horse the fish in. It took about ten minutes to get this thing close, then he jumped. It was a big muskie (the fish of 10,000 casts). It took all I had to get him in and unhook him and raise him up.

Using light tackle, after a fifteen-minute fight, we landed her, the one that didn't get away. After we measured her at 48 inches, she was released unharmed as was Jason's muskie. It was the thrill of a lifetime.

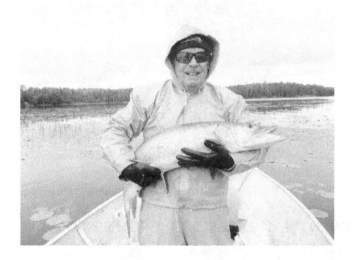

The next day we were in a bay that looked like Jesus made it (maybe he did). Jason lit into a very nice northern Pike, and as he said, he was vindicated. On the very next cast in the same bay at the end of his cast, he felt a big tug also. This fish was way out there. Often though, muskies will strike right next to the boat if, upon retrieving the lure, one does a figure of eight. The fish got hung up in weeds, and I had to clean his rod tip of the cabbage. The sun came out, and I was able to see that it was indeed another big muskie. Then we finally landed this beast and got him unhooked; the expression on Jason's face was what every dad should see. I have it on tape. Both his and my muskie were 48 inches. However, Jason claims his was slightly bigger. No problem, that's how it should be. When I'm up at Century, I always threaten that I'm not going to leave. I'm so at peace there. The Canadian wild is in my soul. One of my biggest wishes is that the Lavender Breast Centers take off, and I can go fishing more often.

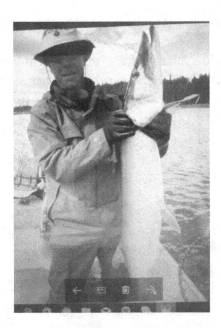

THE TWENTYNINE PALMS AIR GROUND COMBAT STORY

I had some strange experiences covering the ER at Twentynine Palms. The first was when I had been there just a few days. The base holds military exercises that involve about a thousand military personnel from all over. They parachute and fire live rounds from the howitzers they have. It's the only base that is large enough to fire live rounds. Well, this guy was brought in with a fractured arm. He said just cast it, and I'll get back into the action. Then another day of the exercises, they brought in a body that had been decapitated from a helicopter accident. During the same exercise, a Marine was brought in who had coded (doing CPR), and he still had his helmet on. I started a central line and began medications to stabilize his heart. Then someone removed his helmet, and he had no brain in his skull. He had backed into a propeller and sustained a mortal injury.

Later one night, around 3 a.m., a civilian was brought in with a markedly swollen hand and arm. He was drunk and had had an encounter with a rattlesnake, which resulted in it biting his hand. He said, "Don't worry, doc, I grabbed him and bit his head off." I gave him antivenom and sent him to Eisenhower by helo.

Lastly, a Marine was brought in that had a grenade go off near his hand and shattered it and his forearm. I stabilized the bleeding and transferred him. At times the ER there seemed like a war zone. Other times, it was really cool, like when the silent drill team came; it was an unbelievable routine.

During this time, when I was losing everything, the episode of the burning sport utility vehicle and saving Fred occurred. That resulted in my being awarded the Carnegie Medal for an outstanding act of heroism. I received letters of commendation from the Commanding General and the Commander of the Naval unit at Twentynine Palms. It felt good that I received their recognition since they knew real heroes. At the end of my tour, they had a party for me at Kobe's restaurant in Rancho Mirage. They gave me a Twentynine Palms medical unit hat. I wore it with pride until it wore out. It was an honor for me to have served with them and, in a small way, helped me get over the guilt I felt for not serving my country during the Vietnam War.

PRESIDENT REAGAN'S SECRET SERVICE AGENT GOES DOWN

It was the time of year when Ambassador Walter Annenberg (from his home at Sunnylands in Rancho Mirage) held his annual New Year's party. The list of notables and celebrities was evident. Black helicopters flew around, and we were on alert. We had formed a "team" that would essentially be ready at a moment's notice to race into the hospital if something happened to the President. That meant no drinking and notifying people where you were. I didn't want us to get caught by surprise like the docs at Parkland. New Year's passed without incident until about 3 a.m. and the phone rang. One of President Reagan's Secret Service detail was in the ER with abdominal pain. Dr. Kopp and I were there in a flash. After some testing and clinical examination, it was determined he needed an exploratory laparotomy (opening up his abdomen). He had a small bowel obstruction from previous surgery. These surgeries can be pretty tricky with the bowel matted together and the bowel easily torn by even the gentlest of maneuvers. That would lead to infection or worse.

Then to add to the situation, the core of the detail had accompanied their colleague and were obvious strong friends like combat buddies. We said if the patient didn't mind, we invited them in to observe the surgery. Nothing puts hair on your chest and builds character like the Secret Service peering over your shoulder when you're doing a delicate operation and them saying, "Hey doc, what's that?" The special agent did fine. And this operation and the ability to pull it off did not go unnoticed by the White House Physician. This is another example in a building series of my ability and professionalism.

THE WHITE HOUSE

WASHINGTON

January 13, 1985

Dear Doctors Kopp and Bretz:

I would like to thank you both very much for the care and attention afforded Special Agent Dana Brown during his surgery at your facility. We are very appreciative of your care, concern and timely reaction to this situation.

In our travels, to various cities, we are concerned with the capabilities of hospitals. Your expertise has only increased our confidence in Eisenhower Hospital Medical Center to provide care to the President of the United States and his staff.

Again, on behalf of The White House and White House Medical Unit, thank you for excellent cooperation.

Sincerely,

T. Burton Smith, M.D.
Physician to the President

They don't let stumblebums operate on the First Lady and Secret Service personnel. It was extremely gratifying to read the letter from the White House Physician about how they felt about our service and how confident they were in the ability of Eisenhower Medical Center to provide care to the President and his staff. Cool!

THE SAGAS OF DBI, THE COMPASS TREATMENT, TAMOXIFEN, AND LAVENDER

If we start from the beginning, there were really no comprehensive breast centers in 1988. Remember, I had presented Grand Rounds on my arrival to EMC in 1979, extolling the virtues of lumpectomy versus mastectomy. When I got involved with the heart team, my general surgery stopped. After nine years, I thought that all the women were being taken care of with lumpectomies and were living happily ever after. I was dead wrong. And going back to Loyola and the commando procedures we were taught (probably rightly so back then), but remember, I wanted to forge a new path for women. The heart team put that quest on the back burner. After nine years on the heart team, I reviewed the data and found the same 40,000 women were dying of breast cancer and mastectomy still ruled. I decided if I had to do it singlehandedly, I would.

I started DBI in 1988, just before I was unceremoniously dismissed from the heart team. But with DBI, I felt I was home where I should be. My idea of a comprehensive breast center was to have state-of-the-art imaging and committed, talented people who were on the same page as me, all in a non-threatening, inviting setting (with antiques, coffee, and cookies). The live person who answered the phone had to be knowledgeable and inviting to every patient every time. You have read some of the patient letters. I think I hit the mark. That was the bricks and mortar part. The other part was how we, as a team, would approach the patient. The *sine qua non* would be that as the diagnostic person and surgeon, I would only be able to make a diagnosis with a needle biopsy. Then before any treatment, the patient would see the oncologist and radiation therapist. This was significant with the dawn of neoadjuvant chemotherapy (given before any surgery), Before this, the radiation therapist and oncologist never got to see the patient before surgical intervention.

From the first day I opened, patients flocked in, getting away from the hospital's more impersonal and sterile setting, to a doctor they could count on knowing them, being there anytime they needed me, and providing better than cutting edge care. I was seeing over twenty-five patients a day for mammography, in addition to doing stereotactic core biopsies and surgeries. In fact, the chairman of the Department of Radiology at Eisenhower told Dr. Dreisbach that I was the enemy. *What?* Oh well, if the hospital didn't want to provide a setting like mine, that was okay with me. As time passed, I brought to Eisenhower the possibility of incorporating DBI, but each time it was turned down. Stereotactic core biopsy was another first for the valley brought in by me. That is a biopsy procedure performed via the mammogram machine that spared the patient a surgery (open biopsy as in the old days). I had done a lot of stereos and was pretty good at it.

The Tamoxifen clinical trial is detailed in *Sacrificing America's Women II*, but just to glimpse it here, I had joined the largest breast cancer research group, the National Surgical Adjuvant Breast Project (NSABP). When we went up to Canada for the annual meeting that year, I noted that none of their protocols offered anything to prevent breast cancer. It just popped into my head that for many years then, we had been giving Tamoxifen to prevent recurrences. I surmised that if we were asking Tamoxifen to potentially control millions of cancer cells, then it made sense to me (without evidence-based medicine) that if you had Tamoxifen on board in high-risk women, that when that first lone cancer cell appeared, it would snuff it out. Yeah, yeah, I can hear some of you now. What about the side effects?

So, Tamoxifen was the only drug we had back then (1989), and the truth was that most girls could tolerate it well to prevent recurrences, and it was their friend. If you couldn't tolerate it, at least you tried. Well, I was the only one in the country to come up with this idea, and as I said before, everyone thought I was crazy. Ultimately, the government spent $68 million on that idea, and six years later, Tamoxifen became the first drug to be FDA-approved to prevent breast cancer by lowering the risk by 50%. Now we have Evista, which not only helps with bone preservation but also lowers breast cancer risk by 50%. Evista is a selective estrogen receptor modulator (SERM) class drug. But how do you know if you're at higher risk when you have no family history? You can do the breast cancer risk test by Phenogen Sciences. That whole saga is fascinating how it developed a life of its own and what happened and how your tax money is spent. The firsts continue.

I was selected to participate in that vaccine trial. You can see below the company we were keeping. While this didn't work, it launched a new and different path in dealing with breast cancer. I felt as though I/ we were closing in on our prey.

CTL ImmunoTherapies Corp.

Protocol No. 157-165B

A Phase I/II Study of Intranodal Delivery of Synchrovax BPL Vaccine, an Episode Synchronization Plasmid DNA Vaccine, in Stage IV Breast Carcinoma Patients

Principal Investigators:

Dr James R. Waisman
USC/Norris Comprehensive Cancer Center
Harold E. and Henrietta C. Lee Breast Center
1441 Eastlake Avenue, Suite 3440
Los Angeles, CA 90033
Tel: 323.865.3906 Fax: 323.865.0061
Email: waisman@hsc.usc.edu

Dr. Alison T. Stopeck
Arizona Cancer Center
1515 N. Campbell Ave.
P.O. Box 245024
Tucson, AZ 85724
Tel: 520.626.2816 Fax: 520.626.2225
Email: astopeck@azcc.arizona.edu

Co-Investigators:

Dr. George Somlo
City of Hope National Medical Center
Beckman Research Institute
1500 East Duarte Road
Duarte, CA 91010-3000
Tel: 626.359.8111 Ext. 2867 Fax: 626.301.8233
Email: gsomlo@coh.org

Dr. Phillip Bretz and Dr. Philip Dreisbach
Desert Hematology Oncology Medical Group, Inc.
39800 Bob Hope Dr., Suite C
Rancho Mirage, CA 92270
Tel: 760.568.3613 Fax: 760.340.5189
Email: tamdoc@aol.com

Dr. John W. Smith II
Earle A. Chiles Research Institute
Providence Portland Medical Center
4805 N.E. Glisan, Suite 5F40
Portland OR 97213
Tel: 503.215.3655 Fax: 503.215.6841
Email: jsmith3@providence.org

Dr. James L. Murray
MD Anderson Cancer Center
1515 Holcombe Blvd.
Box 0422
Houston, TX 77030-4009
Tel: 713.792.4561 Fax: 713.792.8189
e-mail: jmurray@mdanderson.org

Dr. Paula M. Fracasso
Washington University School of Medicine
660 South Euclid Street, Box 8056
St. Louis, MO 63110
Tel: 314.454.8817 Fax: 314.454.5218
e-mail: fracasso@im.wustl.edu

Version Date: July 15, 2002
May 4, 2002

A STUDY OF TRIAB® (11D10) AND CEAVAC® (3H1) ANTI-IDIOTYPE MONOCLONAL ANTIBODIES IN COMBINATION WITH FIRST LINE HORMONAL THERAPY FOR PATIENTS WITH METASTATIC BREAST CANCER

Protocol   TTP-310-01-01   23APR01

Products: TriAb® and CeaVac®

IND No.:   BB-9453

Sponsor: Medical Monitor:
Titan Pharmaceuticals, Inc.   Harold Keer, M.D., Ph.D.
400 Oyster Point Blvd., Suite 505   Associate Director, Clinical Development
South San Francisco, CA 94080 USA   Telephone: (650) 244-4990, Ext. 282
                                     Fax: (650) 244-4956

Approved By:

_____   ___4/23/01___
Harold Keer, M.D., Ph.D.   Date
Associate Director, Clinical Development
Titan Pharmaceuticals, Inc.

Signature by the Principal Investigator acknowledges that he/she has reviewed the entire contents of this protocol on or before the signature date, and is in agreement with this protocol's conduct, as well as confidentiality.

_____
Principal Investigator's Signature

___5-9-01___
Date

___PHILLIP D. BRETZ, M.D.___
Print Principal Investigator's Name

The next thing was intraoperative radiation therapy (IORT). This was really a quantum leap. For decades we were told that you had to do external beam radiation or there would be occult cancers that would eventually cause a developing cancer. We all swallowed the Kool-Aid of that dogma. Then like I said, APBR came out in around 2004, and I helped pioneered that technology and published my results in ASTRO as you read. I invented a new operation (the Fat Patch) so that many more women could be candidates for APBR. While APBR wasn't a quantum leap in technology, it was just radiation twice daily for five days. With IORT, that was a quantum leap by providing radiation therapy for twenty minutes during the lumpectomy. So, when the patient woke up in the recovery room, she was done with her surgery and radiation therapy.

How is that possible when, for decades, the hierarchy told us that the only acceptable thing was the standard five weeks of daily radiation with a boost at the end? How can twenty minutes twice daily for five days of targeted radiation be better than six weeks? Remember, APBR radiated 1 centimeter around the lumpectomy margin, where about 90% of the local recurrences are found. It just took out-of-the-box thinking (rational thoughts) without evidence-based medicine and utilizing one's experience. Someone thought correctly that you could manipulate breast cancer, enabling a better outcome for all. In this case, targeted radiation. And years later, the people who condemned APBR would have to eat crow (assuming it was performed correctly). As I said, without anyone mentoring me, I did about forty-five cases and never (that I know of) had a local recurrence.

But when IORT came along, that's when the light bulb went off. Not only the light bulb, but it led to the end game I had been searching for. I searched for decades without knowing what the end game was until it appeared. I put the jigsaw puzzle together. I want you to realize the step-by-step enlightenment I went through from radical mastectomy to pioneering neoadjuvant chemotherapy to lumpectomy to cosmetic lumpectomy to authoring the Tamoxifen prevention trial, and from external beam radiation to APBR to IORT and on to the crown jewel, liquid nitrogen. I didn't think it up in my garage. This would allow me to use targeted liquid nitrogen to kill breast cancer in about twenty minutes outside the operating room and outside the hospital, and outside the system altogether. But it wasn't just that revelation. It was the fact that I had put together a method (the Lavender Way) that could find breast cancers ostensibly before they could metastasize (spread), maybe not every time but damn near. That was the real triumph for me. It wasn't that I knew so much more or was way smarter than the thousands of researchers across the country; it was that I had been on a different path that enabled me to see the potential in each method and then capitalize on it (without limitations), for the benefit of women worldwide. The Lavender Way and Lavender Procedure were the keys, and I went straight to work exploiting the idea. To my knowledge, no one was working on or had come up with a way to combine diagnostic capability (especially non-radiation modalities) with therapeutic capability. I knew if a patient was high-risk, we couldn't get mammography or MRIs every six months for G-d knows how long. But I could use non-radiation modalities all day long without affecting the patient while finding ultra-small cancers. This held true even for pregnant women. I had put the pieces of the puzzle together, and I only needed to do it. I was the only one on Earth with these specific modalities in one place. Finding cancer before it could spread and then being able to kill it in twenty minutes outside the system was the key.

As we will read later, the accusations directed at me by the competitor surgeon in town made it sound like I really cooked this up in my garage, fleecing patients left and right. Instead, I was using all FDA-approved (via clinical trials) modalities that had been summarily dismissed by the system as inferior, irrelative, but they weren't. It had taken many years for technology to catch up with breast cancer but it finally did if one bothered to look. Or should I say the reader will decide if what I accomplished against all odds was inferior, irrelative, and inappropriate?

In the end, I will repeat this; I thought we were all in this cancer battle together, each one contributing what he could for better outcomes and further, that in the end, for each patient, they had the right (after all options were discussed multiple times) to choose their own course of treatment. Even if that treatment meant eating nothing but blueberries to fight their cancer. Further, no one or entity would decree what a patient was allowed to choose, only the patient, regardless of whether the treatment wasn't scientifically sound, but I hope the reader will see Lavender was.

And furthermore, that this was a step-by-step process evaluating multiple modalities over decades to bring me to Lavender. Again, this is not something I cooked up in the garage. I was not performing dangerous, unethical procedures in an unprofessional manner. May my soul be damned if I EVER acted in an unprofessional, unethical, or negligent manner over forty years of caring for thousands of patients around the world.

When I started out with founding DBI, I had no idea of how to do anything except follow what I was given as Principal Investigator with the NSABP. After I realized there was nothing on the horizon for breast cancer prevention, I began to think of alternative ways to defeat breast cancer. Looking back, the journey was almost like the poem by Vermont poet Robert Frost, "The Road Not Taken."

In that poem, what is apropos is not only did I take the road less traveled, and that had made all the difference, but in that poem, he has a line about "way leading to way." My journey was just like that. You have the inclination to see what's around the corner (before anyone else) and when you go around the corner, there is a door and then a path to another door, not knowing where it will lead you. Each time I did something new, it was a piece of the puzzle for me to eventually see the whole picture of being able to combine non-radiation diagnostic modalities with a therapeutic modality to kill breast cancer outside the system for a hell of a lot less money. There was no evidence-based medicine here, just common sense, curiosity, and experience. All this would be BS, except I have the cancer-free patients going on seven years out to prove it. On to a lighter note, now.

STORIES OF MY FATHER-IN-LAW (PAPA)

One day (still in high school), Joan had driven downtown to a modeling job with me, and on coming home, we saw a black split-window 63 Vette. It looked cool. As it turns out, driving that Vette was Joan's father, Roy Pedersen. Roy was a car enthusiast and was a race official with the Sports Car Club of America (SCCA), as was his brother, Bill. Papa, as he was later called, told many interesting stories. Like the time when they were trying to smash the atom under Stag Field at the University of Chicago and were looking for some part; otherwise, they couldn't proceed. As fate would have it, who had the part? Pedersen Brothers Tool and Supply, of course. So, to hear the tale from Papa, the first controlled splitting of the atom would not have taken place without Pedersen Brothers providing the critical part.

Papa had a close friend named Ernie Erickson. Ernie had a construction company in Chicago and built skyscrapers. He always had a yellow Porsche. He and Papa raced at Le Mans, France, one year but were heavy into racing locally, like at Road America, which Ernie helped build. Ernie had a big warehouse where the Elva Porsche race car was stored, and they would work on it. His place was right next to Northwestern Golf and the Lava Lamp people. Ernie also had a 550 Spyder and RS 60. Below are a couple of iconic race cars. I was a pit inspector at Road America because of Papa, and could get up close and personal with those cars. The #66 was Jim Hall's Chaparral. In fact, that's Jim in the driver's seat with his checkered flag. That is Ken Mile's Essex Wire #92 (otherwise known as a Ford F-40), the #13 was Carroll Shelby's Cobra, and #64 was Bill Thomas's Cheetah. Ernie Erickson (Papa's racing partner) driving his Porsche, got into a fender bender with Jim Hall's other Chaparral #65. Racing at Elkhart Lake's Road America and because I got to be a "pit inspector" was an experience I'll never forget. It was definitely cool. Then, too, Papa always had bratwurst on the grill.

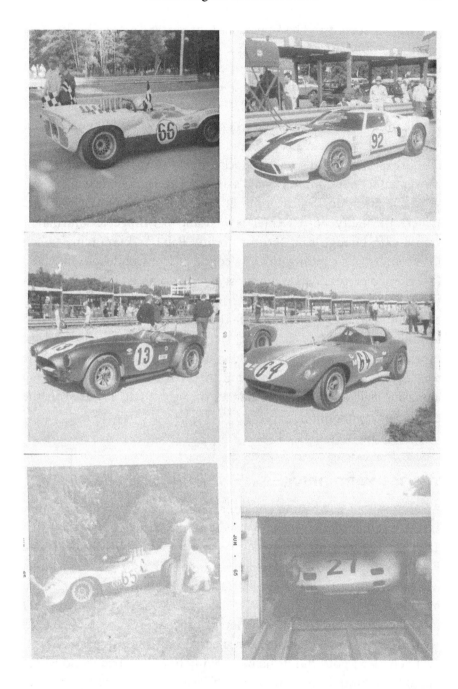

Papa was a pilot and had a plane, a four-seater Cessna. One time, he was flying out west with a couple of buddies, and one owned a twin-engine Beechcraft. While not twin-engine rated, while everyone was asleep, Papa was flying the plane down into the Grand Canyon. Papa was a member of the Evanston Golf Club. Later he would take me to play golf there. It was also the place where we had our wedding reception. All of which was paid for by Papa. As the story goes, Ray Kroc, the founder of McDonald's, had the locker next to Papa and asked Papa if he wanted to invest in McDonald's. If only Papa had done it.

Much later, during my time at Eisenhower Memorial Hospital (where the Betty Ford Center is in Rancho Mirage, California), I would earn enough as a surgeon to buy Papa and Grandma (when his business was winding down) a condo at Ironwood Country Club. It was my pleasure. As I was almost always occupied in the OR, Papa would play golf and became very friendly with the staff in the dining room and bar, mostly the bar. One time I called to make a reservation for dinner and was told sorry, they were full. Then Papa called and got in without a problem. I loved it. One time during his college days, he was asked to play his saxophone at the World's Fair while working alongside Sally Rand the fan dancer of legend and featured in the movie *The Right Stuff*.

Some guys have all the luck.

THE 305-YARD DRIVE

At one point I gave some consideration to becoming a pro golfer. While out in the "Springs," I used to take instruction from Nick Turzian, the pro at Tamarisk Country in Rancho Mirage where Frank lived then on Wonder Palms, more exactly 70588. The street was later renamed to Frank Sinatra Drive. Nick had given me a set of MT Tourney golf clubs. They had a black face on the irons and looked cool. I used to play in amateur tournaments back in college. As years passed as a busy surgeon, I could only play occasionally but every chance I got I did. It helped having homes at Ironwood where I could just jump into my cart and off I went. There were two courses at Ironwood and it was never really crowded. Back then, the north course stretched way back almost to the mountains. I remember on one occasion I was back there and heard a noise. I looked up and there was a Lockheed C-141 roaring out of one of the canyons, I swear, just a few hundred feet off the ground. Man, that was cool. It was like a scene out of *Top Gun*. Besides that, Ironwood had several large lakes. At the time, next to DBI there was a smaller lake that I could fish at will. I kept my fishing rod there and could get in few casts. There were lunkers (largemouth bass) in that lake. When time permitted, I would bring a water cooler with me and transfer the bass from that little lake into the big lakes at Ironwood so we would have breeders there making more bass. There was always plenty of fish and many occasions I brought the kids along so they could learn to fish. That's Christian and me on the left.

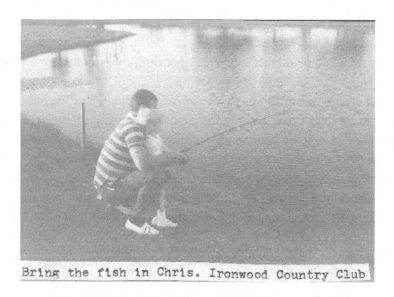

Bring the fish in Chris. Ironwood Country Club

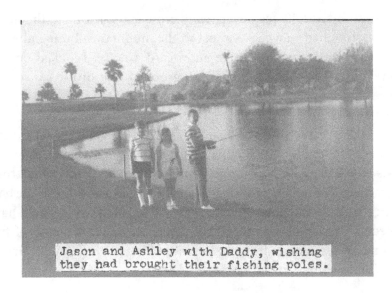

Jason and Ashley with Daddy, wishing they had brought their fishing poles.

Back to the 305-yard drive. One year Jason sent me information on the RE/MAX World Long Drive competition. I was in my sixties then. They had a "senior" division so I figured what the heck, we would go. Upon entering the grounds, there were a lot of people hitting balls. And there a number of club/shaft manufacturers hawking their wares. They were making club combinations on the spot. I had one guy watch me and he offered to make me a special setup right then. Okay. I was hitting the new club really pretty good and decided to use it instead of my own.

While on the tee, you could hear your name blare out over the loud speaker where the actual competition took place down the way. One of the names they called out was "Captain America." Great. There was a guy hitting that I thought was going to eat his club, a big guy. I think the balls he hit are still flying around the earth, he hit a long, long way. This competition was the regional finals from four western states.

I didn't want to wear myself out so we walked down to where the guys were hitting. They had stands in back so people could sit and watch. They had cameras taping each shot. The grid was narrow, about 20 yards or so, but went back over 400 yards. Each contestant got six balls and I think there was a time limit. As we watched everyone, eventually that big bruiser was called. This was the guy whose balls are probably still flying. We were all waiting for the golf balls to fly apart, he hit so hard. I don't know if it was the pressure of people watching, or the TV cameras, but every ball he hit went dribbling off to the right. I thought he was going to break the club over his knee. Poor guy, and during practice with no pressure, he hit them a mile.

Eventually they finished with all the big shots and next were the old men. The old men started at age fifty. Now there is a big difference between someone pushing seventy and someone who just turned fifty yesterday. I had to get that in. My turn came and it was one of the most stressful moments, those six shots. But I did manage to hit on 305 inside the ropes. I came in third. I wish now they had a "super seniors" starting at age seventy-five so we could actually see what's what. I brought one of the balls back that says RE/MAX World Long Drive and now if I have a golfer in the office, I tweak him/her that there only two kinds of golfers, those with this ball and those without.

MICKEY MOUSE CLUB, SPIN AND MARTY, ANNETTE FUNICELLO AND THE RED INK ESCAPADE

Like every kid in America who had access to a TV in the 1950s all looked forward every weekday to the *Mickey Mouse Club* broadcast. I can still remember the song. "Spin and Marty" was a story about boys going to a dude ranch learning to ride and going on "snipe" hunts, etc. What really caught my eye though was a cast member of the Mickey Mouse Club, Annette Funicello. Now Annette was three years older than me (didn't know it at the time). Under the official Mouseketeer costume top the girls wore with their names on it, one could see that beneath that top Annette was blossoming into a young woman, if you get my drift. I could see it anyway and probably like thousands of boys across America I was transfixed.

This went on for some time, my secret crush on Annette. Then I remember I decided to write her. For some reason, I decided to write in red ink. I figured every guy was writing her in black ink so I would be different. As it turned out, she would be the first in a long line of people

I would write to during my career that never answered me. In any case, I decided to write her and the fantasy continued.

The Chicago winters were at times brutal with road closures and snow piling up all over but especially on rural roads like Forest Glen Avenue. At this time the snow fall was about ten or more inches. The streets had developed frozen "ruts," which were created by the cars trying to negotiate Forest Glen Avenue. It was bitter cold, probably around minus 10 degrees Fahrenheit the day I decided to bike to Jefferson Park to Woolworths to buy the red ink. On top of that, it was a blizzard out there. Common sense should have dictated I stay at home safe. However, apparently there is no stopping a pre-pubescent boy from accomplishing his goal.

The sidewalks were not shoveled so I was relegated to ride in the ruts in the street. Jefferson was probably about eight or so miles away and it was all I could do to keep from falling every second on the icy ruts besides cars trying to pass. I managed to get out of their way without getting hit. I made it to Woolworths and bought the ink. The ride back was brutal but I made it. I think I started a fire in the fireplace on my return to warm up. Speaking of fires in the fireplace, every so often when I started a fire when it was very cold, either a squirrel or a duck would drop down trying to warm themselves and they would be in our living room.

It was my first love letter. I'm sorry that back then there was no way to copy it. We did have typewriters but I did it by hand. I imagined in my mind Annette reading it and writing me back with a picture or something personal. Well, some 60-plus years later, I'm still waiting for that replay. Years later Annette would go on to do movies like *Beach Blanket Bingo* with Frankie Avalon. Frankie, who appeared many times on *American Bandstand* (another TV program we all watched), was on a nostalgic tour and came to the desert one year. There was a restaurant in my office complex and while Joan and I were eating breakfast, he came in. Tragically, while I didn't know it at the time, Annette developed multiple sclerosis and deteriorated little by little until she finally died in Bakersfield, California, on April 8, 2013. She missed out.

INTRODUCING PEOPLE TO EVENTS OF HIGHER EDUCATION

Even though one increases their knowledge, only a select few become doctors. Becoming a doctor was the holy grail in the 1960s and 1970s. Fewer actually write papers of clinical trials or the like, but as a consequence of all your work, if people deem your results worthy, you get invited to present your work before a big audience. My biggest was over 2,000 in China. I never lost sight knowing how difficult it was for me to become a doctor. It was mostly because of the "jock mentality" in high school and college that I didn't achieve at the desired level to be accepted into medical school here in the US.

During my time at San Jacinto, I worked with a number of medical assistants (MAs). Most seemed to be content with doing their job and then going home only to start everything all over the next day. There was one guy though, Miguel, who showed strong interest in maybe becoming a doctor someday. I shared with him some of my work and he got to know about DBI, Tamoxifen, and visits to foreign countries to spread the word. As it turned out, I had submitted a paper about infrared helping to diagnose breast cancer and the vision I had of using cryo to treat breast cancer in one day.

I knew that any journey for Miguel would be arduous and prolonged. I wanted him to know the feeling of getting up to speak before people who were dying to hear what you had to say that was groundbreaking. In just those few seconds before you speak when you knew you had done something worthwhile that would benefit mankind, it's a good feeling. I wanted him to know that feeling to help push him forward. You got that feeling because you worked hard to be in a position where you could push the envelope. It's kind of a feeling of elation.

One never has that feeling if you're told to be content with your lot in life and others will do the work. Left unsaid is that the others will make sure they get all the perks and you get just enough to subsist and, therefore, are kept in line.

When my paper got accepted for presentation, I asked Miguel if he would want to present with me. I then included his name as co-author. We went over the particulars and how he would present and what to say. It was a new experience for him to play with the big boys. I'm sure he won't soon forget the feeling. I hope that remembering it will propel him to greater heights and a lifelong pursuit of caring for others while trying to make things better by using his G-D given talent.

ORGANIC HONEY BREAST IMPLANTS

If you're a potential investor or know someone who could, please read on. Breast implants are a $2 billion a year market. One day I walked over to my plastic surgeon's office, who was a master at creating gorgeous breasts using, at the time, silicone or saline implants. He was lamenting that, "We need to find an alternative to the current implant market." As fate would have it, he had bagels, cream cheese and, of course, honey in the lounge room. As I toasted my bagel, I began playing with the wooden handle dipping it in the honey (you know the kind that has at the end a beehive). I immediately noted that the honey mounded up. I didn't know it then but that procedure is called "drizzling." I didn't say anything, but I left and went directly to the store where I encountered about five kinds of honey, mostly variants of "clover." I would later learn that most honey is a "multi-floral" honey, meaning the bees travel to and use multiple types of flowers. I took the jars one at a time and just turned them upside down and watched the bubble rise up to the top. I noted that in some the bubble rose faster and some slower.

I bought the one I thought was ideal consistency and went back to my friend's office. In no time we filled an implant with honey and the first honey breast implant was born. Of course, it seemed heavy but later we learned how to mix it with saline so the viscosity could be changed at will, making the implant more ideal. There are other secrets (not disclosed in the patent) that make it ideal.

That very day I sat down and wrote a patent (having never written one before). We paid the fees and shipped it off to our patent attorney in Virginia. Now as far as I know, you shouldn't be able to patent "natural" products. In any case, months went by and then bingo, my patent number 5,500,017 was issued. I couldn't believe it. I had written my first patent and it was accepted. They didn't change a word. Then we got involved in NAMSA. They are the world's only company 100% focused on medical devices in the preclinical setting. They did stuff for us like bacterial counts, viscosity testing, aging studies and others. We did all the things with them that we knew the FDA would require.

I learned all about honey and the honey associations and producers like Gamber who, in 1957, came up with the iconic bear plastic container we all know. Gamber is located near Lancaster, Pennsylvania. Inside their facility you can eat off the floor it's so clean. At the time we were trying to get funding and we figured what better people to partner with than some of the big suppliers that supply honey for Honey Nut Cheerios, honey dijon mustard, etc. We introduced ourselves to all the national associations of honey producers in the hopes that either one or collectively they would buy in and help us produce the ideal breast implant. Ultimately, it was just too outside the box for them.

While I didn't know everything there was to know about the implant market, I knew that I could reproduce the feel of the human breast (much like silicone does) so it would have the feel of silicone, the safety of saline and something the other two just would never have, and that is sex appeal.

During this time a Dr. Terry Knapp came up with the idea of "soy bean oil" breast implants. I found an article that said he had sold the rights for either $11 or $13 million. That was before any "soy bean oil" implant was marketed. He had a place, I believe, in Switzerland and implanted a few thousand in Europe. Eventually, the problem became, I think, hazardous metabolites via lipid oxidation. All those "Trilucent" implants were explanted.

I contacted Gary Petersmeyer of Collagen Solutions and he signed my non-disclosure agreement (NDA) and I sent him the patent. About a week went by and he called back and I took the phone from my secretary and said, "Hello Gary." Nothing for about ten seconds then he said, "Honey, Phil they would have never come up with that in the laboratory." He said something like, "If I had known about your implant idea, I would have bought that." That was the closest I ever came to an implant company wanting to buy my idea.

Now might be a good time to introduce the reader to the problems of breast implants. Try as they might, manufacturers of breast implants (there are about thirteen companies worldwide) haven't overcome the "capsule" issue. That is, the implants are recognized as a foreign body by the patient's immune system and it tries to wall it off to a greater or lesser extent in each patient. While the implant itself stays soft, the body forms a fibrous capsule around it, which, at many times, can be as hard a feel as a league baseball. This is not a good result as the patient just didn't want bigger breasts but as they said in the movie *Airplane*, "Supple pouting breasts," something a man or woman (depending your sexuality) would want to caress. My formula would prevent this from happening, the capsule formation, that is.

The other complication that has crept in is BIA-ALCL, that is, breast implant associated anaplastic large cell lymphoma. A lymphoma is a cancer of the lymphatic system, like everyone has heard of Hodgkin's disease. There are about 500-900 cases worldwide and about 450-plus in the US (depending on who you read). This is an unsolved problem which, by the way, my organic implants would help solve or prevent altogether. This phenomenon was first reported in 1997 and has increased ever since. It appears to be associated with the "textured" implants. That's why the French outlawed textured implants two years ago. One big company went out of business and was recently acquired by a large pharmaceutical company.

My organic implants would have the feel of silicone, the safety of saline and something all the other implants wouldn't have and that's "sex appeal." If anyone is interested in developing these and freeing women from the problems plaguing breast implants, I'm easy to find. It's a $2 billion a year industry and growing at about 6% a year in spite of these complications. Below are my old patents.

The Commissioner of Patents and Trademarks

Has received an application for a patent for a new and useful invention. The title and description of the invention are enclosed. The requirements of law have been complied with, and it has been determined that a patent on the invention shall be granted under the law.

Therefore, this

United States Patent

Grants to the person or persons having title to this patent the right to exclude others from making, using or selling the invention throughout the United States of America for the term of seventeen years from the date of this patent, subject to the payment of maintenance fees as provided by law.

Bruce Lehman

Commissioner of Patents and Trademarks

Attest

USPTO PATENT FULL-TEXT AND IMAGE DATABASE

| Home | Quick | Advanced | Pat Num | Help |

Bottom

View Cart | Add to Cart

Images

(1 of 1)

| United States Patent | 6,932,840 |
| Bretz | August 23, 2005 |

Implant device

Abstract

A human or animal implant device including a first, inner sealed silicone sheet sac, a second, intermediate sealed silicone sheet sac completely surrounding the first, inner sac, and a third, outer sealed silicone sheet sac completely surrounding the second sac. Each sac has a coating of beeswax on inner and outer walls thereof, and the first, inner sac is filled with a substantially sterile liquid material, preferably of viscosity at least 15 cp. The second, intermediate sac and the third, outer sac are filled with aqueous saline solution.

Inventors: **Bretz; Phillip D.** (Palm Desert, CA)
Assignee: **Absolute Breast Solutions** (Palm Springs, CA)
Appl. No.: **10/935,171**
Filed: **September 8, 2004**

Current U.S. Class:	**623/8** ; 623/11.11; 623/23.34
Current International Class:	A61F 2/12 (20060101); A61F 002/12 ()
Field of Search:	623/7.8,11.11,23.64 524/800

References Cited [Referenced By]

U.S. Patent Documents

3934274	January 1976	Hartley, Jr.
4610690	September 1986	Tiffany
4731081	March 1988	Tiffany et al.
4995882	February 1991	Destouet et al.
5002071	March 1991	Harrell
5500017	March 1996	Bretz et al.

United States Patent [19]

Bretz et al.

[11] Patent Number: 5,500,017

[45] Date of Patent: Mar. 19, 1996

[54] **BREAST IMPLANT DEVICE**

[76] Inventors: Phillip D. Bretz, ▮▮▮▮▮
      Vincent R. Forshan, ▮▮▮▮▮
      Calif. 92260

[21] Appl. No.: 342,054

[22] Filed: Nov. 17, 1994

[51] Int. Cl.⁶ A61F 2/12; A61F 2/02
[52] U.S. Cl. 623/8; 623/11
[58] Field of Search 623/7, 8, 11, 17

[56]   References Cited

          U.S. PATENT DOCUMENTS

  4,157,085   6/1979 Austad 623/8

Primary Examiner—Debra S. Brittingham
Attorney, Agent, or Firm—Dennison, Meserole, Pollack & Scheiner

[57]   ABSTRACT

A breast implant device formed from a polymeric sac filled with a filling material which is a substantially silicone-free aqueous sugar solution having a viscosity of at least 15 cp at 98.6° F. The filling material is preferably honey.

7 Claims, No Drawings

My Russian patent

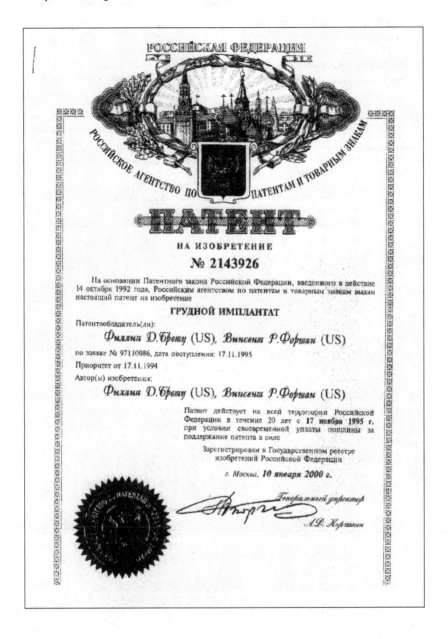

My Chinese patent for Honey Breast Implants

中华人民共和国国家知识产权局

地址：北京市海淀区蓟门桥西土城路6号　　国家知识产权局专利局受理处　　邮政编码：100088

邮政编码：200233
上海市桂平路435号　　　　　　　　　　2G　　　发文日期：

上海专利商标事务所

章鸣玉　　　　　　　　　　　　　　　　　　　1999年6月18日

申请号：95197328. 2

申请号：95197328. 2　　　申请人：　专用乳部填充物股份有限公司

发明创造名称：乳房植入物装置

发明专利申请公布及进入实质审查程序通知书

上述专利申请，经初步审查符合专利法及其实施细则的有关规定，根据专利法第三十四条规定，该申请已在第 **15** 卷、第 **20** 期发明专利公报上予以公布。

根据申请人提出的实质审查请求，经审查符合专利法第三十五条，实施细则第八十二条规定，该专利申请已进入实质审查程序。

注：附公布说明书一份。

提示：

1. 自本通知书发文日起，该申请即进入实质审查程序，自此专利申请人向专利局递交各种专利文件时，应在文件上注明实质审查程序。

2. 根据专利法实施细则第八十六条规定：发明专利申请人自申请日起满二年尚未被授予专利权的，自第三年度起每年缴纳申请维持费。第一次申请维持费应当在第三年度的第一个月内缴纳，以后的申请维持费应当在前一年度期满前一个月内预缴。

申请人未按时缴纳申请维持费或缴纳数额不足的，可在缴费期满之日起六个月内补缴，同时缴纳金额为全额申请维持费的25% 的滞纳金，期满未缴纳的，自应当缴纳申请维持费期满之日起，该申请被视为撤回。

审查员：　　　　　　审查部门：
　　　　　　　　　　　　　初审及流程管理部

2141 — 2

THE LONE RANGER STORY

Like every kid who grew up in the Midwest during the 1950s, we all looked forward to Saturday morning. That was the only time we could see cartoons and it was the only time during the week. Also playing at that time were cowboy serials like the Lone Ranger, Roy Rogers, and Gene Autry. Can anyone remember all three names of the horses that belonged to these guys? I can. I'll tell you a little story about Gene Autry. Joan and I were at the Bob Hope Desert Classic Ball and Joan sat next to Gene. For studs on his tuxedo shirt, he had large gold nuggets. He was imbibing some and got up to head to the restroom but he was a little unsteady and didn't seem to know where to go. I got up and grabbed his arm and said I would help. I told him he and all the other cowboys I faithfully watched taught me the straight and narrow path. I got him back to his seat without incident.

Back to the Lone Ranger. My daughter, Alexandra, had been accepted to CalPoly San Luis Obispo and Joan and I decided for something different we would take the train up there along the coast. It was a very scenic ride. About a half hour out of the Los Angeles area, I was looking out the window and the landscape had changed dramatically to rolling hills with giant rocks, a cool setting. Later, I Googled the area and found out it was indeed so "cool" that Hollywood had filmed many of the westerns there. Back in the day it was called Iverson Ranch located in Chatsworth, California. It comprised about 500 acres. I also Googled the Lone Ranger Rock and sure enough, it was there. It is the opening scene in the show where the Lone Ranger rears Silver up right by the rock and then goes down the hill saying the famous words, "Hi Ho Silver."

At the time, my son, Jason, lived near Valencia by Six Flags. I called him and asked if he would drive over to verify the rock was there. Because if it was, I was going to make a pilgrimage of sorts to visit the iconic site. I didn't know and was interested if that rock formation was real or was it a Hollywood set and taken down at the end? About an hour later he called and said, "Yeah, I'm looking at it and it's still here." So off I go. I get there and indeed, it is there. However, it's in kind of a big gully with earth mounded up in the middle where the rock is. It's also surrounded with all kinds of thicket bushes and snakes. Also, interestingly, is that there are now condos along one edge of the gully. In order to actually get to it takes some time and braving the unknown, as it were.

Once there, you are standing on hallowed ground. So, I touch the rock and was amazed that it has stood the test of time as it appears to be some sort of sand stone. Then I'm looking at it and since Joan wasn't there, I'm thinking I should climb it and stand on top, a feat in itself. I do climb it without much difficulty and I find myself at the top. Then I realized that the top part appears to be almost teetering (look at the picture) and I'm thinking, now what if it disarticulates and falls down? I would have destroyed it. But actually, it's really stable up there. Jason took some pictures that we would later use on our Christmas cards.

Now I try to get down and, of course, it's damn near impossible. Jason starts laughing and says he has a great idea. He will call 911 and they will helo me off the rock and I will end up on the news. That was all I needed. Jason climbed up about three quarters of the way and with him being about six-foot-one, was able to extend his hand to catch my foot as I tried to slide down. It worked and I got down without injury or destroying the rock. Then I'm thinking, let's go to the Long Ranger's grave since it's at Forest Lawn in Glendale. He is among other notables like Walt Disney (about 20 yards from the Lone Ranger), Larry Fine (an original member of the Three Stooges), and John Candy, who is in a crypt just above Fred McMurry. Can you remember the iconic saying of the old gypsy woman played by Maria Ouspenskaya when the Wolf Man dies? It's, "The way you walked was thorny through no fault of your own, but as the rain enters the soil and the river enters the sea, so tears run to a predestined end. Now you will have peace for eternity."

What I did was take a little soil where Silver would have reared up and I later sprinkled it on the Lone Ranger's grave. And yes, I couldn't resist, there are parts of the rock that have fallen off over the years and shattered on the ground so I took some. I've given them to friends who are very appreciative. And there is a member of Pearl Jam who has one. I typed out a certificate of authenticity. They all love it as it's very rare. In the office I have pictures of the Lone Ranger and other memorabilia and if a patient asks about them, I let them touch the rock. I tell the patients to let their husbands know they touched the LR rock and they would be jealous.

Why do I call myself the Lone Ranger? Actually, a patient came up with the idea and as you read in Daphne's article in *Fete Lifestyle Magazine*, it stuck. It should be obvious why some patients refer to me as the Lone Ranger. An interesting fact (if historical records are correct) is that the guns you see the Lone Ranger with are real Colt 45s. They carry a serial number of LR 1 and LR 2. What most don't know is that the first week on the set, someone stole the guns and holster and they were never recovered and never surfaced after all that time. So the guns you see him with are replacements namely, LR 3 and LR 4. Another tidbit, the Lone Ranger drove a Corvette.

I hope I have lived up to the standards he set about conduct and treating his fellow man. He never shot to kill anyone.

THE ANGEL STORY

This story begins with my abstract on the "Compass Treatment" being accepted for a poster presentation at the 5th Annual Multidisciplinary Symposium on Breast Disease held in Rome, Italy in February 2000. Joan and I were enthralled with the eternal city in our brief stay during our honeymoon and we were excited to go back to absorb the history. As a secondary plan, I wanted to meet the Pope, Karol Jozef Wojtyla, better known as Pope John Paul II, and tell him how courageous I thought he was. I thought Dr. Dreisbach with his connections could get me the Pope's fax and indeed he did. This thought occurred to me only a couple of days before we left but I faxed the letter telling him who I was and what I was doing in Rome. *The Shoes of the Fisherman*, which deals with papal conclave of Cardinals to elect the Pope, is one of my favorite movies. We departed before I ever received a reply. We had booked reservations on Alitalia Airlines. I was a little nervous not flying on a more accustomed Boeing.

But in the end, I figured if Alitalia was entrusted to fly the Pope, they were good enough for me. And I thought at least they could find Rome. On the day of our departure, we decided to drive into LAX using a rental car. I stopped to fuel the car in Palm Desert and when I got out of the car and stepped toward the back to begin refueling, I stopped dead in my tracks. There at my feet was an angel about two inches tall, blond hair complete with wings and white robe. She was looking straight at me. I thought, we're going to Rome, might meet the Pope, so what do I do with this angel? Right, I pick her up and put her in my suit pocket. After refueling, I secured her on the dashboard for good luck. One needs all the karma they can get driving into LA. On arriving at LAX, I put her in my suit pocket where she stayed.

The flight over was uneventful but very long. Arriving in Rome, the airport, like most cities, is some distance from the downtown area. We were able to get to the train that takes you into the main railroad station and from there we would catch another train to a station hopefully near the Hotel Cavalieri. On arriving at the main railroad station, we were able to get to a person (no English) who wrote the track number and station where we should get off. It was getting dark and it was almost twenty-four hours since we left California. We got on the train not knowing where exactly we were going and after a couple of stops, I got to know where the names of the stations were. I watched with a keen eye.

We must have stuck out like sore thumbs with Joan carrying the poster and me with the luggage. Finally, there was the name of the station where we were to get off. We did and we were the only ones to get off there.

It was very quiet and dimly lit. We ascended up the stairs into near total darkness. The only thing I could recognize were the street lights from what appeared to be a major street, so we started to walk toward them some blocks away. Once we got to the major street, we felt a little safer. I was able to hail down a cab and we arrived at the hotel without incident. The Cavalieri is located on a hill overlooking Rome, and from there you could see St. Peter's. We checked in and got up to the room and I just flopped on the bed. I was beat. We rested a short while but we hadn't eaten for some hours and went downstairs to the main restaurant. Before that, we stopped by the area designated for the poster presentations and found our spot.

Having grown up in Chicago I know a thing or two about good

pizza. And just to clear up a possible misunderstanding, the idea that Chicago's pizza is nothing but "deep dish," that didn't come along until Uno's started to do it in downtown Chicago near Rush Street in the 1960s. Somehow, the "deep dish" thing stuck. But for years before it was all thin crust with Italian sausage, fennel and usually slightly burned with a lot of tomato sauce and bubbles on the crust. There was a restaurant called El Centro near our house in Chicago and the guy who made those pizzas was from Italy and used to throw the dough high up into the air to get it just right. That guy made the best pizza I ever had until I tasted the one from the Cavalieri. No doubt whoever made that pizza at the hotel knew what he/she was doing. It was damn good. The next morning, we set up our poster and attended the talks. At a designated time, we were to stand by the poster to answer any questions which we did.

After that, we decided to venture out into Rome and see the sights including the Roman Forum, the Sistine Chapel, Trevi Fountain and last but not least St. Peter's. I have to say on entering Vatican City (the smallest country in the world), it's almost like the feeling you get entering Disneyland, like all your troubles are behind you. Regardless of your religion, seeing St. Peter's should be on your bucket list. While I'm not Catholic, I was ready to sign up. St. Peter's is a majestic structure on hallowed ground. Joan got in this time without incident. One of the first things you see is Michelangelo's *Pieta*. Now she is behind reinforced acrylic, but when we first saw her in 1969, you could actually walk up and touch her. A similar thing we encountered at the Louvre in Paris where Leonardo de Vinci's *Mona Lisa* is located. Now she is surrounded by acrylic.

I found out from Dr. Dreisbach that there are hidden stairs by the main altar that winds up to the cupola atop St. Peter's. We found it and proceeded up. The higher you climb, the narrower it gets, not for the claustrophobic. Before you go up the final few steps, there is a rickety platform looking down on the main altar. What a view!

Climbing the last few stairs, the walls seem to close in until you are out and standing within the cupola. From the cupola, there is a commanding view of St. Peter's Square. While enjoying the view,

I suddenly remembered the angel resting in my pocket. I said to myself, if I were an angel, where would I like to end up, in a gas station getting run over by a car or be able to sit atop St. Peter's where I can give out blessings? I waited until I was alone and I took her out. Then I climbed a few disjointed stones until I saw the perfect crevice. I put her deep into it. To remove her you would have to know she's there and try to extirpate her which would be difficult. So now whenever I see the cupola atop St. Peter's, I hope she is there. And like I said, giving out blessings.

After our visit to St. Peter's, we walked around Rome. At one point a woman in beggar clothes came up to me holding a baby. Directly behind her was a little girl about six or seven years of age. The woman rubbed up against me and then left. I don't know what made me do it but I reached in my pocket and my money was gone. I turned around and said in a very aggressive, loud and stern voice, "I want my money back." Meanwhile Joan saw the little girl who actually had the money holding her hands behind her and she went up and forced her to open her hands and there was the money.

At the same time, there was a guy who had been coming up the alley who had turned around. No doubt, this was the final person to pass the money off to. I guess I acted so pissed no one wanted to screw with me. We continued on our way by cab to the hotel to rest.

The restaurants in Rome are kind of semi-hidden, some behind walls and doors. I had obtained the name of a restaurant from Dr. David Kaminsky (my world-class pathologist at Eisenhower) before we left. It seemed no one went to dinner there before eight o'clock. We found this place and had an excellent dinner. When we came out it was around 10:30 p.m. and again we found ourselves quite alone. I could see the Castel St. Angelo in the distance and I knew St. Peter's and the square were a few short blocks away. I wanted to see if the Pope's light was on. His office (when you stand looking at the entrance to St. Peter's) is located in the building to the right and I believe the second window from the right on the top floor. We proceeded toward the Ponte Sant'Angelo (bridge of angels). As we crossed, we were the only ones there. There are five angels on that bridge that were created by pupils of Gian Lorenzo Bernini who was the architect of the bridge. The angels hold objects related to the suffering of Christ.

To be surrounded with such an array of religious renderings is quite imposing. We made our way to St. Peter's Square. The whole area was virtually empty. On arrival there were only a couple of guards and one couple kissing. It was cool being able to stand there virtually the only ones with the lights on in St. Peter's. I looked up and sure enough the Pope's light was on. It was after 11 p.m. Yasser Arafat was in town (the former President of the State of Palestine) and he probably occupied most of the Pope's time. I joked that the light was on in the Pope's office because after dealing with Arafat, he had to write a letter to Bretz before retiring.

We had very much enjoyed our time in Rome and on arrival back home, sure enough, there was a letter from the Pope. The letter thanked me for my comments and he gave me an apostolic blessing. Every once in a while, I think about my angel atop St. Peter's and smile. And now as the folks at Monte Python would say, "And now for something completely different."

THE HUGH HEFNER STORY

While anyone who grew up in America during the fifties and sixties knew who Hugh Hefner was, for those that have no clue, I'll relay a little of his adventure into publishing the "Playboy" credo, including the much anticipated "centerfold" each month. Before *Playboy*, the only place you saw women not fully dressed was in the Sears catalog. While there were some "nudie" magazines out there, the stores kept them well hidden from the general flow of traffic.

When I lost my dad at age twelve, I had no idea what my manhood was for except to take a leak, or as Stanley's father would say, "leave a leak." When *Playboy* was first published in December of 1953, Hugh had borrowed $1000.00 from his mother to start *Playboy*.

But as soon as the first edition came out (which featured Marilyn Monroe as the centerfold), he was off to the races. What separated *Playboy* from the rest was it kind of established an elegant way to treat women, at least that's how I thought of it. As time went on, he was able to acquire the old Palmolive building just off Michigan Avenue. He had the PLAYBOY sign all lit up and with the rotating beacon you could see it a long way off. It lit the way to Chicago's Magnificent Mile as you came in off Lake Shore Drive.

Then in 1960, the first Playboy Club opened. From there it was the huge layout in Lake Geneva, Wisconsin, which Joan and I flew to on a few occasions. It had its own golf course and landing strip. *Playboy After Dark* aired in Chicago on Saturday night. Ostensibly, he would have a party going on and when the elevator door opened, he invited you in. The frosting on the cake though was the "Big Bunny."

It was a DC 9 painted black with the Playboy Bunny logo in white on the tail. As I said before, the call letters for her were 950PB and I thought it stood for Phil Bretz. Of course, I thought I was somehow a quasi-partner along with Hugh which is, of course, absurd. But I was living the dream. As you read, I had my Playboy Card at age eighteen and had my bachelor party there. As years passed and I had become a surgeon and dedicated myself to eradicating breast cancer, I finally wrote him a letter. See below.

By that time, he was in the sunset of his years and he had had a stroke a few years earlier. I just wanted him to know what an impact Playboy had on me and how I learned to treat and revere women, and how I learned to preserve mind, body, and spirit. Having said that, I'll be the first to admit I didn't buy the magazine to read the articles (ha).

I meant what I said in that letter, that using all I had learned about women (at least initially), I was able to convince a centerfold to marry me. While Joan was not an actual centerfold, she easily could have been. She won't let me put in the bikini picture. I sent the letter off and about a week later, Joan went out to get the mail and came back with a letter with the Playboy insignia on it with the initials HH on it. I couldn't believe it. You can read the letter below. The cool part of this letter besides my education from Playboy was Hef saying at the end of the letter, "My best to you and your beautiful wife." That would make her one of the only women on earth who has that said in print, that she is beautiful, from the master. I am in the process of having the letters framed along with the commemorative issue of *Time* telling Hugh's life story, another American adventure like no other.

PLAYBOY

HUGH M. HEFNER
EDITOR-IN-CHIEF

April 13, 2010

Phil Bretz, MD
78-034 Calle Barcelona, Suite B
La Quinta, CA 92253

Dear Phil,

Thanks for your letter. I really appreciate the way in which your initial introduction to Playboy led to a career caring for breasts.

My best to you and your beautiful wife.

Sincerely,

Hef

Hugh M. Hefner

HMH/jn

PLAYBOY MANSION WEST/10236 CHARING CROSS ROAD/LOS ANGELES, CALIFORNIA 90024

How could I not close the book without the famous underwear ad. It's online at "weird underwear ads." There was hell to pay at school, but maybe some of the girls cut it out.

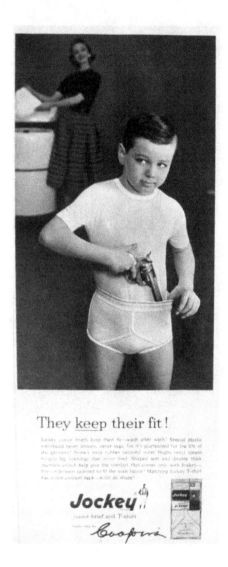

CHAPTER 15

Ending Photos and Final Thoughts

THIS HAS BEEN great for me, reliving my history and adventures. I hope you enjoyed hearing about growing up in the 1950s and 1960s in Chicago and the exploits that followed. I'll say again, it has been an honor and privilege for me to care for each one of the ladies who came to me for help, trusting in me as they did to save them and not destroy them. I hope I lived up to their desires.

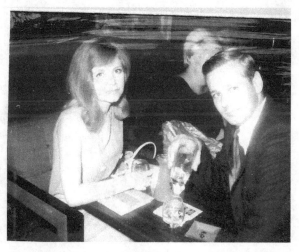

Joan and I at the Playboy Club (under age no doubt)

My bride and her father (PAPA) at our reception.
I promised him I would take very good care of her.

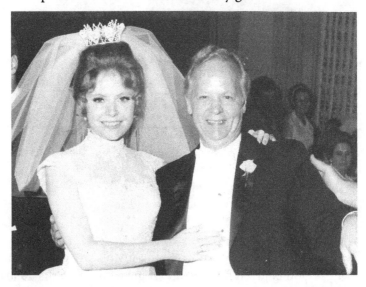

At the wedding. Left to right, Aunt Florence, My Mother, Me, Joan,
Joan's Dad, Joan's Mom, Joan's brother Gary.

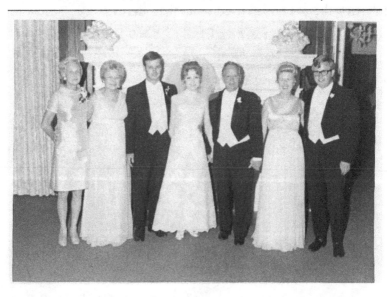

Bernie and I in the backyard at 5533 on my wedding day.

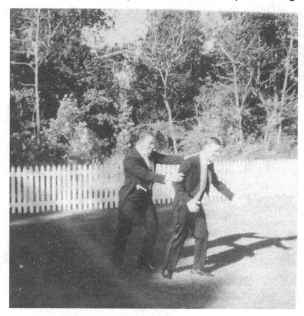

No golfing today.

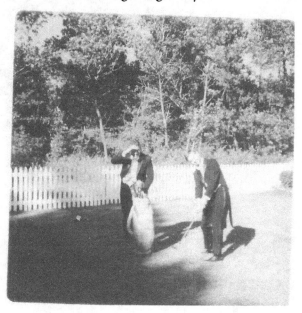

Pam (Joan's best friend) and Chuck at the Showboat in Chicago

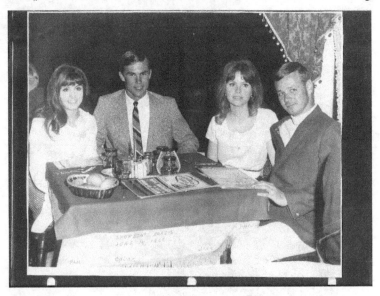

Papa and Howie

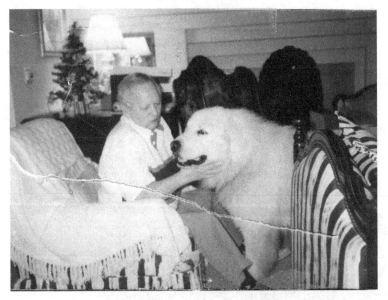

My Bricklin with Jason driving

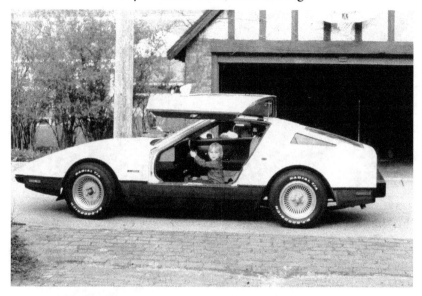

Jason with Howie Long (Hall of Fame defensive end for Raiders)

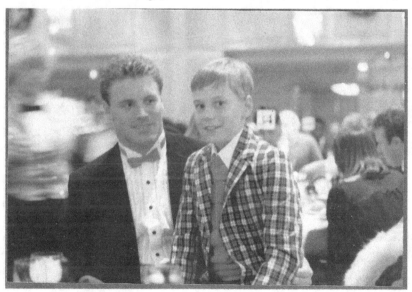

Woodbine in the winter

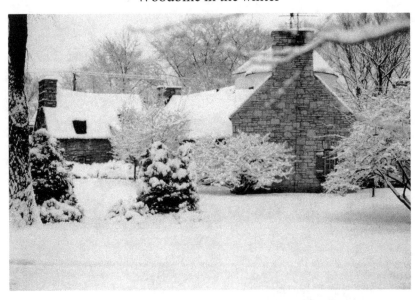

Woodbine in the spring

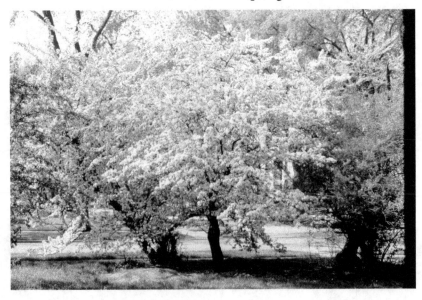

That's me atop the actual Lone Ranger rock.

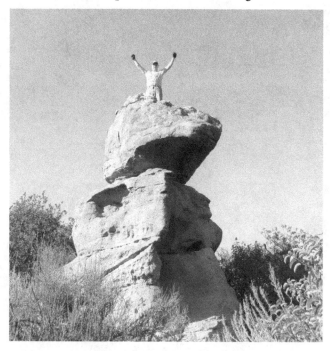

Next is the Lone Ranger rock with the real Lone Ranger filmed in the 1950s at Iverson Ranch in Chatsworth, California. Most of the old westerns were filmed there and most of the film sites can still be found.

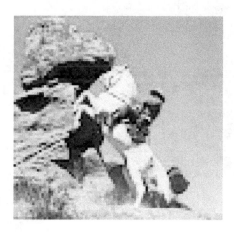

This is me at the Forbidden City which seemed to go on forever.

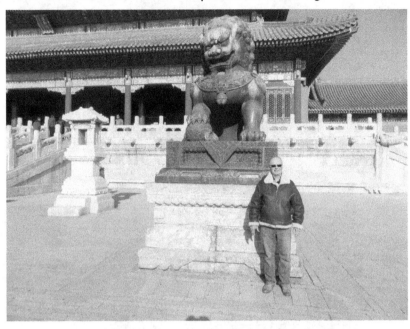

I'm sure a rare sight, the Great Wall with no one around (December 2017).

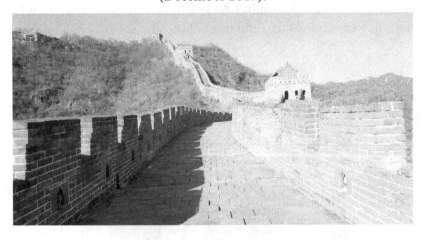

I wasn't going to include this photo of the nursing class, but when I read what my mother wrote, it's priceless. Every guy's dream.

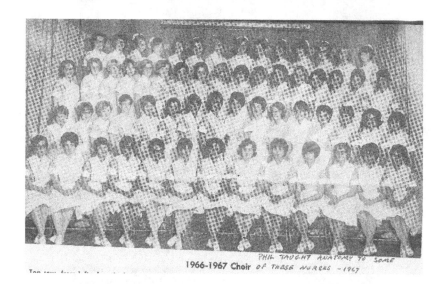

1966-1967 Choir *of these nurses - 1967*
Phil taught anatomy to some

The below two works of art were made by a patient (Carol, whose letter is in the opening of the book) and another surgeon in town who is also a sculptor. Both these people know me and what I accomplished and stood/stand for. Both took time to create these two works. The surgeon told me it was an honor to have made that sculpture and present me with the 'Pinnacle,' because I had reached it. These kinds of things are far more important than any certificate. Big Horn sheep are ubiquitous in the mountains of our community. Would they really have done all this for an unscrupulous, unethical, unprofessional, negligent surgeon? I don't think so, do you? I guess Granite Company was right after all, CHARACTER MATTERS.

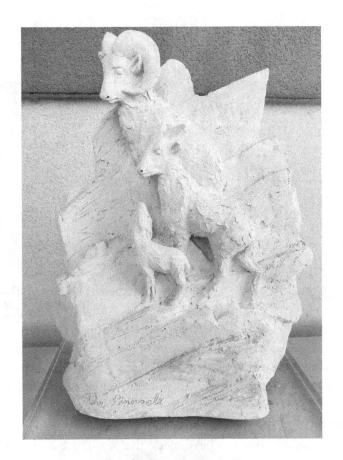

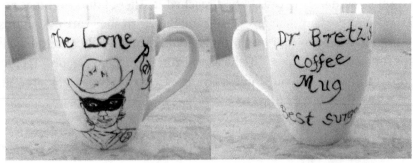

An image of the Coachella Valley

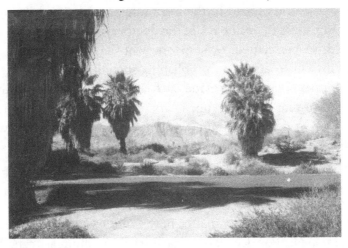

Below is a letter I received from Dr. Rasa, which she didn't have to do, however, it was very much appreciated.

♛ ColumbiaDoctors

AZRA RAZA, MD
Chan Soon-Shiong Professor of Medicine
Director, MDS Center

177 Fort Washington Avenue, 6GN-435
New York, NY 10032
212-305-0591 Clinic Appointments
212-305-6891 Fax
azra.raza@columbia.edu

February 3, 2020

Dear Phil,

Thank you for reading The First Cell so carefully. I was honored to sign the copy of the book you had mailed me and sent it back the same day in the envelop you so kindly provided. I hope you have received it.

I think we agree on many things about what ails the cancer paradigm today. I am delighted to hear that you are considering the leadership of the breast cancer program in Vietnam. More power to you! Wishing you the best in this venture. Unfortunately, I don't know anyone who would be interested in such a partnership with you.

Finally, I wish to once again thank you for your service to patients and applaud you for the courage you have consistently shown in standing up for the patients. I am confident you will continue to uphold the moral high ground. I would not describe you as the wounded warrior but as the warring hero. Recognition by others is not important. "To thine own self be true..."

Sending best wishes,
Sincerely,

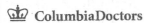

Azra Raza, M.D.

So now you have the whole story and the other side of the coin from my perspective. As I said in the beginning, I must leave it up to the American people to decide if I'm the doctor whose case should not be reopened, so persecuted, or someone who has worked tirelessly for women my entire career, accomplishing something of note? It's up to you if you so choose to provide such an outcry to change things in California so that the Governor hears of it (and he reopens my case, using different people). I know without that, and with the new edict from the Board of being in non-compliance (actually non-practice), with no end in sight, I will not be able to practice beyond September 30, 2021. I thought we were all in this together, trying to find a cure for cancer, especially breast cancer, which has wrought so much devastation to so many no matter how you do it, assuming we didn't hurt the patient. For decades we have tried to kill breast cancer with innumerable drugs and have been unsuccessful. If we were successful then with breast cancer, no one would be dying. Perhaps Lavender Way/Procedure is just another way no one has given credence to? What I mean for you to remember is, it's not just the ability to kill breast cancer in twenty minutes in the office. It's the Lavender Way which, when practiced right, can find nascent tumors before they have the ability to metastasis. It's the *combination* of the two.

I guess they thought I was wrong in trying to find a cure outside of the "system." No matter what you say about me, you can't wipe out my cancer-free patients who might have something to say if asked.

If my case is not re-opened, the least and just thing to do is to open a case against the competitor surgeon in town who didn't have the guts or courtesy to just call me to avoid all this, but wrote to the Board with untruths and half-truths and threatened the patient with harassing phone calls and told her she was going to die. What the hell kind of doctor is that? How can the Board tolerate this aggressive, irreverent, and unprofessional behavior by this surgeon? In Mrs. Smith's case, I have not participated in her care and am unable to reach her. Whatever happened after all this time may have been different if I had been involved.

Lastly, I'll say it again, it has been my privilege to utilize all the talent I possess that G-D gave me to care for the thousands of women worldwide. They entrusted their lives to me and I hope, if you ask anyone of them, they will respond that I lived up to my promise to be a voice for those who don't have one and to persevere until I found a way to rid us of this disease. In the last days now as many patients as we can see are coming in before I can't be their doctor. What was very touching to me has been their uniform response. Almost everyone cried, especially the ones I have been seeing for thirty years. It was very heartwarming to know they cared that much for me and Joan. Like I said, I told each one that I am very honored and privileged to care for each one of them. What was especially gratifying was that I was able to reach a station in life where beautiful girls (they're all beautiful) have come to me from all over the world to help them traverse very difficult times.

My heart, of course, is in this but they won. The question is, did you benefit from my demise? Or again, am I the doctor you wish you had?

G-Dspeed.

Here is Alexandra with her baby.

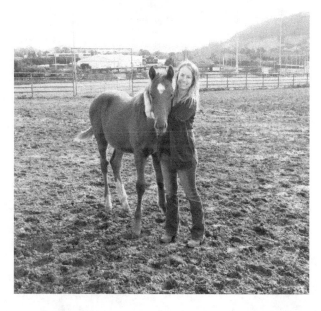

A one in a million shot of a uma inornata or Coachella Fringe-toed Lizard. He is surevying his kingdom, at least he has one.

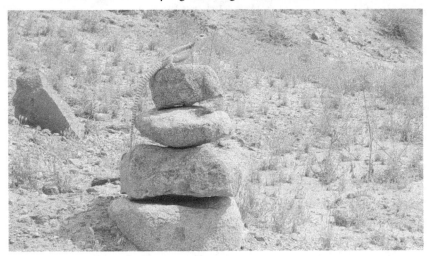

EPILOGUE

Original Article: PDF Only

A Randomized Trial of Robotic Mastectomy versus Open Surgery in Women With Breast Cancer or BRCA Mutation

IT SEEMS EVERY time I try and put the pen down yet another egregious article confronts me. This one is from *Annuals of Surgery* dated June 27, 2021. I picked it up in *General Surgery News* and they had a photo of a supposed women surgeon standing next to the robotic machine like it was some sort of victory. I can see the ads run by hospitals now, "Come to our open house and see our robotic mastectomy machine in action." How dare these people turn to this method instead of trying to find less invasive means. I just don't understand. You can bet it's an ego trip (all unsaid of course), for some surgeon who wants to be known as the "robotic mastectomy king/queen." And I'm sure that those robotic surgeons will be beating the bushes for patients telling unsuspecting family doctors how great robotic mastectomy is. That's the latest and greatest girls. Who will line up first?

I had to include this new article. It seems like a never-ending flow doesn't it? Again, it's the kind the public never sees, but this epitomizes the problem all women have when diagnosed with breast cancer. This one takes the cake though. It is hot off the press of *General Surgery News,* October 2021, Volume 48, Number 10. The article was intitled "In a Patient's Shoes." It was written by a woman breast cancer surgeon who had practiced for twenty years and she "Rethinks 'What Quality of Care' Really Means After Becoming a Patient Herself." After finding a stage 3 breast cancer diagnosed as a lump in her breast, she ended up with neoadjuvant chemotherapy, a mastectomy, radiation and a reconstruction implant (which she had removed later). Three years later after losing her breast, and all but the kitchen sink being thrown at her, she ends up with a local recurrence. Because of the local recurrence, she had to have additional surgery and more radiation. The side effects of all that caused reduced arm range of motion which forced her to retire. That portended possibly hundreds of patients missing out on her expert surgical care. The other thing she says is in all those years, she focused only on "outcomes."

For example, she always told patients who asked about hot flashes, "you'll be fine." But she relates that she had no idea just how devastating it all can be from the surgery, chemo, radiation, hot flashes, arm pain, and the list goes on. She goes on to say, "How great it would be if in addition to telling our patients what the side effects of their treatments are, we tell them how to manage these side effects." In other words, without knowing about Lavender Way, she wants the Lavender concept for all women. You see I was right that treating breast cancer is not like changing a tire. It involves, besides the physical component, a psychological component that must be addressed but isn't by most surgeons. They just move on to the next case as in, it's someone else's problem. You see how a dedicated breast doctor who sees hundreds of women with these problems can really aid in the understanding of these issues of which hot flashes are just the tip of the iceberg. And remember, with Lavender, many of these issues that plagued women for eons are eliminated. She continues talking about what patients need beyond a good outcome to maintain quality of life. Another very important thing she discusses is that breast cancer recurs in about 30% of patients. And if the patient doesn't know how to spot a local recurrence and "if their primary care physicians don't know the warning flags, we're doing our patients a disservice." Having read this book now and knowing how the Lavender Way is set up, the reader knows that all this is a moot point because all this would be covered by your dedicated breast surgeon. Your "forever care" would not be entrusted to a family or primary care physician. You'd be seeing your DEDICATED breast surgeon WAY before any problem arose and you would have had the genetics test and individualized imaging to find ultra-small breast cancers which permits the Lavender Procedure to make surgery, chemotherapy and radiation possibly all unnecessary.

This just typifies the entire situation all women find themselves in (just like the lady in New York that I spoke to on the phone and received that email from), which is the reason they are being sacrificed. My comment is, "What?" In this article we have not just an unaware woman who finds a lump in her breast, caught off guard as it were, but an honest to G-D veteran breast cancer surgeon with twenty years' experience and she ends up with a large lump? I'm sorry but to my way of thinking, something untoward happened (meaning she didn't come in for regular mammography and exams) or the system somehow missed it and on a breast cancer surgeon no less. Remember, a 1-centimeter (about dime size) breast cancer has been there on average for about ten years growing. Our technology, if given a chance, can and should detect breast cancers well before they become a palpable mass. Here we go with national guidelines again and their shortcomings. Being a breast cancer surgeon herself, I'm sure she was treated "differently" than a "regular" patient, yet she found her experiences to say the least, I think, disheartening. Here we had a female breast surgeon who, because of the standard of care treatment and its attendant complications, can no longer save lives. That's just great. What do you think?

The whole thing needs to undergo radical change as called for in my paper. Again, there is only one person in this land who could bring Lavender to every woman almost overnight. You know who that is, the President of the United States, creating a separate entity, The Lavender Breast Centers, answering only to the President. Change the name if you want. It just crushes me to think that even a learned breast cancer surgeon had to undergo such a horrendous treatment when my Lavender girls have played eighteen holes of golf immediately after with their breasts intact and are cancer-free going on eight years. Makes me wonder just who is in charge to change things? At least a pilot study would be in order to test whether my results can be duplicated, which is part of the scientific method.

Remember, my results were of someone with no experience in cryoablation and basically self-taught. I never got the opportunity to really hone my talent (if I had any). Yes, there are a number of existing national breast center societies, but one doesn't HAVE to join them and one doesn't HAVE to do what they preach especially when it's all just a variant of the same old system. And with the implementation of some national guidelines about breast imaging that supposedly covers everyone, how can we turn this ship around? Again, the only answer I see is the President of the United States.

Whoever is in charge or gets to be in charge, I sincerely hope they have more vision than the director of cancer prevention for the National Cancer Institute when we met in Frank Young's office (then assistant secretary of HHS under Luis Sullivan) when I was told my vision to work with the Soviets was too big. Was the thought of conquering breast cancer too big as well? This all boils down not to me but to the women of our great land (ALL OF THEM) collectively saying enough is enough and starting to put breast cancer disfigurement and deaths in the history books.

Thanks again, it has been an honor and a privilege. Make sure you visit the website (thelavenderproject.net, assuming it hasn't been taken down), to view the videos of the girls who looked breast cancer in the eye and won beyond belief. Make your voice heard if you want far better treatment for ALL women.

Just out of curiosity, I Googled "Why are doctors leaving their profession." I won't make you read the result here, but there is a thing now called the "drop-out club," where over 38,000 frustrated doctors get advice from others about leaving their profession. Remember, becoming a doctor is a lifelong commitment and whatever is causing these doctors to want to leave must be pretty bad and who is to blame? Come on, you know and if you don't, I have failed. Want further proof? Why is your doctor thinking about leaving medicine after years of commitment or calling? Here is one glaring example of outrageous demands by "functionaries." Again, these edicts were nowhere to be seen when I first started practice in the 1970s, but now would take up your doctor's entire day trying to understand everything they demand. The real problem is that this is from just one insurance company but there are many and they all have their own edicts coming into the office almost daily. Then there are the monthly "bulletins" each insurance company sends plus the quarterly newsletter from the Medical Board and countless other things that make it so your doctors are so frustrated they want to quit. Let's look at these demands of the provider (ha).

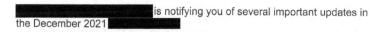

███████████████████ is notifying you of several important updates in the December 2021 ███████████

- Clinical Practice and Preventive Health Guidelines
- Case Management
- Coordination of Care
- An Overview of our Medical Necessity Review Process and Language Assistance Services
- Member Rights & Responsibilities
- Pharmacy Updates

Check the provider website quarterly for pharmacy updates (first of the month for January, April, July and October), and throughout the year for additional updates on Clinical, Behavioral and Preventive Health Guidelines. If your office does not have Internet access and you would like a printed copy of ████████, please contact your network relations representative.

Note, ████████ is published monthly, and you can find each issue online at

Excuse me! Clinical Practice and Preventive Guidelines? The real kicker is "Case Management and Coordination of care." In my day, no one dared to tell me as someone's "doctor" how I should manage a case or coordinate care of my patient. That's what the hell I and your doctor went to medical school for. And, of course, let's not forget the ever present "Member Rights." Why isn't there an edict about "doctor" rights? In my day one didn't need member rights because the doctors who practiced with me at Eisenhower treated their patients like they were family. And as I have said before, sacrificed themselves daily for years to make sure the patients at EMC were treated with the utmost care. It's wasn't just EMC, it was probably most doctors in our country back then. I think there was a different mindset when I practiced that is almost undefinable. I hope you can see the intrusion on a colossal scale never before seen. Couple this with the constant badgering of the entire population with these ridiculous TV ads for various drugs every ten minutes. They hammer home to the public, "Make sure you ask your provider about this new drug."

Don't worry about all the side effects (like anaphylaxis that is sometimes fatal) that many times are worse than whatever symptom you're trying to relieve. I especially like the one about a patient taking a mental health drug and your mind is better but now because of that drug (instead of trying to straighten out your life by yourself and not creating a dependency on drugs), you have uncontrolled involuntary movements. But don't worry, we have a drug for that also. Never mind the side effects which are compounded because now you're on two drugs with side effects instead of no drugs and being raised right by your parents to deal with life or seeing your pastor, priest or rabbi.

But don't worry about that either because you can drown your sorrows with a pizza or liquor that can be delivered right to your door. Dr. Rick Bradshaw had a saying back in the day about "instant gratification." The problem with "instant gratification" is it only lasts for an instant instead of immersing yourself in an environment that builds "character" enough to sustain you throughout life.

Why is your provider (sorry force of habit, doctor) wanting to leave the profession? Come on you should know the answer. If you don't, I have failed.

Below is an email I received on January 7, 2022 from a lady in a Middle Eastern country. Grammar and layout are as I received it. It seems this breast cancer issue and how women should be treated is a problem all over the world. This one is hard to believe. In the garbage, come on man.

"I guess the lump i feel is scar tissues.
I tried speaking to few people,
they are closed minded.
And so Stupid.
I spoke to well know surgeon he used to be friend since long time, i visited him in clinic recently to show the paper.
He said this is noway this tech works for you
You should do mastectomy.
Bastard!
How easy for them to say it.
Another stupid one, said you have to remove the breast and themrow in the garbage.
Group of Ignorants.
I will try to approach another one."
I guess we all have some work to do, don't we?
See below

588   Phillip Bretz M.D.

 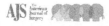
FULL LENGTH ARTICLE | ARTICLES IN PRESS

A contemporary reassessment of the US surgical workforce through 2050 predicts continued shortages and increased productivity demands

Wendelyn M. Oslock ⚬ ✉ • Bhagwan Satiani ✉ • David P. Way ✉ • ... Timothy M. Pawlik ✉ •
E. Christopher Ellison ✉ • Heena P. Santry ✉ • Show all authors

Published: July 22, 2021 • DOI: https://doi.org/10.1016/j.amjsurg.2021.07.033

✺ PlumX Metrics

Highlights

- Surgeon shortages were identified for nine specialties in 2030 and eight specialties in 2050.

- Clinical productivity would need to increase by 7–61% addition RVUs to overcome shortages.

- General surgery may have the worst deficit with a gap of over 25,000 surgeons by 2050 if trends --- not addressed.

Like I said, almost every day I have to read about some egregious assault on my profession and here is another one. I'm including this because it is so apropos to the discussion of intrusion into the medical profession of forces that have nothing to do with the art of medicine. This article is taken from *The American Journal of Surgery* and came to me by way of Doximity. It was published on July 22, 2021. I just printed the first page down a bit. The problem I have with these types of articles is everyone already knows about this surgeon shortage and have been echoing this sentiment for decades. It offers *no* solution, but someone in charge knows how to fix it and they don't because they count on and know that surgeons will be there to their last breath no matter the indignation served up to them. As I have said, who reads these articles and who has any authority to change anything? Then why the hell don't they change things? It brings up a very important point, like years from now you may find yourself in an emergency room at 3 a.m. and need lifesaving surgery only to be told they have no surgeons. It might happen. As we have seen throughout this book, I try to back up what I say with other physician authors' papers to point out I'm not the only one. All this suppressed anger will eventually surface.

Apropos to this immediate discussion is a response from a lowly general surgeon out there who has probably saved more lives than you can count. That would be Emil Shakov and he says, "Maybe when there is not enough general surgeons, we can get paid a fair amount for our tireless and lifesaving work." There you go, but these discussions never see the light of day. As said in the article, by 2030 the shortage across nine surgical disciplines will increase work load 10-50% and by 2050 7-61%. What they don't say is that work load will be on the poor bastards that are still left trying to save lives yet still having to make sure the EMR is right or else. Being a doctor, I know the old joke that one can never read a doctor's handwriting. I will give the functionaries that, that at least a typed version of a progress note is easier for one to read, but otherwise, as far as I'm concerned, you can pull the plug. We didn't need all that back in the day. We just took care of patients properly. This paper was arrived at with the authors going through twenty-one years of American Medical Association (AMA) Masterfile data, which was used to predict the problem of surgeon shortage until 2050. If you don't want this to happen, then raise your collective voices and make it so doctors and surgeons in particular have an environment they want to practice in for their entire career.

An interesting tidbit I just learned from *The American Journal of Medicine* which, of course, the public is never privy to. It is Volume 134, Number 12, December 2021. The article is entitled, "The Language Game: We Are Physicians, Not Providers." While we won't explore the entire article here, I will bring to light just what the system thinks of us as doctors. "Some may salute "providers" as a neutral term of inclusivity, wrapping all members of a "health care team" in a cloak of equality in purpose, independent of specific functions within the team. And here is the irony of "providers." The term was first introduced by the Nazis in the 1930s when trying to debase German physicians of Jewish descent." Just great. I hope everyone's happy now.

Here are a couple of my pragmatic thoughts on things that could help our country a great deal, I think. The first centers around a doctor's DEA number. For those that don't know, your doctor can't write a prescription for narcotics without a DEA number issued by the Drug Enforcement Administration (founded by Richard Nixon). Whenever a doctor calls the pharmacy to call in a prescription, the pharmacist always asks what their DEA number is. It's like the holy grail. A doctor's DEA number is like a ribbon on the gift that was his/her medical diploma. A DEA number separates your doctor as one of the only people on Earth who can legally write narcotic prescriptions.

Having said that, everyone knows the problem with addiction and deaths from prescription narcotics. I remember reading somewhere that a death from prescription narcotics occurs every nine minutes. Michael Jackson is a name everyone remembers who was one of those statistics. Well, I have a solution that could be easily done that would help in large part to eliminate the problem. What's that? And because a doctor's DEA is important, we let them keep it as issued. However, when the time comes for renewal or as a first-timer, they simply check the box on the application that says: "By checking this box you will be issued your DEA number but the assignee will NOT be able to write prescription narcotics." For my part, although I signed up for a DEA number, I hadn't written an Rx for narcotics for many years even though there were many many people (especially in the urgent care setting) who would come in asking. A real common excuse was they needed a refill on their Vicodin as their nephew flushed their prescription down the toilet and that they needed the meds because they have been on it for years. Then instead of getting into an argument, they just went away when I said I couldn't write one.

So, in essence, by just checking the box on the DEA application that says you get your number but can't write for narcotics, any doctor who signs up will be helping with the cause to eliminate the problem of addiction and deaths. I know it's deeper than that and there are patients legitimately who need narcotic pain relief, say after a surgery. But this would help, I think.

Lastly, here's an idea that would help alleviate ongoing suffering for people across our great land. The President would have to bring it into existence. That would be ASERT, which stands for America's Surgical Emergency Response Team. Does anyone remember Hurricane Katrina? There were hundreds of people basically without food and water around the Superdome in New Orleans. Do you remember the movie *The Andromeda Strain*? The plot goes that a deadly organism comes to Earth on a comet and all the people in this town die except a drunk and a baby. Then the authorities find out about the select people who are on the scientific team to isolate the organism and find a way to treat it and are called into action right then with their beepers going off at parties.

Well, imagine, if instead of being stranded by some disaster for days with nothing, that real help in a matter of a few hours would come, with the sky dark with helicopters bringing much needed aid, food, water, and medical assistance able to handle anything just like a MASH unit. It would be a very demonstrable way for the government to show it does really care about its people. Then there wouldn't be delays with FEMA people arguing about what needed to be done. The ASERT group would be in charge and the responsibility would fall squarely on their shoulders.

You could probably easily staff ASERT with volunteers of retired doctors, surgeons and the like who would probably jump at the chance to be part of the select team. They would get a uniform and a certificate from the President extoling their selfless volunteerism. I guess that is too pragmatic though. After Katrina, I came up with this idea and sent it to multiple people on Capitol Hill, nothing. If I had been elected to Congress, that is one of the things I would have tried to get passed.

Acknowledgements

FIRST, BEFORE I get in trouble like Ray in *Everybody Loves Raymond* sitcom where, in his speech after being awarded an honorary degree, he fails to mention his wife. Let me first thank my wife of fifty-two years and counting. As cliché as it is, she is my best friend and the only one who actually knows my daily struggles with what drives me and what assaults me. There probably isn't a question she could be asked about me that she couldn't answer. Her willingness to review my manuscript is much appreciated, as what Dr. McCoy said on Star Trek, "Damn it Jim, I'm a surgeon not a secretary" is all too true in my case. It's not just editing the book; she has been the backbone for Visionary Breast Center being the Office Manager and she is the first to talk to a patient when they call the office. As you read in the patient letters, she is praised by all our patients for her caring demeanor and promptness in carrying out all the needed details of patient reporting.

I suppose to acknowledge all the people who made it possible for me to achieve what I have, the list would have to start with my parents and my Aunt Florence. Next would be Ms. Plagge, my kindergarten to third-grade teacher, who apparently saw in me the possibility of taking on responsibility as a patrol boy at age eight. From there we can go down the list of teachers at NPA like Rev. Magnuson, who was like a second father to me and instilled in me the spiritual foundation I would find necessary to carry out life's demands. And those involved with teaching me the "art" of medicine from the UAG to Loyola. For me, it was like standing on the shoulders of giants; Drs. Piffare, Freeark, Pickleman, Greenlee and Folk, thank you. You were there no matter what.

And while I lost my dad early on, as an adult, I came to realize just what it took for him to accomplish all the things he did. Using his code of conduct, it gave me the wherewithal to forge new trails in the diagnosis and treatment of breast cancer. My mother's chocolate cake didn't hurt either. She taught me how a family should behave and grow together. I hope I used that knowledge in bringing up our four children. Although Joan did most of it with me in the operating room.

Then there are those in my profession that help me succeed. Particularly the doctors who helped me at EMC, who together, we really did work like a band of brothers. Those early years at EMC were the last gasp of medicine as it should always be practiced. That is, the patient first, not some computer screen or the doctor forced to accept increasing regulation from some HMO or insurance company. A special thanks to BG Richard Lynch, DO, who instilled in me his work ethic and taught me everything I know about mammography and imaging, and to Dr. David Mantik, who helped forge new pathways in radiation therapy with me. To Drs. Philip Dreisbach, David Kaminsky and Doug Bacon, I also owe a debt of gratitude for believing in my theory about Tamoxifen to prevent breast cancer and contributing to its goal of finding that it does lower the risk of breast cancer by 50%. It was a big deal that we did this. In more recent times, Dr. David Conston (radiologist) has helped me a great deal reviewing ultrasounds and as an independent reviewer of all my mammograms and doing the follow-up core biopsies on the Lavender girls. Dr. Conston probably has the most experience in the country on follow-up of these cryoablation patients.

I can't leave out Steve DeLateur, who has helped me with the Honey Breast Implant project and entrusted me with the care of his family members. Jay Ash, who served our country in the Korean War, was for years doing our billing and since became a great friend.

The people at Gatekeeper Press, Eden, my editor, Kathryn, Tony, and Rob (CEO), they were there for me from the beginning to the end and deserve credit making this work right and helping me design the book, jacket, and contents. If you are considering self-publishing, these are the folks you should contact.

Lastly, to all four of my kids, who turned out to be everything I'd hoped, thanks for being better than me, a father's joy to behold. Christian and Jessica (his significant other) have created a cool VR/PC game called *Alien Dawn*. Jessica created the poster below. You can buy *Alien Dawn* now. Just go to voyagervr.com or Steam. Jason is married to Susan, a nutritionist, and he continues to be an assistant film editor in Hollywood. You can IMDb him. Alexandra has a master's degree in animal science, and at this time is deciding between jobs at the zoos in Seattle and Los Angeles. Her significant other, Brandon, is an aerospace engineer. Ashley continues to do interior design and home renovation (House of Stiles) and husband, Justin, is a real estate investor and volunteer coach for little league and football in Seattle while raising my two grandchildren. Mr. O. at age eleven can throw a league baseball over 60 mph and with his love of sports may well end up an MLB pitcher. Harrison at age six is fixated on discussing medical cases with me—maybe in twenty years he can reopen a Lavender Breast Center.

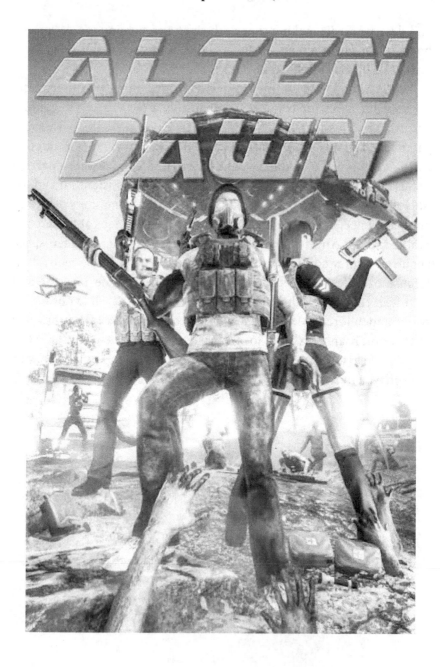

I guess the US Postal Service knew who the real breast surgeon was in the Coachella Valley (ha)

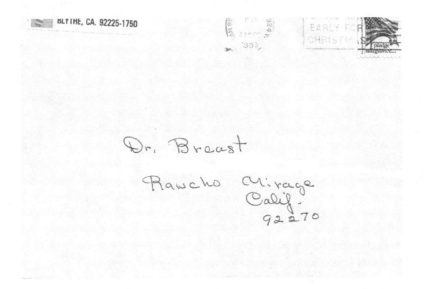

Take care. Joan and I are already missing all of you, especially our beloved patients. We hope you enjoyed reading about our lives and our commitment to all women. It is our hope that this book will unite all women to demand much needed change.

Please visit the website: thelavenderproject.net

Remember: LAVENDER IS THE NEW PINK!

Best and G-Dspeed.

ITE, MISSA EST

Phil

CPSIA information can be obtained
at www.ICGtesting.com
Printed in the USA
LVHW080736051222
734550LV00015BA/1051